Why Wellness Sells

Why Wellness Sells

Natural Health in a Pharmaceutical Culture

COLLEEN DERKATCH

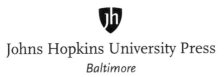

Johns Hopkins University Press
Baltimore

© 2022 Johns Hopkins University Press
All rights reserved. Published 2022
Printed in the United States of America on acid-free paper
2 4 6 8 9 7 5 3 1

Johns Hopkins University Press
2715 North Charles Street
Baltimore, Maryland 21218
www.press.jhu.edu

Library of Congress Cataloging-in-Publication Data is available.

ISBN 978-1-4214-4528-1 (hardcover)
ISBN 978-1-4214-4529-8 (ebook)

A catalog record for this book is available from the British Library.

*Special discounts are available for bulk purchases of this book. For more information,
please contact Special Sales at specialsales@jh.edu.*

For Isla and Nathan, always

CONTENTS

ACKNOWLEDGMENTS

My first and most significant thanks go to the forty research participants who shared how they think and feel about wellness and natural health. Their vulnerability and open-minded reflections on their search for both health and care made this study possible. Many participants spoke candidly of living with difficult and painful health conditions, and others recounted traumatizing experiences both in and outside healthcare; I thank them for trusting me with their experiences and hope I have returned their kindness with a fair and illuminating analysis.

I am grateful for substantial institutional support over the years of writing this book. My research was supported by two consecutive grants from the Social Sciences and Humanities Research Council of Canada, for which I want to thank especially Iain McQueen and his team and the reviewers whose feedback helped me clarify my goals and arguments. I am also grateful for financial and other assistance from my home institution, most notably the Department of English and the Faculty of Arts. The successive chairs of English Nima Naghibi, Andrew O'Malley, and Anne-Marie Lee-Loy provided important professional and moral support over the years I researched and wrote this book, and I am fortunate to have had them to lean on. I am also grateful to my former research assistants, who helped me with a wide range of tasks at various stages of this project: Natasha Ferraro, Jennifer Fraser, Christine Frim, Fergus Maxwell, Julie Morrissy, Allison Munday, Preeti Pasupulati, Shaun Pett, Ryan Phillips, Stacey Seymour, June Scudeler, and Tanya Tan.

The most rewarding and fun part of my job is working with students, and I am deeply grateful to all the students who have thought along with me as I incubated this project. A few dozen graduate and undergraduate students took chances on strange-sounding English seminars about "wellness" that analyzed artifacts such as fitness magazines, diet books, supplement bottles, and online quizzes. I cannot name you all here, but my thanks to each of you: your creativity and generosity continue to astound me, especially when, even years later, you reach out to tell me about cool wellness artifacts you have found. I hope you continue to find meaning in reading and thinking critically about the culture of wellness around you.

The second-best part of my job is working with other scholars, and I am lucky to be part of a field with colleagues who are generous with their time and their ideas. Indeed, the generosity of the rhetoric of health and medicine (RHM) community makes it difficult to name everyone with whom I have discussed this project at conferences, symposia, workshops, and other gatherings, and so I would like broadly to thank participants of events that include the RHM Symposia, the Greater Toronto Area Science and Technology Studies Symposia, the International Health Humanities Conference, and Writing Research Across Borders. I would also like to thank members of the following organizations: the Association for the Rhetoric of Science, Technology, and Medicine (ARSTM); the Canadian Association for the Study of Discourse and Writing (CASDW); the National Communication Association (NCA); RhetCanada; and the Rhetoric Society of America (RSA). Additional thanks go to the wonderful scholarly community I have found on Twitter, which has enriched my scholarship more than I could have anticipated.

In addition to members of the events and organizations above, I do want to acknowledge and thank certain people in particular. Everyone associated with the Health Communication series at Johns Hopkins University Press has been incredible to work with, most notably acquisitions editor Matthew McAdam, but also Joanne Allen, Adriahna Conway, Kyle Kretzer, and Julie McCarthy. Extra thanks go to Robin Jensen, the series editor, and to the full series board for being psyched about this project from the beginning and for remaining magnificently supportive throughout, as well as to the two anonymous reviewers for taking the time during a global pandemic to engage with and improve my work. Derek Gottlieb created this book's superb index, for which I am grateful. I also am sincerely indebted to many wonderful colleagues who have reviewed and otherwise responded to, poked at, or cheered on my work over the course of this and related projects: Mono Brown, Jennifer Burwell, Laura Fisher, Scott Graham, Naomi Hamer, Jenell Johnson, John Lynch, Lisa Melonçon, Alan Richardson, Mollie Stambler, Christa Teston, Monique Tschofen, and Lyn Uhl. Special thanks, forever, to Amy Koerber, Lisa Keränen, and Blake Scott for being extraordinary mentors over the years and to my nearest and dearest colleagues, Philippa Spoel and Judy Segal, without whom I would be doing something entirely different. I am also grateful to Nili Benazon, Lauren Campbell, Mai Ly, and Evelyn Rubin for keeping me in one piece as I wrote this book.

My greatest debts are, rightly, to my friends and family. Thank you to the Ballshawskis and my other Annex/Seaton Village compatriots, who appreciate my intensity and share my love of living-room dance parties. For helping me incubate this project with thoughtful conversation, whisk(e)y rankings, and garden tours, I thank John Blazina and Amanda McConnell. To my ride-or-dies, Wynn Deschner, Kim Duff, and Heather Latimer: thank you for steadying me. My parents have always been my biggest fans, and I am so fortunate that they have been mine. My mom, Dorothy Berg-Derkatch, did not live to see my first book in print, but she inspired much of this one by shaping my thinking about what it means to live in and be a body. My dad, Jim Derkatch, and my stepmom, Sheri Derkatch, offered unfailing enthusiasm about this project, even when I droned on. Most importantly, I would like to acknowledge and thank my daughter, Isla Whitford, and my husband, Nathan Whitford, who put up with a lot while I worked on this book and still love me anyway. They are the best. This book is for them.

Portions of my article "The Self-Generating Language of Wellness and Natural Health," from *Rhetoric of Health & Medicine* 1, no. 1–2 (2018): 132–60, appear, in substantially revised and expanded form, in two paragraphs of the introduction and in the first two sections of chapter 1, courtesy of the University of Florida Press.

Why Wellness Sells

Introduction

In March 2020, when the World Health Organization declared the global coronavirus outbreak a pandemic, my university in Toronto, Canada, closed its campus and pivoted immediately to emergency remote instruction. Over the eighteen months that followed, I received periodic emails from my employer reminding me to look after my health and well-being. The first few of these messages were comforting: no one knew how the pandemic would unfold, how many people would die, or when it would end, so it was reassuring to hear my employer express concern about me and my fellow faculty during a scary and stressful time. Our everyday lives had been upended as our in-person classes moved online, our kids' schools and daycares closed, and most services and businesses were shuttered. By summer, as it became clear the pandemic would persist for the foreseeable future, the university president announced a new well-being campaign branded "Recharge," which for faculty meant suggesting limits to the length and timing of videoconference meetings (fifty minutes maximum; none after 6:00 p.m., none on Fridays or weekends) and email availability (weekdays only until 7:00 p.m.). This announcement gave me pause: if reducing meeting length and keeping to business hours were the university's marquee measures implemented to "recharge" stressed faculty during a global emergency, what had been its expectations before?

Six months after the university closed, over the pandemic fall semester, it became clear that expectations had not changed much from what they were in years prior. I taught the usual number and size of courses, and even though I received some extra teaching assistant hours, my workload increased substantially as I prepared dozens of video lectures, managed online learning and discussion spaces, and did the important work of meeting with students who rightfully were upset, stressed out, and unable to meet course deadlines. I was grateful to be able to work safely at home with secure employment while healthcare and other essential workers risked illness to keep my city running, but it was still a slog. Even in the midst of a pandemic, faculty life continued apace, all while my family was also at home, competing with me for both time and internet bandwidth. By this point, the university's insistent reminders about my wellness began to grate.

As with so many employees across institutions and sectors, my job required me to carry on, mostly as usual, while the entire planet struggled to reckon with an airborne pathogen devastating populations. By November 2020, my irritation had grown as the university implored me, via email: "Please keep your wellbeing top of mind and make sure you are balancing work and time away as best you can." How can I take time away from work when it is in my living room? When my job is far more demanding than it has ever been? When my work is constantly interrupted by my loving kid, who is home all day and needs my help because her teacher is not here? When I am shepherding 160 students through a difficult and new form of learning while their lives fall apart? When I spend hours on Zoom each day, when I have a book to finish, and when the psychic burden of disaster looms inescapably over everyone, everywhere, all the time? Others' burdens were far greater than my own, but by the following pandemic spring, a year into the crisis, my frustration about my employer's messaging about my well-being had blossomed into anger. My well-being needed real respite, not reminders. A plan, not platitudes.

Wellness and well-being are frequently invoked as catchall solutions to problems in contemporary life. Most of these problems are not easy to solve. For example, as a public institution, my university could no more pay for universal course release for faculty than it could stop the pandemic. The university could have meaningfully reduced workload in other ways, without additional cost, but reminding employees to look after their own well-being is both cheaper and faster. When I received each of those reminders, I felt like I was being told to take a relaxing bubble bath or to meditate while my house was burning down.

I did try to take time away from work, turning like so many others to Netflix, carbs, and cocktails, and that did help to some extent. However, I would never have called myself *well*. I was simply getting by, which was about the best anyone could ask, given the context. But working and living through the coronavirus pandemic confirmed and amplified my deep and long-standing misgivings about wellness in contemporary Western culture, particularly because it is a fix that is not solely reserved for global crises. Wellness is ubiquitous in everyday life: at big-box stores we can buy wellness teas, juices, cereals, advice books, aromatic tinctures, candles, magazines, and yoga sets; online we can follow wellness Instagram accounts, podcasts, and YouTube channels. To enhance our wellness, we can visit specialty clinics, spas, and retreats, and we can take our pets to animal wellness centers. To stay productive, we can enroll in workplace wellness programs and visit university student wellness centers. And to protect our wellness, we can take dietary supplements, tracking on our smartphones the products we consume along with the details of our diets, exercise habits, moods, and even sex lives. Wellness is ever present in lives increasingly lived in crisis, and crises not just on a global scale but for each of us as we try to be healthy, to protect ourselves, to be productive, and to be good people.

Wellness as a Self-Generating Rhetoric

In this book, I explain how the idea of wellness came to saturate contemporary Western life, particularly in the United States and Canada. *Wellness* generally refers to the optimization of an individual's daily life across multiple domains (physical, psychological, social, and spiritual), emphasizing function over dysfunction, agency over passivity, and overall well-being over mere bodily health.[1] Many conceptions of wellness incorporate an element of reflexivity, figuring the "well" individual as one who is aware of and deliberate in their performance across these domains.[2] The twin emphases on multidimensional well-being and self-awareness exhort individuals without illness symptoms to monitor bodily states such as digestion, mobility, energy, cognition, and mood and to intervene on perceived suboptimal states largely through the use of complementary and alternative medicine, including natural health products, also known as dietary supplements.[3] These practices of surveillance and intervention are undergirded by recent redefinitions of health as a "semi-pathological pre-illness at-risk state" that must be mitigated through health-protective behaviors and by larger cultural rhetorics of self-improvement that frame individuals as socially and morally responsible for maintaining their health, well-being, and productivity.[4] These rhetorics may seem targeted to the most economically and socially privileged among us, but their effects reach far beyond that core demographic, affecting us all.

Recent scholarly and public commentaries on wellness products and services offer entertaining exposés of the excesses of wellness culture and provide important insight into the potential problems of its global ubiquity.[5] Critiques of celebrity health advice such as Timothy Caulfield's *Is Gwyneth Paltrow Wrong about Everything?* and manifestos against the medicalization and overtreatment of aging such as Barbara Ehrenreich's *Natural Causes* helpfully illuminate the many ill effects and errors of wellness culture. However, because these texts aim to critique wellness rather than to understand and explain how it works as a socio-rhetorical phenomenon, they lack the power to explain why wellness is so pervasive and what it does both for and to us. Similarly, Carl Cederström and André Spicer's wonderfully provocative and nuanced analysis in *The Wellness Syndrome* generates significant insight into wellness culture's complex moral and cultural effects, but since it figures the lucrative wellness market as a problem in and of itself, it is harder to see how the prevalence of wellness is also a symptom of a broader underlying problem. Wellness culture is not the product of any one agent—not celebrity health gurus such as Gwyneth Paltrow and Dr. Oz; not journalists and editors peddling the latest health "hacks"; not advertisers, marketers, institutions, or public health agencies.[6] Wellness is much broader, and more insidious, as it invisibly penetrates and fundamentally reshapes our lives and affects even those of us who consider ourselves immune to its influence. So long as we do not understand the core drivers of wellness culture, we have little hope of intervening in its most harmful effects.

To find out what those drivers are, we need to ask "prior questions" about wellness culture, questions that come before those usually asked in conversations about wellness. The concept of the prior question comes from rhetorician of health and medicine Judy Segal, who observes that humanities scholars are particularly well positioned to ask questions that are conceptually prior to questions often asked about health.[7] In the realm of wellness, for instance, instead of asking "Do wellness products and services actually work?," a prior question would be "What makes those products and services so appealing in the first place?" Relatedly, if wellness is a sales pitch, as previous analyses have illustrated it is, how does it work? What is the promise wellness makes to us? Why is it so effective—even, often, when we know it is a sales pitch?

The answer, I suggest in this book, is that the proliferation of wellness discourse is rooted not only in commerce, as previous critiques suggest, but more significantly in rhetorical-cultural processes occurring at the level of language. Wellness constitutes a language that circles back on itself, appearing to empower individuals to take charge of their health outside of an illness-centric pharmaceutical model of medicine while reinstalling them anew in that same system. In this system, what it means to be "well" is forever just out of reach: there is always more we could or should be doing for our wellness—there is always a new book to read, a new supplement or diet to try, a new clinic to visit, or a new app to download.

The concept of wellness is mercurial, taking on different, sometimes conflicting significations even while it maintains and accrues cultural and rhetorical significance as a health state worthy of aspiration. Over the course of this book,

I show that this mercurial movement between meanings in fact propels discourse about supplements and natural health. I use the word *propel* deliberately here to note a strong momentum among different meanings of wellness as its threshold ever recedes, remaining always just over the horizon. The rhetorical power of wellness lies in its ability to move fluidly, and invisibly, between seemingly contradictory and yet mutually reinforcing significations that are driven by opposing logics of health that cycle into and amplify each other. I term these the logics of *restoration* and *enhancement*: people who seek wellness products and services seek, often simultaneously, both to restore their bodies, perceived as malfunctioning, to prior states of ideal health and well-being and to enhance and optimize their bodies to become "better than well," to borrow bioethicist Carl Elliott's well-known phrase.[8] For example, someone experiencing insomnia might use natural health supplements to restore their sleep but then continue to use them even when their symptoms abate, slipping seamlessly from the logic of restoration into enhancement because one could always sleep *better*. The tension produced in this movement between logics furnishes wellness discourse with the ability to spiral and grow, generating rhetorical force as it also draws upon and reproduces its own cultural significance.

My core argument is that the rhetoric of wellness is *autopoietic*, or self-generating, because the tension between the logics of restoration and enhancement creates an essentially closed rhetorical system wherein wellness is always a moving target. In making this argument, I draw on rhetorician Lisa Keränen's investigation of autopoiesis, or self-reproduction, in rhetorics of terror preparedness and viral apocalypse, which offers a model for illustrating how some forms of discourse become essentially self-generating rhetorical systems.[9] Keränen draws the concept of autopoiesis from social systems theory, which in turn drew it from biology to characterize living systems as closed, autonomous, self-replicating units (*auto* means "self"; *poiesis* means "creation"). Sociologist Niklas Luhmann appropriated this concept, somewhat metaphorically, to describe how social systems operate and reproduce apart from individuals with independent agency.[10] For Luhmann, communication is at the heart of autopoiesis because, as Keränen explains, "social systems exist by generating more communications, which further the system's evolution and reproduction."[11] Importing the concept to rhetorical studies, Keränen employs autopoiesis as a heuristic for examining how rhetorics of terror preparedness and viral apocalypse spiral and grow as risk discourse expands: heightened levels of perceived risk lead to expanded efforts toward surveillance and security; expanded surveillance and security in turn lead to heightened perceptions of risk; and so on.[12]

The concept of risk similarly undergirds the language of wellness, particularly in the logic of restoration, wherein risk of illness becomes a "symptom" that warrants treatment. For instance, I may not currently be sick, but I could potentially *become* sick, so I might seek immune-boosting supplements to lessen that risk. Or, I may feel less productive than usual, so I might seek natural health products to help with concentration or energy as a means of preventing burnout. Within broad cultural matrices that valorize the mitigation of illness risk, individuals who believe they are at increased risk of becoming ill may seek ever-elusive, ever more qualified interpretations of wellness. Because there are always more steps we can take to support and enhance our wellness, wellness is reconstituted, in part, as a risk state that must be surveilled and managed as if it were an illness, leading various cultural critics and scholars to characterize wellness as a "sickness," a "syndrome," or even an "epidemic."[13]

The concept of risk tells only part of the story about how the language of wellness self-generates and grows, however. While *risk* (of illness) is a central driver of biomedical discourse and its associated institutional, regulatory, and commercial rhetorics, its effects are amplified when it is paired with its seeming opposite, *optimization* (of health). This is the core principle that underlies the logic of enhancement, where being "well" is not an end point or mode of being but a state of constant, self-reflexive activity. One does not simply find wellness and stay there: wellness is a process of self-perception and interpretation that calls upon individuals to continually assess and adjust their performance across different domains. In the logic of enhancement, there is always room to improve, and so failure to optimize constitutes its own type of risk that brings us right back into the logic of restoration. And so it goes.

Applying the concept of autopoiesis to wellness discourse illustrates and expands the explanatory power of autopoiesis within rhetorical studies and helps to explain how wellness discourse has become so forcefully persuasive among North American consumers. Over the course of this book, I develop my argument that rhetorics of wellness are self-generating, or autopoietic, by tracking the logics of restoration and enhancement within and across six key vectors of wellness to explain the different cultural currents that wellness taps into and fuels as public interest in wellness takes hold and spreads.[14] These vectors, which are the subjects of the book's six chapters, include the framing of wellness as a form of (1) *incipient illness*, a state of pre-disease that requires monitoring and care; (2) *self-management*, the regulation of the body under neoliberal logics of health citizenship and choice; (3) *harm reduction*, the use of natural health products to counteract everyday "toxic" life; (4) *survival strategy*, to mitigate the exhaustion of daily living; (5) *optimization*, the drive to become maximally well by becoming more effective and more efficient; and (6) *performance*, the self-conscious enactment of self, identity, and virtue. By examining the self-generation of wellness rhetoric through these six vectors, I show that the idea of wellness sells because it taps into broad cultural anxieties that are reproduced, often invisibly, through the very language we use to talk about wellness, health, illness, and ourselves.

Viewing wellness as an autopoietic rhetoric shifts our focus beyond individual, intentional agents of persuasion to the powerful ability of organizational and institutional discourse, such as medical-pharmaceutical rhetoric, to shape human life in ways we may not immediately recognize. Therefore, the power of wellness discourse is not that it operates at the level of individual or institutional rhetors—such as gullible consumers or predatory marketers, as earlier works have suggested—but that it operates at the level of systems. Accordingly, the appropriate point of critical intervention in the proliferation of wellness discourse does not lie primarily in consumer-directed debunking of wellness trends but in broader networks of power such as legislation, professional and commercial regulation, public health and social support systems, and health professions training and policy. Analyzing the culture of wellness from a discursive-systems perspective allows us to understand a key way that arguments function in public discourse and explains how wellness has accrued the cultural force that it has.

A systems perspective explains how wellness culture is not (or at least is no longer) solely the province of the privileged. Because wellness discourse self-generates, it spirals and grows far beyond the white, wealthy world we typically associate with Westernized yoga, cleanses, and organic food, fundamentally reshaping all human life in the United States and Canada. One need look no further than the online retail juggernaut Amazon's introduction in May 2021 of its "WorkingWell" program for employees, which, according to its news release, is "a new comprehensive program providing employees with physical and mental activities, wellness exercises, and healthy eating support that are scientifically proven to help them recharge and reenergize, and ultimately reduce the risk of injury."[15] This story broke at a time when Amazon workers across the US were sharing stories about inhumane working conditions, including wage theft and having to relieve themselves in water bottles and plastic bags because Amazon's algorithm does not account for bio-breaks for its human workers.[16] The *pièce de résistance* of Amazon's new wellness program was the introduction in its warehouses of "Mindful Practice Rooms," phone booth–sized boxes in which employees can take a momentary time-out before returning to their insecure and underpaid work. Amazon excitedly posted about its "AmaZen" chambers on social media but quickly deleted the posts after widespread public outcry. As a crackling article on Vice.com noted with contempt, "A worker is not a robot with a battery that needs to be charged. A worker is a human who needs things Amazon simply does not provide its workers."[17]

Amazon's WorkingWell program illustrates the far reach of wellness culture as it moves beyond its seeming roots in bourgeois-hippie culture to shape our very conditions of life, most particularly for racialized and low-wage workers. The idea of wellness informs workplace and government policies that assume and expect that each person has the resources of time, wealth, energy, and knowledge, as well as the inclination necessary to seek constantly to restore and enhance their wellness. Even those who do not or cannot actively participate in wellness culture are affected by it.

To investigate the rhetorical workings of the language of wellness, I focus on dietary supplements, or natural health products, because they are at once both substantially like and unlike pharmaceuticals. Like pharmaceuticals, products such as echinacea, St. John's wort, and glucosamine sulfate are typically synthesized and produced in laboratories by large corporations and consumed, often in capsule or pill form, to effect a change in the body. Here, importantly, we can bracket off the question whether and how these products affect the body because for the person taking the supplement, the intent is the same regardless of whether its effects are "real." People take supplements because they believe they will restore and enhance their wellness.

While natural health products are similar to pharmaceuticals in many respects, they remain distinct in several key ways. Most significantly, natural health supplements are regulated differently than pharmaceuticals in both the United States and Canada. In the US, supplements are regulated under the 1994 Dietary Supplement Health and Education Act (DSHEA), which effectively classifies supplements as food products rather than drugs, which means that supplement manufacturers do not need approval from the Food and Drug Administration (FDA), nor are they required to show evidence of a product's safety or efficacy.[18] The situation in Canada is fairly similar, although natural health supplements are classified as "therapeutic products," a category that also includes pharmaceuticals, personal care products, and disinfectants. Natural health products do require approval from Health Canada, but there are two routes to approval—one for products for "traditional use" and one for use based on "modern health claims"—and only the second, less common route requires formal scientific evidence of safety or efficacy.[19] In general, supplement producers in both countries are limited to making claims related to the structure or function of bodily systems (e.g., "supports cardiovascular health") rather than to disease or its treatment (e.g., "lowers cholesterol"). The limits on the types of allowable claims regarding natural health products help differentiate them from pharmaceuticals because consumers largely interpret supplement claims as wellness claims, distinct from both medicine and illness. As a participant in one ethnographic study of supplement use in the US explained, "One of the main reasons for my supplement use is just to feel better—because I am doing something for me, for my wellness, not just my illness."[20]

Beyond regulatory differences, those who use natural health products perceive those products as oriented to wellness rather than to illness because the products circulate so differently in culture. People perceive supplements as more natural than pharmaceuticals because they conspicuously contain botanical and mineral substances. Their marketing is also distinct: even though natural health products are most often sold, as pharmaceuticals are, as pills in bottles, their packaging and promotional materials (display cases, advertisements, websites) often feature symbols of nature, such as leaves and flowers. Supplements are differently available as well: while they can be purchased widely in big-box stores and pharmacies, they are also readily accessed through natural food stores, natural health practitioners, and online wellness stores. Finally, people who use natural health products also often experience them as more empowering to use than pharmaceuticals because, as consumer goods that do not require a doctor's prescription, they give users greater agency regarding when, how, and why to use them.[21] Because natural health products so closely mirror pharmaceuticals even while they simultaneously seem so distinct, they provide a useful lens for examining how the two logics of wellness interact with and reinforce each other.[22]

The interweaving of the two logics of wellness occurs, for example, in discourse surrounding bioidentical hormone treatments for menopause, which involves a combination of "natural" hormones and other supplements intended to alleviate menopause-related discomfort, as I discuss in chapter 4. Popular writings on menopause, such as those by former *Three's Company* star turned wellness guru Suzanne Somers, often frame bioidenticals in emancipatory terms as a means of wresting control from doctors and pharmaceutical companies over "the uncomfortable and unhealthy symptoms" of menopause.[23] Somers describes bioidentical hormones in terms of restoration and enhancement, often at the same time. Her claims are founded on the very grounds upon which conventional pharmaceutical hormone treatments are based: that menopause is an illness requiring medical intervention. For instance, Somers explains that post-menopause "I was no longer making my full complement of hormones. Because of that, I had no life-restoring nutrients feeding me metabolically. My organs were shutting down from lack of nutrients."[24] Here Somers describes menopause *in terms of* illness, of bodily dysfunction, rather than as part of the natural course of an aging body. Similarly, she frames arguments about natural hormones *in terms of* pharmaceuticals, as she seeks not only to support and enhance the well body but to correct and repair the ill one. And yet, Somers also explains throughout her books that bioidentical hormones enhance her body, so that she becomes "ageless"—strong, sexy, balanced, and joyful—regardless of the number of candles on her birthday cake. Natural health products have so enriched her life that she effuses, "I have never felt better or been happier in my life. I love my age."[25] In Somers's case, the logic of enhancement upholds the logic of restoration, both logics working together to reinforce the ultimate conclusion that menopause is best managed with bioidentical hormones.

By mapping the entanglements of the wellness model of enhancement with the medical-pharmaceutical model of restoration, we gain greater insight into the rhetorical means through which public discourse can "smuggle values" into itself from the very frameworks it seeks to disclaim.[26] Because the values embedded in public discourse are imprinted by dominant ideologies and can influence human action, tracking how values manifest in particular cases such as wellness discourse can illuminate their broader cultural implications. In the chapters that follow, I show how the transformation of wellness into a multibillion-dollar industry has occurred largely at the level of language, framed within idioms of illness and optimization that situate wellness as always close by but just beyond our grasp.

Wellness as Ambient

The discipline I am writing from is rhetoric. Like *wellness*, *rhetoric* has many different, sometimes conflicting significations. At its root, rhetoric is a critical-hermeneutic and empirical practice that centers on persuasion, examining all the ways we influence one another and ourselves, both consciously and unconsciously, through various communicative means.[27] Rhetoric first emerged in the Western tradition in ancient Greece, as figures such as Socrates, Plato, Aristotle, and others sought to understand and teach effective communication in the public realm. Later systematized by Romans such as Cicero and Quintilian, rhetoric evolved over the intervening centuries into a rich tradition that has variously theorized specific rhetorical arts (e.g., preaching, letter writing); elements of style; reason and empiricism; composition and public speaking; and more recently, broadly interdisciplinary understandings of how people are moved (or move themselves) toward certain actions and away from others. These more recent approaches include rhetorical-cultural scholarship that combines close attention to principles of persuasion with the insights and methods of cultural studies,[28] studies of individual texts and text types (or genres), visual and material rhetorics, and more.

It is not my aim in this book to align myself with any specific mode of rhetorical analysis, although there are many; indeed, I draw on a range of approaches without explicitly calling attention to the specific modes I am working in at any given time. My interest is not to stake a claim in debates within rhetoric about what rhetoric is or should be but to explain, in the specific case, how the language of wellness contains within itself the resources for its own self-perpetuation. To illustrate how this self-generating process works, I move fluidly between close-up analyses of language (words, phrases, linguistic patterns, arguments), genres (magazine and newspaper articles, nonfiction books, television shows, YouTube commercials, Instagram posts, websites, internet comments, interview transcripts), objects (pills, plants, apps, biological tests, drinks, IVs), and practices (coping, managing, shopping, tracking, diagnosing, treating, hacking, performing), and I likewise move fluidly between modes of inquiry (empirical analysis, critical appraisal, philosophical and sociological engagement, personal reflection). I also shift the focus of my critical gaze throughout to remain dually attentive to my objects of analysis and to what that analysis means for the argument I advance in this book. I focus largely on language because language reveals the conceptual entanglements between the logics of restoration and enhancement. To show how wellness persuades not only at the level of individuals but also at the level of systems, I therefore work from a wide-ranging, integrative perspective that incorporates a range of tools from rhetorical criticism as well as insights and approaches from other fields that intersect with my topics and methods of study, including anthropology, sociology, philosophy, critical health studies, and science and technology studies.[29]

Even if my approach is broad, it is not unsystematic or unprincipled. At its core, this book is a work of biocriticism, a concept that Keränen characterizes as "a sustained and rigorous analysis of the artifacts, texts, discursive formations, visual representations, and material practices positioned at the nexus of disease and culture."[30] Echoing Michel Foucault, Nikolas Rose, and other scholars who have written on the politics of life, or "vital politics," Keränen argues that the aim of biocriticism is to understand how these "discursive formations and material practices comprise 'life' by investigating 'vitality,' the politics, possibilities, and perils of 'making live.'"[31] Keränen's interest lies in mapping the movement of pathogens across populations and in the corresponding implications of this movement for national preparedness and security and the management and treatment of bodies. I extend biocriticism beyond the pathogenic realm by examining the politics of life in its most optimistic form, wellness, a concept in which vital politics becomes a politics not only of risk avoidance and mitigation but of human flourishing. Underneath all the pills, products, gurus, clinics, and mantras that wellness culture comprises is a drive to access some approximation of what we perceive as the good life. The good life, as Lauren Berlant explains it, is a "fantasy" we each strive toward, in which our lives have purpose and meaning, we have what we need, we want what is attainable, and we can become the people we really are.[32] Taking a biocritical approach to wellness allows me to situate my analysis within larger scholarly conversations about life-politics that consider bodies and health within and in relation to broad networks of power, knowledge, and privilege, principles of self-determination, and everyday conditions of living.

By showing how the discourse of wellness contains within itself the resources for its own self-perpetuation, this book expands the field of rhetoric beyond studies of how individual rhetors, groups, genres, materials, and situations advance arguments over time and across contexts by explaining how specific rhetorics themselves accrue and generate momentum, independent of those who advance those rhetorics. My approach therefore aligns with a range of recent innovations in rhetorical studies, such as Thomas Rickert's description of rhetoric as "ambient." Considering rhetoric as ambient is an approach that encompasses our "material, spatial, and environmental" surroundings and affective engagements and relations that necessarily de-centers the individual listening and speaking subjects who have been so valorized over rhetoric's history.[33]

A particularly salient element of Rickert's understanding of rhetoric as ambient is his notion of the rhetorical "dwelling place," which considers "how people come together to flourish (or try to flourish) in a place, or better, how they come together in the continual making of a place; at the same time, that place is interwoven into the way they have come to be as they are—and as further disclosed through their dwelling practices." Importantly, Rickert argues, when we inhabit these dwelling places, "performing rhetorical acts does not require completely grasping all that is entailed in the performance."[34] This is an important idea for this book because it moves the study of rhetoric away from calculated, deliberate acts (and agents) of persuasion and toward feeling and modes of being in the world. Wellness rhetoric is not the product of any one persuasive agent but instead is the product of wider cultural forces that both produce and shape persuasive situations. Rickert describes these wider forces as ambient, whereas other scholars frame them in similar terms as "distributed assemblages" of human and nonhuman actants and "networked," "ecological," and "percolation" models of rhetorical circulation.[35] However we describe these approaches, collectively they illustrate that rhetors do not act within systems as actors on a stage; rather, as rhetorician Dan Ehrenfeld observes, "systems *cocreate* with rhetors."[36] Wellness is therefore ambient: it is simply "in the air," and it deeply affects who and how we are.

Jenny Edbauer provides a useful frame for understanding how a given rhetoric cocreates systems along with rhetors through shared "contagions and energy."[37] In a parallel of my organization of this book into six viral "vectors" through which wellness accrues cultural significance and strength, Edbauer writes:

> A given rhetoric is not *contained* by the elements that comprise its rhetorical situation (exigence, rhetor, audience, constraints). Rather, a rhetoric emerges already infected by the viral intensities that are circulating in the social field. Moreover, this same rhetoric will go on to evolve in *aparallel* ways: between two "species" that have absolutely nothing to do with each other. What is shared between them is *not* the situation, but certain contagions and energy. This does not mean the shared rhetoric reproduces copies or models of "original" situations (any more than the shared C virus turns a cat into a baboon). Instead, the same rhetoric might manage to infect and connect various processes, events, and bodies.[38]

Examining wellness rhetoric from a systems perspective as autopoietic therefore allows us to see more clearly that within a pharmaceutical culture in which doctors can prescribe drugs to grow thicker eyelashes or eliminate unwanted hair growth, even the worst excesses of wellness trends, products, and services are not aberrations but logical consequences of rhetorical influence elicited by both "audience and material situation."[39] Within wellness discourse, individuals take up the terms and framings of biomedicine, which so often transform problems of normal human experience (such as hair that is too sparse or too thick) into medical problems that require pharmaceutical intervention, and (re)enact those terms and framings as wellness.

Examining wellness discourse as autopoietic allows us to see how interest in wellness may in part be an expression of broader public concerns about health and healthcare that are not addressed by doctors, public health agencies, or legislators as we collectively work longer hours, get less sleep, live under increasing financial strain, and spend much of our lives sitting (mostly in front of screens), all in the name of productivity. These impacts are compounded for queer people,

people with disabilities, and Black, Indigenous, and other people of color, who live under the additional weight of individual and institutionalized discrimination, marginalization, economic disadvantage, and personal and intergenerational trauma. It should be no surprise, then, that people would be attracted to the idea of wellness at precisely the same cultural moment when we have shrinking institutional and structural supports for our ever-failing bodies. For health studies—a broad topic area that includes health humanities, critical public health, health professions education, social studies of health and medicine, and related fields—this book offers a nuanced account of how language, belief, behavior, experience, and persuasion collide to produce and promote wellness, which is among the most compelling and possibly most harmful concepts that govern contemporary Western life.

Before I preview the specific topics, texts, and methods of analysis in the individual chapters to come, I want to briefly account for my own subject position and perspective on wellness and natural health. I am squarely in the target demographic for natural health products: I am a white, straight, cisgender woman and mother in her mid-forties with a stable salary. This does not mean I take my own subjectivity as my orienting perspective in this book, however, because a target is only a central point of focus and not the full field of play. Wellness companies seek constantly to expand their markets, find niche audiences, and appeal to consumers' individual identities. Further, those whose literal business is wellness are only part of the broader systems that make wellness sell, so if wellness is ambient, we need to go beyond markets to look at wellness where it is. Additionally, while wellness has skewed historically toward middle-aged white women, this is increasingly less true, as calls for diversity and inclusion have meant sweeping shifts in wellness culture that range from including a broader range of body types, sizes, and colors in media and advertising to financial initiatives that include free or sliding-scale facilities and services to allow patrons to pay in accordance with their income. It is tempting to view such shifts as important moves toward equity, but as I suggest over the pages to come, equity and market expansion can be tricky to pull apart.

With these considerations in mind, I often speak about wellness in this book using first-person plural terms such as *we* and *our*. I do so not to suggest that my observations and arguments are universally shared by all (including you, reader) but to indicate that they are pervasive, that they affect us as collectives, and that I am personally implicated in them. The *we* I address in this book does not refer to all of us all the time but rather to most of us most of the time. I may be precisely in the center of the target wellness demographic, but the target is deliberately very wide.

Regarding my own perspective on wellness and natural health, I hold two positions that may seem contradictory but that I bring into harmony over the course of this book: first, that most wellness products, such as natural health supplements, probably either do not work or do relatively little; and second, that people who use those products are neither gullible nor (usually) ignorant of science. This book is therefore not a polemical "gotcha" takedown of wellness culture and the wellness industry, nor is it a defense. I do think wellness culture can potentially be harmful and often does more to line corporate pockets than to help human health, but I also think it provides a crucial sense of support, motivation, empowerment, and care to those who seek it. My interest is therefore not in investigating whether natural health products really do work. If we want to understand why wellness has the cultural force that it has, we must engage with wellness on its own terms to see what it can tell us.

Chapter Previews

The book is organized into six chapters, each of which corresponds with one of the core vectors of wellness: incipient illness, self-management, harm reduction, survival strategy, optimization, and performance. Each chapter situates its corresponding vector in relation to the logics of restoration and enhancement. Some chapters emphasize one logic over the other, but the tension between the logics is the central thread running through the book as a whole. While each chapter can stand on its own if necessary, they build on one another as the book progresses, so the ideal approach would be to read the chapters sequentially. For readers who prefer an à la carte approach, please note that I discuss my two main datasets in chapters 1 and 2, respectively, so consulting the early pages of those chapters will clarify how I assembled, managed, and analyzed those materials.

The artifacts I analyze encompass a range of discourses, genres, objects, and practices that collectively produce, refract, circulate, and enact ambient rhetorics of wellness, both over time and across rhetorical domains.[40] These artifacts originate about equally in Canada and the United States. My two main datasets, which comprise interviews and a corpus of online petition comments, are from Canada, whereas the bulk of the wellness products and services I discuss are from the US, although they circulate globally. Rhetorics of wellness operate virtually identically in both countries even though Canada's publicly funded system of single-payer universal health care stands in sharp contrast to the complex patchwork in the US of competing systems and programs, and private and public insurance. The comparable circulation of wellness rhetoric despite these national differences may be the result of the countries' proximity, their sociocultural, political, and economic similarities, and the influence of American marketing, advertising, and cultural production within Canada. Additionally, wellness products and services have similar regulations in both countries and they sit in approximately the same relation to mainstream biomedicine with respect to where and how they are accessed and consumed. Given these important similarities in the wellness cultures of Canada and the US, I focus on both countries at once, except in cases where differences between the countries become relevant to my analysis. The most significant relevant difference between nations is that natural supplement users in Canada often frame their choice to use supplements partly in terms of wanting to bypass the publicly funded health system, which they do either to protect it by reducing usage and costs or to avoid it because they perceive it as inadequate.

I begin in chapter 1 by examining wellness as a form of incipient illness, while I provide at the same time an overall foundation for my theoretical account of wellness as a self-generating discourse. I outline the core principles of the logics of restoration and enhancement in wellness discourse generally by showing how these logics self-generate and spiral in interviews about wellness and natural health that I conducted with forty research participants in two Canadian regions in 2015 and 2018. These interviews offer insight into how ambient rhetorics of wellness are distilled in the language of everyday people. I show that wellness is frequently mapped conceptually in public discourse onto a medically oriented illness model that reframes wellness as a risk state that requires active monitoring and intervention. For example, when the interview participants were asked to describe wellness as an abstract concept, they framed it positively as a means of enhancing their health as a multidimensional whole (e.g., body, mind, spirit), but when asked to describe how they manage their own wellness with natural health products, they slipped seamlessly into a language of restoring the ill body through symptom monitoring and treatment. This chapter shows that the language of "wellness" frequently resembles that of the illness model it is meant, partially, to replace, and therefore this language often invisibly embodies the very values it disavows and locks individuals into the same patterns of thinking and acting they seek to avoid.

Chapter 2 examines wellness as a form of self-management that emerged out of larger shifts in cultural understandings of bodies and health over the last several decades that download responsibility for health from the state onto individuals. My analysis draws on public comments on a Canadian parliamentary petition against new regulations of natural health products that were proposed in 2008. This petition amassed 24,339 signatures and 8,585 public comments over a five-month span. In these comments, petitioners grapple with the role that both government and the market play in how they, as individuals, make and manage choices about their health and the health of their families. I argue that the petition signatories view themselves as consumers within a health marketplace where wellness is a commodity to be freely bought and sold. Their comments assert their rights and responsibilities as individual health citizens, but as I show, the emphasis on individual responsibility for self-care in wellness culture inadvertently short-circuits potential opportunities for systemic change in the landscape of illness, health, and wellness. As citizens take on increasing duties of self-care, wellness may not represent empowerment as much as it does abandonment by redefining wellness as an ongoing project of self-management we are morally obligated to perform. This vector of wellness discourse is driven largely by the tension between both logics of wellness, as good health citizens must aim both to restore their health and to enhance or improve it.

As I outline in chapter 2, neoliberal policies of self-governance establish self-care as an act of individual consumer responsibility, foreclosing possibilities of collective-systemic action to solve social, health, and environmental problems. In chapter 3, I argue that in part this foreclosure of collective action personalizes risk, so that wellness becomes, in part, an exercise in individual harm reduction.[41] I focus on how the language we use to discuss risk largely transposes rhetorics of *contagion* with rhetorics of *contamination*: no longer is it sufficient to guard against specific agentive forces such as pathogens, as we now must also fight against poorly defined but imminently harmful threats that lurk undetectably everywhere in our everyday lived environment. Drawing on a range of primary sources that include the interviews from chapter 1 and the petition comments from chapter 2 as well as a pair of bestselling popular books from 2009 and 2013 about how to detoxify our lives, I show that although consumers often understand toxins in only abstract terms, they are nevertheless well trained to recognize their prevalence and to know how they, as smart, empowered consumers, can and should avoid them. In chapter 3 I track how consumers use natural health products to avoid risks of pharmaceuticals and to rid their bodies of accumulated toxins, processes that draw on both logics of wellness simultaneously, as they seek to restore themselves to a state of purity and to proactively build up their bodies' defenses. Ultimately, I show that although toxins may be invisibly everywhere, beyond our control, the possibilities of remediation in wellness discourse remain radically individualized, focused not on their point of origin but on the point of their consumption. This narrow focus leaves little space for responding collectively to the threats we face.

In chapter 4 I take up the ways wellness functions as a strategy for survival in lives defined by exhaustion. Drawing on sources that include the interviews and petition comments, as well as advertisements and commercials for a range of natural health products that appeared between 2015 and the present, I explain how wellness supplements offer consumers a means of restoring themselves even when they cannot carve out space or time for true rest and repair. Products such as energy-boosting supplements, stress-reducing tinctures, intravenous vitamin infusions, and herbal hangover remedies offer consumers a sense of agency even when they are at the limits of what they can manage by providing a cushion against the burdens of everyday life. This is the vector of wellness that drives discourse about "resilience" and work-life balance, leading to lunchtime meditation seminars and pep talks, or pandemic "recharge" initiatives to limit nighttime emails, rather than providing reduced working hours, better pay, or more realistic expectations. While much of the marketing language surrounding this vector of wellness operates in terms of enhancement ("boosting," "energizing," "supercharging"), its underlying motivations are fueled instead by a will to restoration. By examining how wellness culture transforms resilience from a state of being into a consumer good, I illustrate that wellness may not positively redefine our experience in the world so much as simply patch us up so we can continue on.

Chapter 5 moves squarely into the logic of enhancement by examining wellness as a form of optimization. Within a culture that frames self-improvement as a moral and social obligation, wellness becomes, for many, a means of becoming the best, most effective, most efficient, most productive, strongest, healthiest version of themselves they can be. I examine two interrelated processes through which people seek to enhance their wellness, tracking and hacking. Wellness tracking involves using technologies of self-surveillance such as apps, wearables, and laboratory testing of blood, urine, or stool, which offer users information about their bodies to inform strategic wellness optimization using specific natural health products. To examine wellness tracking, I survey several at-home laboratory tests that consumers can use to test their hormone levels and gut microbiomes and to optimize them with supplements. Wellness hacking involves adopting novel, individually customized solutions, or *hacks*, to correct perceived weaknesses or problems that are often discovered through tracking but also through intuitive self-observation and interpretation. Wellness hacks are largely undertaken in the name of efficiency and optimization. In natural health this often means either using a broad base of supplements to allow the body to flourish or targeted supplementation to improve a particular body system, such as using supplements to enhance gut health or balance hormones. I examine hacking by analyzing how individuals who participated in the interviews and the "Stop Bill C-51" petition use supplements to hack their wellness. I show in this chapter that rhetorics of optimization rest primarily on the logic of enhancement but then circle back to the logic of restoration by rendering the human body infinitely improvable by natural health supplementation.

In the sixth and final chapter, I examine how the previous five vectors of wellness are animated in individual performances of wellness. Contextualizing my analysis in theories of ritual performance from the field of performance studies, I explain how wellness performances are scripted by cultural pieties about what is appropriate to say or do in the name of wellness. For example, in the genre of what I call "the daily wellness routine," individuals recount in varying detail the steps they take each day to restore and enhance their wellness. Natural health products are typically the centerpiece of these narratives, as individuals outline what products they take daily and when, how, and why they take them. I argue that these routines function as rituals whose significance often goes beyond the properties of the supplements themselves, most notably by offering the potential for self-transformation through reverence of nature, medicine, and the self. I examine the interviews and petition comments as well as Instagram posts, product websites, and other popular sources from the last decade to illustrate how the performance of wellness becomes a marker of who we are as individuals, as health citizens, and as fundamentally good people—as people, that is, who *are* well.

I conclude by reflecting on how this book enhances our understanding of autopoiesis, or self-generating arguments, in rhetoric and how viewing wellness rhetorics as autopoietic enhances our understanding of wellness culture, and with it, our understanding of health and medicine. In the book as a whole, I offer an explanatory model of how wellness discourse operates not merely at the level of individual or institutional rhetors, many of whom stand to profit by selling the idea of wellness, but also at the level of systems. By shifting focus toward systems-level rhetoric, I reveal more subtle and diffuse patterns of communication that interact with, extend, and resist the many spheres of influence that shape how we live, think, and feel. I conclude by suggesting that wellness discourse ultimately preempts or circumvents possibilities for real, large-scale, lasting change and that it is therefore important to consider wellness as potentially an obstacle to our personal and collective flourishing. Wellness may be a syndrome, as Cederström and Spicer put it, but it is also a symptom, and we need to pay attention to the underlying illness, or set of illnesses, that symptom represents. Until we do, no product or service—no workplace wellness program; no specialty clinic; no podcast, supplement, gym class, or meditation session—will ever provide more than a fleeting glimpse of what wellness might be.

CHAPTER ONE

Wellness as Incipient Illness

In the home health handbook *The Wellness Prescription*, Walter George Smith urges readers to practice what he calls daily "wellness monitoring."[1] When readers wake up each morning, Smith advises, they should survey their bodies methodically by checking their breathing to determine if it is without strain and free of tightness; checking their throat, mouth, and eyes to see if they feel dry or gritty; and checking that their morning urination is comfortable, with nothing out of the ordinary. He recommends scanning the digestive tract for appetite or nausea and feeling for abdominal tenderness, as well as making note of their body temperature to ensure it is where it should be. Smith then encourages readers to examine whether they are free of stiffness and pain and to ask themselves, "How energetic are we feeling this morning? Refreshed and ready to go, or a bit sluggish? . . . Are we looking forward to today's planned activity?" Finally, he asks readers to compare their bowel movements to the previous day's to make sure their movements are regular and normal. Once this wellness scan is complete, Smith invites readers to reflect on their findings by asking themselves, "Are we happy with the information gathered in response to these questions? Have we discovered something that requires corrective action?"[2] If readers find anything out of the ordinary, he recommends further investigation through a process of "ailment recognition" to identify the source of the symptoms and then, if necessary, "ailment amelioration" with natural health supplements and various alternative health remedies.

The level of self-monitoring suggested in Smith's handbook is as mundane as it is all-consuming. Wellness culture exhorts individuals to continuously engage in self-surveillance by closely observing how they feel, how they move, how they sleep, and what they are able to do in the course of a day and to intervene when they fall short in any of these areas. For those of us who (like me) wake up in the morning like the cartoon cat Garfield—disheveled, stiff, cranky, with bleary eyes that barely open—Smith's wellness monitoring routine spells trouble. Ordinary sensations such as feeling tired or stiff are re-coded as ominous signs of hidden ailments, turning the body into an object of scrutiny and even suspicion. Although Smith's book did not see high circulation or uptake,[3] his advice is entirely in keeping with broader cultural messaging that constitutes wellness as a risk state that must be actively surveilled and managed with external interventions. Active surveillance and intervention in turn transform wellness into potential illness.

This first chapter serves a dual purpose: it provides an overall foundation for my theoretical account of wellness as a self-generating discourse, and it serves as the first plank of my argument. In what follows, I outline the core principles of the logics of restoration and enhancement in wellness discourse, which operate in tension, in different ratios, across each of the six vectors of wellness examined in this book. More specifically, I show here how these logics self-generate and spiral in the first of these vectors, wellness as an incipient illness. In this vector, the logic of restoration dominates the logic of enhancement, as those who use natural health products to strengthen and improve their wellness often figure wellness instead as a deficiency state that requires repair. Drawing on qualitative interviews with individuals who are actively interested in wellness and natural health, I show that wellness paradoxically involves the monitoring and treatment of bodily states that are framed in the very terms of illness that wellness is intended, at least partly, to supersede. I argue that this paradox is central to rhetorics of wellness as a whole because the idea of wellness itself depends on its simultaneous continuity and discontinuity with biomedicine. That is, although many of us are drawn to wellness because it appears to offer something new and different from conventional medicine, at the same time, wellness offers a comfortable familiarity because it operates largely in the same idiom of illness we are used to.

Let me unpack that last idea. Wellness-oriented products such as supplements appear to free us from pharmaceutical ways of thinking and being because of their cultural associations with nature (not chemicals), self-healing (not artificial or superficial interventions), self-determination (not paternalistic authority), and health (not illness). However, as this chapter illustrates, natural health products may not liberate us from pharmaceutical ways of thinking and being as much as they reinforce and replicate the norms of pharmaceutical culture by shifting our dependence laterally, from one set of external health interventions to another. In contemporary public discourse, the idea of wellness frequently slips from an optimistic notion of wellness as a "generalized self-perception of health" into something more pessimistic—what medical sociologist David Armstrong calls a "semi-pathological pre-illness at-risk state" that requires ongoing, active intervention.[4]

For example, the individuals I interviewed for this book typically spoke about the concept of wellness in positive terms of action and surplus, of stimulating and rejuvenating the body, but when they discussed their own use of supplements, they instead framed wellness in negative terms of deficiency and dysfunction, often using medical diagnoses. These individuals languaged wellness using what anthropologist Joseph Dumit describes as the "grammar of illness, risk, experience, and treatment" characteristic of pharmaceutical culture. This grammar figures the human body as "inherently disordered" and invites us to view ourselves as requiring treatment.[5] Within this grammar, the goal of treatment shifts from remedying actual illness to reducing the risk of illness. In the realm of wellness, this shift from illness to risk of illness means that feeling stiff or sluggish in the morning is not merely a signal of a potential health problem but becomes a problem itself and therefore requires treatment. As I show below, positive activities aimed at enhancing the well body slip frequently, and invisibly, in wellness discourse into a negative framework focused instead on restoring the ill body. This slippage between logics helps fuel the rhetorical power of wellness and natural health.

My analysis in this chapter, as in much of the rest of this book, is based on forty interviews about wellness and natural health that I conducted in 2015 and 2018 in two large Canadian cities (ten per city in each year), one on the west coast and one in the east-central region.[6] The goal of the interviews was to understand key terms that constitute wellness discourse and how those terms intersect with discourses of illness and health. Further, I wanted to learn how these key terms are taken up by individuals as they decide whether and how to use natural health products to manage their wellness. I advertised the study to prospective participants who consider themselves actively interested in wellness and who use natural health products regularly. The individuals who took part in the interviews aligned well with the demographic of natural health product users in the general population in both Canada and the United States, the majority of whom are educated women.[7] Participants ranged in age from 18 to 75, with an average age of 41. Thirty-three participants self-identified as women, six as men, and one as nonbinary, and most participants had at least some postsecondary education. I did not ask participants about their income, but their range of careers indicates that most were at the lower to middle scale of earnings. Eight participants were full-time students, four were retired, and the remainder were split fairly evenly among the service industry, office administration, education, and health care.[8]

Each interview was conducted by a research assistant who followed a set of standardized, open-ended questions about wellness and natural health that I designed to elicit rich, spontaneous, idiosyncratic responses and to ensure comparability of questions across participants. Participants were asked to reflect on what it means to be well—how wellness differs from illness, how it is distinct from health, and how it can be maintained and enhanced through the use of natural health supplements. Although the questions were pre-scripted, when participants responded with only a single word or phrase, the interviewers followed up with prompts such as "Can you say more?" or "How so?" to elicit a more detailed response. The interviews were audio recorded and lasted an average of forty-two minutes, with a range from seventeen to seventy-nine minutes. The recordings were transcribed verbatim by a research assistant and checked by another research assistant and by me.[9] I analyzed the transcripts using the qualitative data analysis software package NVivo, employing a mix of inductive and deductive approaches.[10] While I draw on a range of other sources in this book, the interviews offer a focused sense of the language that individuals use when thinking and speaking about wellness and allow comparison across different individuals' responses to the same questions. Comparing across responses illuminates instructive patterns in how people take up and (re)produce the language of wellness.

I illustrate in this chapter that wellness sells at least partly because it taps into the same rhetoric of cure advanced within Western pharmaceutical medicine, which increasingly primes us to see ourselves as candidates for medical intervention. As writer and disability activist Eli Clare writes in *Brilliant Imperfection: Grappling with Cure*, "The medical-industrial complex taps into our desires, promising us so much. Through cure, it assures us that we can control and reshape our body-minds; restore them to some longed-for, imagined, or former state of being."[11] This is the logic of restoration—although, as Clare points out, the self we seek to restore in wellness is not always an actual past self but is at times an imagined ideal self. In the first section below, I unpack the concept of wellness by illustrating how those who took part in the interviews defined wellness in relation to illness and health. In the second section, I explain how wellness works as a self-generating discourse that moves fluidly between the logics of restoration and enhancement. I close the chapter by situating wellness as an incipient illness within broader scholarly conversations about medicalization and the pathologization of everyday life.

Wellness in the Illness Model

Several years ago, writer Nicole Cliffe mused on Twitter that "the person who came up with 'wellness' as a product adjective is probably living in a castle carved out of gold right now."[12] This tweet is funny because it is true: wellness is a powerful branding technique, one that has an almost horoscopic quality in that it invites consumers to project onto it their desires for self-determination, flourishing, and the good life. The idea of wellness marshals these desires into a seemingly productive form by giving us a project, a set of concrete steps we can follow to realize our hopes and needs for our bodies, minds, and lives. However, as Lauren Berlant reminds us, the "good life" is always a fantasy, an imagining about how life *could be* that we can never quite realize.[13] Here, in calling wellness a fantasy, I tip my hand: while some approximation of wellness may be possible under entirely different conditions of living, I do not believe the promises of wellness culture have any bearing on our contemporary present. As I illustrate below and in the chapters to come, wellness is ultimately an object of what Berlant terms "cruel optimism"—something we ardently desire that, in our seeking it, becomes an obstacle to our flourishing.

To illuminate the rich range of meanings of wellness, I explain in this section how the individuals I interviewed understand the concept and its connection to the related concepts of health and illness. When asked during the first stage of the interview about wellness as a general idea, participants overwhelmingly defined it in positive terms as maintaining health rather than treating illness, a perspective that accords strongly with dominant characterizations of wellness in both Canada and the United States as the absence or opposite of illness, centered on enhancement or optimization of the healthy body, rather than treatment of the ill or diseased body.[14] The participants similarly situated natural health supplements in binary opposition to pharmaceuticals because they viewed supplements as intended to support wellness rather than treat illness and also because they believed supplements to be natural (rather than chemical or synthetic), safe (rather than dangerous), self-determined (rather than prescribed), and protective (rather than defensive). Viewing supplements within this positive frame, participants described feeling empowered to preempt illness rather than merely to react once illness occurs. Although the participants later framed wellness more negatively when they were asked to explain the concrete steps they take to support their wellness, their candid reflections on wellness, health, and illness in the early parts of the interviews allow us to see how wellness operates on a closed rhetorical circuit, particularly as an incipient illness.

What Wellness Means

I began each interview with a deliberately open-ended question: "When you hear the term 'wellness,' what do you think it means?" I asked this question first because I wanted to capture participants' candid descriptions of wellness in their own words, before we started discussing more specific interpretations of the concept. The interview participants uniformly felt they had an intuitive understanding of wellness but most struggled to define or describe it in concrete terms. For example, Donna, a retired social worker in her late fifties, began by characterizing wellness as a balance among physical, emotional, mental, and spiritual factors but then interrupted herself with a laugh, saying, "I don't know how else to explain it. I'm probably going to struggle with words here."[15] Some participants offered only brief explanations of what wellness is, even after further prompts. Trav, a salesperson in his early thirties, stated: "I think it means holistic health."[16] Maria, a student in her early thirties, was similarly succinct, defining wellness as "having a sense of, like, stasis or thriving within the body."[17] Other participants offered rich explanations that sifted through different layers and significations of wellness. Clara, a retired dance instructor in her late fifties, detailed in almost a thousand transcript words how wellness constitutes a form of "optimal health."[18] More pragmatic assessments of wellness were offered by some participants, including Steve, a retired business person in his early seventies, who said: "Well, very often, companies use the term 'wellness' as a marketing tool. They're trying to reach out to people. . . . Wellness is a vague marketing term."[19]

Collectively, the interview participants' definitions of wellness were thoughtful but nonspecific and often circular, with frequent pauses, false starts, and self-interruptions. This response from Suri, a graduate student in her mid-twenties, is typical of the interview dataset, with pauses noted with ellipses and filler words preserved to illustrate Suri's significant efforts to articulate her ideas: "Um, . . . I think [wellness] means, . . . um, . . . kind of . . . a state of . . . well-being across, um, . . . like, cognitive, . . . emotional, . . . and . . . physical, . . . um . . . domains. So, . . . I guess . . . not just the lack of . . . something bad going on . . . but in fact . . . wellness, . . . I think, is, you know, . . . a state of well-being or, . . . you know, . . . everything's working properly."[20] Note the tautology here of defining wellness as "a state of well-being," a pattern that recurred in many participants' responses. Anjali, a nutritionist in her mid-twenties, similarly described wellness as "a feeling of well-being," and still others defined wellness more specifically as "eating well," "living well," and "looking well" and being able to "sleep well," "feel well," and "get well."[21] Steve explained that "wellness means basically people want to be well," which in his view is why it is such an effective marketing strategy.[22] The concept of wellness is slippery enough that even those who are passionate about wellness have difficulty defining it.

The problem of defining wellness may be due in part to the inherent ambiguity of the term itself, particularly given that it encompasses multiple domains (physical, psychological, social, and spiritual) and contexts of use (personal, professional, medical, commercial). However, as I explain later in this chapter, this difficulty may also be a product of the fluid movement in wellness discourse between the logics of restoration and enhancement, creating a kind of definitional impasse for those trying to pin it down: it is difficult, if not impossible, to explain in concrete terms a dynamic and multidimensional concept that generates different meanings as it moves between logics. This difficulty was reflected throughout the interviews; participants explained wellness more easily in relation to other concepts or specific behaviors than on its own terms. This was perhaps because the act of comparison temporarily anchors wellness in a fixed relation to the two logics. In any case, this definitional ambiguity may ultimately be a key rhetorical resource for wellness as a self-generating discourse, as it can mean different things even at the same time.

Despite the difficulty participants had in defining wellness, their responses revealed two significant trends that illustrate how they understand wellness in optimistic terms of enhancement. First, nearly all participants described wellness as foremost a state of balance across different domains that supports feelings of contentment, as in the following examples:

> I think of [wellness] like a balance between a lot of aspects in life. . . . It's about balance between all our aspects and [to] find an equilibrium and all of that.[23]

> I think [wellness] means a sort of harmony between your mind and body and soul, and sort of in relation to your expectations and reality in life.[24]

> I think [wellness] means health but not just physical health. It means physical, spiritual, and emotional health. It's all—the whole package.[25]

> [Wellness is] a balance in life. Health both mentally, physical, and emotionally.[26]

> Wellness incorporates a whole range of things: physical health, mental health, spiritual, emotional, cognitive, social. All of those things to me are a package of wellness.[27]

Participants frequently invoked synonyms of balance to define wellness, such as *harmony*, *homeostasis*, and *equilibrium*, as well as terms that evoke a similar idea of integrating multiple domains, such as *holistic* and *synergy*.[28] All these examples characterize wellness as the ability to juggle the different parts, roles, and demands of one's life. The study participants therefore conceived of wellness as a state of perpetual activity, always just beyond their grasp as they tried to balance the different, often competing domains of wellness. What is more, all participants felt that they must accept and assume responsibility for trying to achieve that balance, even if it remained elusive.

A second, related way participants defined wellness was as a state of functionality, of being able to succeed despite the demands of hectic, stressful lives. For instance, Gene, a construction worker in his fifties, described wellness as being "able to get through a day and . . . be able to endure stresses physically or mentally," and Jordana, a graduate student in her late twenties, characterized it similarly as "a state in which the body can manage daily existence."[29] For Clara, the dance instructor, wellness meant not needing coffee or medication to get through the day, being productive, and having the energy to do everything you need and want to do.[30] In every participant's response, *wellness* signified above all the ability to maintain and enhance productivity, with each person being "optimized" for their "particular range [of] functionality," as Lance, who is in his early fifties and works in marketing, put it.[31] Notably, the participants' overall emphases on responsibility and productivity reflected a particular ideological position about wellness vis-à-vis capitalist production that seemed to escape most participants' notice; I return to this ideological positioning in later chapters (most notably chapters 2 and 5).

Wellness versus Health

The second interview question prompted participants to compare wellness with its sister concept, health. Participants found this question almost as difficult to answer as the first, although several important patterns nevertheless emerged in their responses. These patterns further illuminate participants' understandings of wellness as optimistic and oriented to enhancement. First, participants felt strongly that the concept of health focuses solely on the physical body, whereas they view wellness as holistic and focused on the "whole entire person," as Jenisa, a first-year nursing student, explained.[32] Deanna, a doctoral student in her forties, indicated that she understands wellness as a form of "holistic well-being" that balances different aspects of a person's life, including "emotional and psychological and bodily" factors, whereas, for her, *health* refers only to the body.[33] For several participants, the emphasis in wellness on holism distinguishes it from health because it goes beyond pharmaceutical-based medicine, as Jasmine, a public policy professional in her early thirties, explained: "When I think of health, I think of a very, kind of, clinical model. I think 'health' is doctors, more of a science based approach to medicine. Wellness seems to be more holistic so I think wellness takes into account, certainly, physical health but also emotional, mental, . . . spiritual, . . . your sense of belonging or your purpose in life."[34] Kayla, a 30-year-old tech worker with a doctorate, similarly felt that "wellness is a little bit more natural so it's about natural products as opposed to only Western-based medicine."[35]

Some participants described physical health as a prerequisite to wellness: without a healthy body, they argued, one cannot be well. However, many other participants understood the two concepts as related but distinct. Marilyn, a school support worker in her late fifties, for instance, explained that in her view one could be physically healthy but still not well because "wellness . . . encompasses everything. Mind. Body. Soul. Spirit. Everything. So if one part of you is not functioning well, then I would say maybe your wellness is not a hundred percent. Even though your physical being—you know, you might be feeling physically okay."[36] For most participants, distinctions between wellness and health run both ways: just as a person could be physically healthy while not well overall, one could be physically ill but remain essentially well. People living with chronic illness or cancer, for example, may be able to balance their physical illness with their psychological, social, and spiritual health to feel holistically well. Many of the interviewees live with ongoing, challenging conditions; wellness is important to them because it allows them to understand and support their well-being in multidimensional terms.

The second pattern I found in participants' distinctions between wellness and health is that they see wellness as an active, conscious state, pursued deliberately and strategically, whereas health has more to do with bodies and doctors. For Erin, a nutritionist in her mid-twenties, motivation is a key factor because "wellness means that you've taken your health into consideration and *you're looking to be a better or healthier person* in some shape or form in your life."[37] Overwhelmingly, participants felt that although doctors may provide an impetus for improving one's health, only individuals can assess and advance their own wellness. Andrea, a mid-forties nonprofit administrator, put it this way:

> Health is more, like, kind of standardized and . . . what doctors would consider healthy. Right? So they might say, "Your blood pressure's fine, your cholesterol is fine. You're within all [the recommended] ranges. . . ." But then when I think of wellness, I just think of it as more, like, it's just a broader term so I think it's more

individual too. . . . Like maybe wellness also is about the things that you do to take care of yourself. . . . Health would be more [related to] tests [that] say that you're healthy but wellness is more, "Do you feel well? How do you feel?" On paper it all looks good but maybe, when you're exercising, you get tired or maybe you're not eating well or or maybe you get stressed easily. . . . So I think wellness is kind of like a broader term.[38]

The participants uniformly viewed wellness as each person's own responsibility, which they fulfill primarily through their choices as consumers, buying natural health products and paying out of pocket to visit alternative health practitioners such as naturopaths, as well as through other personal choices, such as diet and exercise, spiritual and religious practices, and so on. According to the interviewees, people who want to be well must consciously decide to do so, and then they must carry out that decision in the choices they make.

A third pattern in how participants understand wellness vis-à-vis health is that they view wellness as inherently self-reflexive, a state of self-perception and interpretation rather than an external state that can be observed or measured by others. Jenisa, the nursing student, explained that health is "more biological, . . . like pathogens or like diseases, but wellness is your state, like *how you view yourself*."[39] Anjali similarly described wellness as "a sort of harmony between your mind and body and soul, and sort of *in relation to your expectations and reality in life*," whereas valuations of health are more external and objective.[40] Some participants, such as Lance, tied the difference between wellness and health to different health professions, arguing that medical doctors consider only physical health, such as the "mechanical or chemical aspect" of heart function, whereas practitioners such as naturopaths are concerned with a person's overall state.[41] In sum, participants understood wellness as distinct from health, existing outside mainstream medicine, concerned with the whole person (not just the body), and something that individuals must monitor and actively maintain for themselves.

Wellness versus Illness

Participants evinced a much stronger sense of what wellness is, and is not, when they considered it in relation to illness. Lee, a nonbinary nonprofit administrator and salesperson in their mid-twenties, struggled to put into words their understanding of wellness both on its own and relative to health, although they did note that health is more measurable than wellness. When comparing wellness with illness, however, Lee found wellness much easier to define; they felt that because illness refers to a specific "inability," or a verifiable limitation, wellness is, by extension, more of a feeling than a reality. Giving a laugh, Lee concluded: "I guess I have a more clearly defined idea of illness than I do of wellness."[42]

The fact that participants found wellness easier to define in dialectical relation to illness indicates the extent to which idioms of illness organize our lives. We have become habituated to understanding our bodily states, our functioning, and even our moods in terms of illness, thanks to the creeping trawl of medicalization, a socio-rhetorical phenomenon that transforms ordinary problems of living into medical conditions that require treatment.[43] When medicalization tells us that poor attention or fatigue or stress is a sign of illness that must be ameliorated, wellness becomes, in relief, marked by the absence of those signs. Accordingly, the two most common ways participants related wellness to illness were that wellness is the absence or opposite of illness and that wellness exists on a continuum with illness. Both responses presuppose an essentially spatial relationship between wellness and illness wherein, as the nutritionist Erin put it, "one's over here and," gesturing in the opposite direction, "the other one's over here."[44]

Whether participants viewed wellness and illness as "polar opposites," as one interviewee put it, or on a spectrum, they generally viewed the concepts in tension with each other: the higher the value of one becomes, the lower the other falls.[45] Kaia, a creative arts therapist and fitness instructor nearing 30, described this tension as a type of seesaw relation: "If you're lower on the wellness [scale], you don't really take care of yourself too much, then illness would be higher," and vice versa.[46] Graduate student Suri considered all three terms—*wellness, health,* and *illness*—in direct relation to one another: "I think about illness anchoring one end of the spectrum, and then health at 50%, and then wellness at a 100% on the other end of the spectrum. Illness is a state of things not working properly, whether that's cognitively, emotionally, or physically."[47] In this example, wellness and illness sit on a spectrum with the definite boundaries of zero at one end, which is presumably the most ill a person could be, and 100 at the other end, a sort of "maximal wellness."

Overall, participants imagined wellness as a kind of math problem: the goal is to get and remain as close as possible to 100, with any value below that requiring intervention. In this impulse to quantify wellness there are traces of biomedical emphases on numeracy and measurement, which sit at odds with the principles of holism and balance central to most understandings of wellness. More significantly, this idea of striving for maximal wellness, of being "at one hundred percent," as Marilyn put it, is pivotal to my overall argument in this book: all participants acknowledged that reaching a maximal state of wellness is perpetually tantalizing, always just out of reach, and yet they felt compelled to continue reaching for it all the same.[48]

That wellness is an "ideal type" seems to be the defining idea of wellness discourse. As graduate student Jordana explained it, "It's not something that's actually in existence or something that's achievable but rather something that you can compare your current situation to."[49] Donna, the retired social worker, used a metaphor of a gas gauge on a car to explain that we cannot reach true wellness because the tank never remains full. Like a gas tank, she explained, "you're half full or you're empty or you're full. You know? And so wellness is at one extreme and illness is at the other. And so, the balance I guess is in the middle and [you're] always trying to have the car three-quarters full on the gas gauge, right?" With a laugh, she said that while "it would be nice to have it completely full," the wellness tank requires constant refilling because we get sick, we get run down, and we do not always get sufficient rest or nutrition.[50] In both of these examples, wellness is an aspirational state that prompts constant activity just to maintain the status quo, regardless of where one falls on the wellness spectrum. There is a parallel here with broader cultural redefinitions of health as a risk state, where even the healthy are reframed as merely healthy *for now*, particularly in the face of elevated disease risk (real or perceived) and expanded diagnostic screening programs, which, for all their positive effects, transform the healthy into the (pre-)ill.[51]

Ultimately, for the interview participants, as for all the other primary sources I examine in this book, wellness is not a state to be enjoyed but one to be vigilantly observed and maintained. Wellness is fundamentally precarious, requiring continuous recalibration and intervention. And so, consider again the multidimensional nature of wellness as participants initially defined it: "Wellness . . . encompasses everything. Mind. Body. Soul. Spirit. Everything. So if one part of you is not functioning well, then I would say maybe your wellness is not a hundred percent."[52] Given the low odds of someone successfully and sustainably balancing all these factors (mind, body, soul, spirit), and given that attaining 100 percent wellness depends on achieving that unlikely balance, there is virtually always something else the wellness seeker could or should be doing to improve it. There is always more room in the wellness tank. This may be one of the reasons why participants found wellness difficult to define: because wellness is an ideal state rather than a lived reality, we never experience it firsthand. As I illustrate in later chapters, this state of perpetual seeking is a defining component of "good" citizenship within neoliberal imperatives of self-care and self-improvement, and these imperatives create the rhetorical conditions under which wellness discourse self-generates and grows.[53] These rhetorical conditions emerge out of the tension between the two logics of wellness.

The Two Logics

In the previous section, I analyzed how participants conceived of wellness as an abstract concept. Here, I examine how that concept manifests in the specific ways those individuals described using natural health products to support and enhance their wellness, including why and how they use those products and how they assess the products' effects. I show that the language of wellness and natural health draws simultaneously on the argumentative resources of two seemingly contradictory and yet mutually reinforcing logics, a pharmaceutical-centric model of illness (the logic of *restoration*) and a natural health–centric model of wellness (the logic of *enhancement*). In the interviews, these two logics operated on a loop wherein participants slipped seamlessly, and seemingly unknowingly, from one logic to the other. I begin this section with the logic of restoration, then consider its apparent opposite, enhancement, and close by showing how the logics are intertwined in the language of wellness and how they reinforce each other in a spiraling fashion.

Restoration

When considering wellness in the abstract, all interview participants perceived it in optimistic terms as the absence or opposite of illness, centered on enhancement and optimization of the self. However, when they were asked about their own specific wellness behaviors, their descriptions were structured largely on a pessimistic model of illness, centered on dysregulation and dysfunction. This is the logic of restoration, wherein the goal of using natural health products is to restore the damaged or impaired body to a perceived prior state of functionality. For instance, when participants were asked which natural health products they used and why, they referred to something going wrong in the body that requires external intervention:

Instead of Polysporin for a cut, I have natural papaya stuff that I use.[54]

If I have pain, need pain relief, I use arnica.[55]

If I get a yeast infection, I don't go out and buy Canesten. I'll use boric acid.[56]

[For colds, I use] oil of oregano tincture, which is supposed to be antiviral and antifungal.[57]

I take [colloidal] silver . . . to rinse my mouth because it kills bacteria.[58]

I had a bladder infection, or a UTI, once and I took cranberry pills for a little while.[59]

In the first example, the body has been breached by a cut and needs to be protected with an external product. In the remaining examples, the body is figured in an aberrant state of pain or infection that requires an external remedy to return it to its former, functional state. In the final example, the participant Suri's self-interjection is particularly noteworthy: in an appositive set off in the text by commas, she reframes the colloquial expression *bladder infection* in medical terms using a specific diagnostic category, *UTI*, or urinary tract infection. This act of translation between colloquial and specialized medical language illustrates how biomedical ways of thinking and speaking have been imprinted on Suri's everyday experience of her body.

In the logic of restoration, natural health products are figured as roughly co-equivalent with biomedical interventions, although participants prefer to use natural products because they perceive them as more natural and safer. For example, the participant who described taking boric acid for yeast infections, Leigh, a media technologist in her early forties, explained that while she believes that boric acid and commercial antifungal preparations are equally effective, she prefers not to use an antifungal such as Canesten because "it's messy, it's gross, and it's not natural." Leigh further explained that she prefers not to use pharmaceuticals in general because "I think there's just more chemicals in them. There's more side effects. They're more harsh. It's just, the chemical components of them. I'd rather take something that's plant-based, natural, rather than made in, like, a science lab."[60] Erin described her preference for white willow bark over ibuprofen in similar terms: "Advil's . . . an extract of white willow bark made in a lab with other ingredients, whereas white willow bark is just the pain reliever that Advil's from. So, quite a difference in two products."[61] In both examples, natural health serves as a proxy for biomedicine, a one-to-one replacement for interventions that participants view as necessary but unnatural. The participants see natural health products, which they use in place of biomedical pharmaceuticals and which they perceive as having fewer risks, as essential for restoring the body.

There is a certain irony in participants' beliefs about natural health products. Although they see those products as freeing them of unnatural and potentially dangerous effects of pharmaceuticals in an illness-centric culture of biomedicine, the logic of restoration that underlies their beliefs is based squarely in that same culture. This logic casts the body as always at the edge of illness or failure and in need of external intervention to maintain function.[62] That is, wellness-oriented behaviors such as taking natural health products often rely on processes of surveillance and intervention that come directly from a pharmaceutically oriented model of illness. Participants described observing their bodies, their minds, and their moods closely and intervening when they perceived any kind of dysfunction, but instead of reaching for pharmaceuticals, they reach for natural health products. Ultimately, although participants believed that their use of natural supplements freed them from dependence on pharmaceutical culture, their dependence seems instead simply to shift laterally from one type of external health intervention to another.

Furthermore, within the logic of restoration, even the risk of illness requires remedy. In keeping with broader shifts toward the medicalization of risk, wellness discourse pivots on a potential for illness that, like illness itself, needs to be surveilled and managed.[63] For example, participants reported taking natural supplements to treat perceived risks, including kelp to prevent thyroid problems, nettle tea to prevent liver problems, and oil of oregano to prevent acquiring infections on public transit, such as colds.[64] Additionally, as I discuss in chapter 3, participants viewed natural health products as a form of "harm reduction," a means of decreasing risk in a world they perceive as increasingly toxic and harmful to health. For instance, Cassidy, who recently completed a graduate degree, attributed recent rises in public interest in natural health products to "the growing number of health problems . . . that people are having and especially in this more stressful urban environment. People need ways to deal with this stress and the impact it has on your body."[65] For Cassidy, risk caused by stress and urbanization becomes itself a symptom that warrants treatment, just as if it were an illness. Other participants cited similar risks, such as pollution, poor nutrition and chemicals in food, fatigue, and poor concentration as problems to be mitigated with natural health products. As I close this chapter, I return to the logic of cure, which expands from actual illness (cuts, urinary tract infections) to include a broader spectrum of human experience. First, however, let us turn to the logic of enhancement.

Enhancement

Of the two logics of wellness, the logic of enhancement is by far the more rhetorically present in public discourse. Perelman and Olbrechts-Tyteca define rhetorical presence as the art of making immediately felt or perceived, "by verbal magic alone, what is actually absent."[66] Presence renders a particular perspective "foremost in our minds and important to us."[67] The logic of enhancement dominated the interview participants' perceptions of wellness, which were premised on positive valences of health and well-being that cast those who use natural health products as empowered and responsible health consumers rather than ill patients in need of care. For the participants, natural supplements are a value-added way to optimize their bodily systems and processes to become "better than well."[68] For example, Erin remarked, "I think [wellness is] an all-encompassing holistic approach to *being the best you can be in all aspects of your life.*"[69] The rhetorics of self-governance, self-improvement, and responsibility inherent in the logic of enhancement resonate with similar rhetorics at work in contemporary culture at large, where individuals are implored, often in the imperative mood, to become the best possible versions of themselves.[70] Such imperatives are playfully manifest in the title of Weston Kosova and Pat Wingert's 2009 *Newsweek* article critiquing wellness advice on the television talk show *Oprah*: "Live Your Best Life Ever! Wish Away Cancer! Get A Lunchtime Face-Lift! Eradicate Autism! Turn Back The Clock! Thin Your Thighs! Cure Menopause! Harness Positive Energy! Erase Wrinkles! Banish Obesity! Live Your Best Life Ever!"[71]

Interview participants invoked the logic of enhancement by using positively charged language that conveyed a sense of activity, engagement, and empowerment. This language was most prevalent in the first half of the interviews, when participants reflected on the meanings of wellness, health, and illness, but it also occurred in their descriptions of their own wellness activities, as in these examples (emphasis added):

[I use] Biosil, which is a *collagen builder* for hair, skin, and nails. Which is really amazing, by the way.[72]

Vitamin C has a *boost on my mental health.* Somehow the NAC [N-acetyl cysteine] has a *boost on the mental health.*[73]

[For] seasonal change, I always take *immune boosting* herbs. . . . Because if your immune system's strong, generally everything's okay.[74]

There's herbal tinctures which I take and have found helpful . . . in terms of *stimulating the immune system.*[75]

Bell [Lifestyle] Products . . . have this cell stimulator that is said to help *rejuvenate* your cells, so periodically . . . I will take that. It *stimulates your cells* and *builds the red blood cells.*[76]

The Omega[-3 supplements] I take because I want to *feed my brain.*[77]

In these examples, participants describe dietary supplements as enhancing their health rather than treating an illness—"boosting" the immune system or mood, say, rather than alleviating a cold or depression. They describe the products' effects using vibrant, punchy verbs such as *boosts, builds, rejuvenates,* and *stimulates,* which convey a sense of spirited and bountiful activity. These emphases on enhancing function rather than treating dysfunction can be traced at least partly to Canadian and American legislation that limits the claims supplement manufacturers are allowed to make about their products, which can only refer to the structure or function of the body (e.g., "supports immune health") but not to disease symptoms or treatment (e.g., "prevents/treats influenza").[78]

Participants also praised dietary supplements for fostering attributes in the body that presumably increase in value as they increase in quantity, such as collagen, energy, "good" bacteria, immunity, and oxygen in the blood.[79] Within the logic of enhancement, if a little extra energy or oxygen is good, more is even better. The ceiling of wellness—or what measures "full" on the wellness gauge—retreats further beyond reach because in the realm of enhancement there is always room to improve our energy levels, cognition, digestion, mood, physical strength, immunity, bone health, heart function, and so on. If nothing else, we will always be progressively aging. And so, although the logic of enhancement promotes a sense of agency among users of natural health products by appearing to liberate them from medicine, doctors, the pharmaceutical industry, and commercial enterprise, this logic ultimately circles back in on itself and becomes entangled with the illness-oriented logic of restoration.

The Two Logics Intertwined

As I have illustrated thus far, the participants I interviewed invoked the two logics of wellness separately at different points in the interviews, moving fluidly between them over the course of the discussion. But these logics were also frequently intertwined in a single response. Individuals who at first described their use of natural health products in positive terms of balance, action, and surplus often slipped, almost imperceptibly, into negative terms, shifting to an idiom not of balance but of imbalance, not of action but of reaction, and not of surplus but of deficiency. Participants who praised supplements for addressing the root causes of illness to prevent illness from occurring then described their own use of these products precisely in terms of reacting to illness and relieving its symptoms. What is most striking about the two logics of wellness, therefore, is that they often operate on a loop or circuit: when individuals deplete the rhetorical resources of one logic, they can shift seamlessly into the other.

The following example illustrates how the logics of restoration and enhance-ment circle back in on each other. When Marilyn, a school support worker in her late fifties, described which supplements she uses and why, she began with this explanation:

> I found out about this product called Bell [Lifestyle] Product, I don't know if you've ever heard of it? Bell Product. And I found this in the *Vitality* magazine and they have . . . this cell stimulator that is said to help rejuvenate your cells and all of that so, periodically, I will say, "Okay, I'm going to buy and maybe take [it] for three months and stop." And then, you know, maybe another time. So, periodically, I will take that. That stimulates your cells and builds the red blood cells and things like that.

Here Marilyn draws on the logic of enhancement by using positively inflected verbs such as *stimulate, rejuvenate,* and *build.* In her view, the product helps op-timize her red blood cells to strengthen and even renew her body. As Marilyn continued speaking, however, she shifted fluidly into an idiom of illness as she explained how she decides when to take the product: "If, say, for example, my iron is low or something, say if I go to the doctor [and the doctor says], 'Well, the iron is low. You need to build it up,'" then she will think about taking it.[80]

Marilyn worries about becoming anemic because she is vegetarian. A vegetar-ian diet can result in low blood iron levels, which can inhibit the production of red blood cells, which oxygenate the body's tissues. She explained that if the doc-tor tests her blood and "says it's not at a critical stage, then I'll go and get the Bell Product" rather than a conventional iron supplement. In this example, what Marilyn at first framed as a positive wellness activity (taking the product to op-timize her red blood cells) shifts into a framework of dysfunction and deficiency as a treatment for low iron or anemia, which is an illness claim. She explains that she decides whether to take the product based on her doctor's advice, following a medical diagnostic procedure (a blood test). And yet, as Marilyn continued, she clarified that her decisions are not based solely on medical advice, either: "If I wanted to really build [blood iron levels] at a faster rate, if the instructions say [to] take one in the morning and one in the afternoon, I may decide, 'You know what? I will take two and two.' Because I know it wouldn't do me any [harm] but it will maybe get the process going faster. So if it's just for ongoing maintenance, I'll take [the dosage recommended in] the instructions, one or two times a day. . . . It depends on the situation."[81] By this point in her response, Marilyn has cycled several times between the logics of restoration and enhancement, returning now to enhancement by describing her efforts not only to regain lost levels of iron but to build up a reserve by taking more than the recommended dose since more is better in the logic of enhancement.

While participants often alternated between the two logics of wellness in a single response, as in Marilyn's case, sometimes both logics were overlaid in a single statement. For instance, Ariel, an alternative health practitioner in her early thirties, reported: "I'm taking ashwagandha, which is an Ayurvedic herb to help tonify your kidneys and adrenal glands from stress."[82] Here the goal of taking the product is to tone her organs—a wellness claim that refers to making more energy available to them—but she explains the need to do so as a consequence of stress, which is an illness claim based on a condition resulting in heightened cortisol production in the adrenal glands. Similarly, the construction worker Gene explained his reasons for taking a turmeric supplement this way: "It's supposed to calm down any inflammation or be good for your liver and your general circulation and the whole body, . . . [to] stimulate the immune system, help fight fatigue." He reported that he knows it is time to take the supplement "when I feel a lot of fatigue, run down. And when I feel better . . . or when I kind of feel a return to my energy, I stop taking it."[83] In this example, Gene draws on both logics of wellness simultaneously, linking illness-oriented symptoms of inflammation and fatigue with wellness-oriented structure-function claims about supporting circulation, immunity, and liver function.

To summarize my analysis thus far, participants moved fluidly in the interviews between the seemingly opposing logics of illness and wellness, of restoration and enhancement, each of which casts the idea of wellness in a different light. Although the participants initially asserted that wellness and natural health occupy a realm distinct from illness and biomedicine, they described their own wellness beliefs and behaviors using a language of symptom surveillance and intervention that comes directly from biomedicine. Interviewees spoke about monitoring states such as immunity, mood, alertness, and aging, much as one would illness-predictive factors such as blood pressure and cholesterol, and about treating those states with external interventions if they were below a certain perceived threshold of performance. The main difference for the participants in my study is that instead of using prescription or over-the-counter pharmaceuticals, they reach, at least initially, for natural health products.

Wellness is therefore both a part and a product of a pharmaceutically driven culture of overtreatment, an environment in which diagnostic categories expand to include not just illness but pre-illness, and so individuals increasingly seek health interventions that may be unnecessary or even dangerous.[84] Within this culture, wellness becomes the responsibility of individuals to surveil and address on their own using interventions aimed at restoration and enhancement. Consider again, for instance, Marilyn's decision to take the cell rejuvenator, which was driven by two simultaneous impulses: to raise her depleted iron levels to a healthy level (a restoration claim) and to "stimulate" and "build" her blood cells "for ongoing maintenance" (an enhancement claim). In this example, the two logics cycle into each other in a spiraling fashion that positions the product as the only appropriate choice, regardless of whether it functions as a remedy for low blood iron or for ongoing cell maintenance. In wellness discourse, taking action is always the right answer.

A New Form of Illness

Although the concept of wellness appears to empower individuals by offering independence from an illness-oriented biomedical model, contemporary understandings of wellness instead often expand the ways we can be ill (or pre-ill); this expansion of illness correspondingly expands the extent and forms of intervention we require. For Marilyn, natural health products are appealing because they allow her to manage her own blood iron before she gets to a "critical stage." However, to avoid conventional iron treatments, she must surveil her body even more closely than she otherwise would and intervene even sooner if she detects anything amiss. Here, natural health remedies become a one-to-one replacement for conventional treatments: Marilyn swaps out one diagnosis (anemia) for another (nonoptimal red blood cells), as well as one intervention (iron supplementation) for another (a red blood cell stimulant). Importantly, though, she must react even more swiftly by lowering the threshold for what she considers acceptable, thereby transforming a state that would not yet count as illness into a condition that requires treatment. I take the phrase *lowering the threshold* from sociologist Peter Conrad, who argued in his landmark book, *The Medicalization of Society: On the Transformation of Human Conditions into Treatable Disorders*, that as medicalization occurs we see "the threshold for treatment decreasing and becoming more inclusive," which results in expanded diagnostic criteria, higher levels of treatment, and more intensive medical surveillance.[85] The idea of wellness may ultimately do as much to medicalize people as it does to liberate them.

Let us return to how I began this chapter, with Walter George Smith's home handbook *The Wellness Prescription*. The level of self-scrutiny encouraged by Smith's practice of daily "wellness monitoring" seems at least as likely to compound concerns about one's health as it is to foster a sense of wellness. For me, when I wake up in the morning, it usually takes a while to clear out the cobwebs and get moving. Whereas I might otherwise assume that waking up groggy and a little stiff are ordinary conditions of living for a busy, sometimes stressed-out parent and academic in her mid-forties, Smith would encourage me to view my grogginess and stiffness as "ailments" to be ameliorated. Following Smith's prescription for wellness, I would therefore need to take steps to improve how, and how well, I wake up. I might need to take a sleep supplement to get a better night's rest, perhaps, or to use an energy-boosting supplement to get me going in the morning. (For the record, my preferred method is to stare into space with a cup of tea until I am awake enough for coffee.)

Smith's wellness prescription includes various alternative health approaches, such as Ayurveda, chiropractic, herbal medicine, homeopathy, reiki, and traditional Chinese medicine, as well as mainstream biomedical treatments. Tellingly, nowhere in his book does he suggest that problems such as my morning grogginess might be products not of my own failings but, rather, of social or structural factors beyond my control. Financial strain, workplace stress, gendered care expectations, and other social determinants of health such as food and housing insecurity, discrimination, inadequate health insurance, and lack of affordable and accessible birth control and childcare are all eclipsed in wellness culture by rhetorics of personal empowerment and lifestyle choice. It could also just be that my own biological rhythms do not square with contemporary ideals about working hours and productivity. In any event, Smith is not alone in his position that our health and wellness are primarily within our own control, as we are surrounded in our daily lives by alarmist claims about how much we should sleep, move, and work, what we should eat and drink, how energetic we should be, and how we should feel. The overall message is that if we fail to meet those benchmarks, we cannot be well.

Recognizing Symptoms

When Marilyn described early in the interview how she understands wellness, she pointed out that physical health alone is insufficient for wellness because "wellness . . . encompasses everything. Mind. Body. Soul. Spirit. Everything." Like other participants, Marilyn considers wellness in mathematical terms, adding up the scores for each of the independent factors that make up wellness to arrive at a total, summative score: "If one part of you is not functioning well, then I would say maybe your wellness is not a hundred percent. Even though you might be feeling physically okay."[86] When Marilyn wants to assess her wellness, she must therefore monitor the different dimensions of her wellness à la Smith's *Wellness Prescription* to determine how she is faring in each category—mind, body, soul, and spirit. The problem, of course, is that it is unlikely anyone would achieve a perfect score in all of those categories at the same time to arrive at a total wellness score of 100 percent. Feeling preoccupied or inattentive (mind), tired or stiff (body), unvirtuous or guilty (soul), or angry or blah (spirit) would alone be enough to knock your total score below the maximum possible, and you would have more wellness work to do. While wellness enthusiasts rightly point out that conventional medicine is often reductive in its focus on physical health, the expansion of health and well-being beyond the physical does mean widening the scope of surveillance and intervention to a broader range of human states and experiences. It also means there is more that can be wrong, and more that must be fixed.

As we cycle through the logics of restoration and enhancement, there are always more steps we can take to address our wellness deficit, thus reframing wellness in terms of pathology. Even within the logic of enhancement, the threshold for treatment plunges because a good wellness score still merits intervention under the guise of "maintenance" or "optimization." To put it simply, wellness has become medicalized, requiring ever-increasing surveillance and earlier, more intensive treatment. Importantly, however, the medicalization of wellness is not the product of any one agent; as Conrad explains, medicalization is a product of collective action. For wellness, this collective action occurs in many ways: supplement manufacturers mimic the pharmaceutical industry's marketing and promotions; popular media narrativize wellness within the contours of standard illness stories; advertisers piggyback on the values sold in lucrative pharmaceutical ads; individuals extend dominant medical frames of thinking and acting to other parts of their lives. Caught in the web of these and similar forces, wellness seekers are essentially stuck because even when they try to move beyond the realm of medicalization, they largely remain suspended within it. In wellness, medicalization is so powerful that it transcends "the medical."

When Marilyn decides whether to take the cell-stimulating supplement, for example, she engages in a process of what Dumit terms *facilitated recognition* of her body's condition and needs. Dumit argues that one of the ways that pharmaceutical companies determine what health is and how to get it is by facilitating particular interpretations of how we feel, move, and function, which transforms our experiences into symptoms that need treatment. Sensations we might otherwise have dismissed as normal become causes for concern. Similarly, wellness culture invites people to scrutinize their lives in specific terms that come from "a specifically pharmaceutical language and worldview" that causes us to ask of an ever-increasing array of situations, "Is this a symptom?"[87] For Marilyn, who is nearly 60, feeling tired is a symptom that prompts her to use the cell rejuvenator before her fatigue gets to a point where she needs to see the doctor. Her recognition of fatigue as a problem to be fixed is facilitated by pharmaceutical grammars of illness and risk that figure her as always incipiently ill.

These grammars shape Marilyn's experiences to such an extent that she admits that she will never reach 100 percent on the wellness scale because "I can always still do better." With a sighing smile, she elaborated: "I think when I reach that point and say, 'You know what, I can't do any more than I'm doing,' then I think that's sufficient for me. But I think, for me personally, I always think that I can do better. So I haven't reached [wellness] yet."[88] By recognizing different elements of her wellness as targets for restoration or enhancement, Marilyn must continually take action to reach her goal of becoming "well."

Enacting Cure

Dumit argues that pharmaceutical marketing has cultivated a language and worldview that aims to convert attention to health to concern or worry.[89] By shifting attention to concern, he argues, people are moved to act by taking preventive measures to ensure their continued health, which is always necessarily failing. The lines between sickness and health therefore shift and blur, resulting in a phenomenon that Dumit terms the *prevention paradox*, wherein larger numbers of people need to engage in greater amounts of treatment to prevent increasingly less prevalent disease.[90] Dumit asks an important question: does taking preventive drugs mean that a person is sick, because they are at risk of illness, or healthy, because they are reducing that risk? He observes that as the realms of illness and illness risk expand, the culture of prevention likewise grows, poising people to follow lifetime courses of treatment. Within this paradox, Dumit argues, *healthy* risks becoming a "legacy term, one that no longer has meaning."[91] Natural health products emerge out of this rhetorical ecosystem as pharmaceutical understudies for people who want to restore and enhance their wellness, and want to do it without drugs.

Marilyn, for instance, works to manage her red blood cell production on her own using a natural "cell stimulator" before her iron gets low enough that she needs to see the doctor because she wants to avoid iron supplements. Even though iron supplements are regulated as natural health products in Canada, where the interviews occurred, Marilyn sees them as interchangeable with pharmaceuticals, presumably because they are recommended by her doctor, they are used to correct a physical deficiency, and they are kept behind the pharmacist's counter. However, pharmaceuticals and natural health products are more similar than Marilyn and other study participants allow.

Leaving aside their specific chemical contents, even regulated pharmaceuticals such as aspirin and ibuprofen are interchangeable in several important ways with their apparent natural counterpart, white willow bark (*Salix alba*). All three come as liquids or pills synthesized in labs and are bottled, distributed, and sold by large, for-profit corporations. All three aim to correct a problem in the body, which in this case might be pain, inflammation, or fever. And the use of all three is facilitated by a process of surveillance and intervention that begins with recognizing a problem requiring treatment and ends with the act of taking the product into the body. If we suspend the question of whether natural health products have any measurable physiological effects, by choosing to use them wellness seekers can avoid pharmaceuticals and have their medicine too.

Natural health products tap into and expand the rhetoric of cure advanced within Western pharmaceutical medicine. Recall, for instance, Eli Clare's argument at the beginning of this chapter that the notion of cure "assures us that we can control and reshape our body-minds; restore them to some longed-for, imagined, or former state of being."[92] Writing in the context of disability studies, Clare urges us to reassess the medical-industrial complex's promises of cure because those promises are premised not on past or present reality but instead on a fantasy of an other-bodied future. This is a fantasy in which we are, in effect, not ourselves. Here is Clare, in a vital passage from *Brilliant Imperfection*:

> The desire for cure, for the restoration of health, is connected to loss and yearning. What we remember about our body-minds in the past seduces us. We wish. We mourn. We make deals. We desire to return to the days before immobilizing exhaustion or impending death, to the nights thirty years ago when we spun across the dance floor. We dream about the body-minds we once had before depression descended; before we gained twenty, fifty, a hundred pounds; before our hair turned gray. We ache for the evenings curled up in bed with a book before the ability to read vanished in an instant as a bomb or landmine exploded. We long for the time before pain and multigenerational trauma grabbed our body-minds.
>
> We reach toward the past and dream about the future, feeling grief, envy, shame. We compare our body-minds to friends and lovers, models in *Glamour* and *Men's Health*. Photoshopped versions of humans hold sway. We find ourselves lacking. The gym, diet plan, miracle cure grip us. *Normal* and *natural* won't leave us alone. We remain tethered to our body-minds of the past, wanting to transport them into the future, imagining in essence a kind of time travel.[93]

Wellness is a form of time travel in the same way Clare outlines here, with the promises of natural health products constituting a cure not just for illness but also for everyday living. For this reason, wellness and natural health are deeply ableist because they center normative, able-bodied, autonomous, privileged subjects. The well you is the one who is free of stiffness and grogginess in the morning, who is free of fatigue, pain, stress, and worry. The you whose trips to the bathroom are uneventful, whose wallet can manage the cost of an expanding array of supplements, and who has the time and mobility to visit health food stores and natural health practitioners, to hit the gym, and to take yoga classes. The well you does a careful mental scan for ailments each morning and, like Marilyn, sometimes takes supplements in higher than recommended doses for an added wellness boost. The well you is, fundamentally, not actually *you*.

As I have illustrated in this chapter, wellness has no ceiling because the language of wellness cycles endlessly between the logics of restoration and enhancement. Even if I were to find a way to restore myself so I would wake up chipper and bright in the morning, I could easily slip from restoration to enhancement, since one can always wake up happier, or earlier, or even more raring to go. In wellness culture, if you are not irrepressibly energetic and efficient and sharp-minded and mobile, you have work to do. In the next chapter, I explain how the language of wellness transforms wellness work into a condition of responsible citizenship, with each of us becoming personally responsible for ensuring that we and our families are as well as we possibly can be—even while we are at the same time, inescapably, incipiently ill.

CHAPTER TWO

Wellness as Self-Management

In the first vector of wellness discourse, wellness sells by expanding the domain of illness to include a broader range of symptoms, conditions, and treatments; in the second vector, the subject of this chapter, wellness sells by tasking those who seek it with their own self-management. Figured in wellness discourse as health subjects always necessarily on the edge of illness, we become responsible for an ongoing project of restoration and enhancement. Recall, for instance, the interview participants I discussed in the previous chapter, who overwhelmingly asserted that they alone were responsible for their wellness. They described their efforts to balance the different domains of wellness and to make good choices in support of their well-being by buying organic food, visiting natural health practitioners, using natural health products, and more. The participants outlined their strategies for restoring their wellness when they experience a rough patch, as well as how they optimize their wellness when they would like an extra boost. As the participants moved fluidly between the two logics of wellness, they also inadvertently demonstrated that because wellness has no ceiling, wellness work never ends. In what follows, I examine a new set of primary texts to illustrate how wellness converts interest in natural health products into an obligation of good citizenship: individuals must accept and assume responsibility for their own and their families' well-being, absolving the state of its duty to care for its citizens.

My focus in this chapter is a public petition from 2008 that protested Canadian legislation introduced in Parliament that year to increase the power of Health Canada, Canada's federal health regulator, to enforce existing legislation regarding the safety of foods, cosmetics, and a new legislative category called "therapeutic products."[1] The bill, known as Bill C-51, would have articulated clearer guidelines in Canada's Food and Drugs Act for licensing, inspection, clinical testing, and postmarket monitoring of all health-related products, along with increased penalties for violations. Bill C-51 was a fairly mundane piece of legislation, representing not a shift in Canadian health policy but simply an effort to add bite to previously "toothless" regulations intended to protect consumers.[2] The bill seemed poised to pass the first reading in Parliament and eventually become law, but it instead ignited a firestorm of debate in Canada about the rights of individuals both as *patients* who receive medical interventions and as *consumers* who choose their own interventions within an open wellness market.

The debate about Bill C-51 centered on the new category "therapeutic products," which includes drugs, medical devices, and human cells, tissues, and organs. This category subsumes natural health products such as herbal remedies, high-dose vitamins, and other plant and animal extracts under the subcategory "drugs." Over its sixty pages, Bill C-51 refers directly to natural health products only three times, and never specifically regarding supplement regulation or enforcement. Nevertheless, thousands of Canadians quickly mobilized against the bill, fearing that it would drastically restrict their access to natural health supplements. One online petition against the legislation, "Stop Bill C-51," quickly generated more than twenty-four thousand signatures,[3] while fifty-three Facebook groups formed in opposition in the days following the reading of the bill. The Facebook groups, some with memberships in the tens of thousands, all echoed one group's framing of the bill as placing individuals' "health at risk" by impinging on the overall "rights and freedoms of Canadians." The group argued that this legislation would result in the "erosion of democracy," when "simply possessing herbs would become illegal."[4] Similarly, a website set up in protest of Bill C-51 warned that the bill would result in restrictions of Orwellian proportions, enabling the government to conduct "search and seizures without warrants," in which "no evidence will be required" for levying "up to $5,000,000.00 fines if you are caught growing, preserving, or sharing an unregistered natural health product (Garlic, Vitamins . . .)." Ultimately, the website claimed, the proposed law would "apply crack house style of enforcement to the natural health industry," under which even parents giving herbs such as chamomile to their children would face fines and possible jail time.[5]

The case of Bill C-51 is pertinent to my argument in this chapter, as well as to my larger argument in this book, because the outrage sparked by the bill was so wildly out of proportion with its comparatively innocuous mandate, which was simply to add enforcement to existing regulations regarding all health-related products in Canada, not just natural supplements. The discrepancy between Bill C-51 and the resulting public outcry evinces the significance accorded to products such as oil of oregano and white willow bark by those who use them. For these individuals, natural health products have accrued such deep cultural and personal meaning that losing access to them would be tantamount to an attack on democracy itself. In the petition against Bill C-51, for example, commenters frequently asserted that supplements should be freely available without restrictions because individuals have the right and responsibility to care for themselves without government interference. The opposition to Bill C-51 can therefore help to illuminate what is at stake, both publicly and politically, in rhetorics surrounding the production, regulation, and consumption of supplements and other wellness-oriented products. Bill C-51 was ultimately dropped following the first reading, although portions of it have since been reintroduced under several other Canadian bills.[6]

In this chapter, I draw on public comments on the "Stop Bill C-51" petition to examine wellness as a form of self-management that emerges out of larger shifts in cultural understandings of bodies and health that download responsibility for health onto individuals. Supplement use in both Canada and the United States, as well as in much of the rest of the Western world, is rooted in and facilitated by an illness-oriented neoliberal ideology. Individuals are charged with responsibility for elements of health that could more effectively be addressed through state-level initiatives such as public health and nutrition interventions, programs for affordable food, safe and accessible housing, living wages, health and sick leave benefits, and physical activity programming. Instead, individual people are exhorted, as "good" health citizens, to seek actively to manage both their own health and that of their families.[7] This model of citizenship assumes that people have the time and financial resources to self-manage, which privileges the already privileged. Further, as citizens take on increasing duties of self-care, health self-governance may not represent empowerment as much as it does abandonment, especially as individuals are invited to manage their wellness in the same fashion one might manage illness. By tracking the logics of enhancement and restoration through the lens of wellness as self-management, I illustrate in this chapter how the discursive processes that underlie self-governance and the politics of health have come to reshape how we think of our bodies and our health within a biomedical framework—even when we believe we are acting outside of that framework, as in wellness and natural health.[8]

The "Stop Bill C-51" petition amassed 24,339 signatures and 8,585 public comments over a five-month span in 2008. From those 8,585 comments I extracted a randomized sample of 368 comments and imported them into NVivo for analysis. I initially analyzed the comments by topic,[9] and then I worked back through that analysis to identify salient patterns that illuminate how wellness constitutes a form of self-management. While the petition is from 2008, it provides important insight into Canadians' health beliefs and behaviors, particularly regarding the impact of government and the market on their health choices. The arguments advanced within the petition resonate with all the more recent cultural artifacts and datasets I analyze in this book, including those from the United States and other countries, with the added advantage that the petition includes thousands of people all commenting on exactly the same thing, which provides a rich site for understanding the range of ways people responded to the proposed legislation.

I begin this chapter by outlining how the petitioners envision Canadians' core responsibilities and rights as individual health citizens, and then I examine how they view themselves as consumers within a health marketplace where wellness is a commodity to be freely bought and sold. I close by considering how neoliberal emphases on individual responsibility for self-care can short-circuit opportunities to meaningfully shift the landscape of illness, health, and wellness by occluding the possibility of systemic change. Before I begin, I want to point out that my goal in this chapter, as in the rest of the book, is to examine what people believe is true about wellness and natural health, not to determine what is necessarily true. In the petition comments, for example, Lyse and others argue that the government should only "monitor quality" of natural health products, as Lyse put it, without restricting access, when in fact legislation in both Canada and the United States prevents even that level of regulation. Neither country requires testing for safety or efficacy before approving natural health products for sale, and health agencies in both countries can only respond to aftermarket complaints of harm.[10]

To engage with wellness as an autopoietic discourse, we need to engage with prevalent arguments about natural health products as they circulate, rather than focusing solely on essentialized underlying truths about such products, because those prevalent arguments have persuasive effects regardless of their fact status; whether or not they are true, these arguments move people to belief and action. Overwhelmingly, the materials I engage with in my analysis indicate that people believe that natural health products should, and do, come straight from nature to those who use them and that they are safe and effective. We need to begin with those beliefs and seek to understand them.

The Good Wellness Citizen

Over recent decades, responsibility for health has shifted globally from the state to individuals as governments increasingly call upon people to manage their own health as good health citizens.[11] This shift ushered in a "civic-moral imperative of healthy living" that reframed people as citizen-consumers who fulfill their obligations of citizenship through informed individual choices and behaviors.[12] Governments in countries with publicly funded health systems seek to reduce costs and heed calls for greater patient autonomy by creating self-service tools such as free at-home medical handbooks, websites, and twenty-four-hour nurse lines for individuals seeking health information, all of which aim to reduce costly visits to clinics and hospitals. Employers and insurers in private systems such as in the United States use similar self-serve options to reduce healthcare costs and premiums that, in the case of employers, aim also to reduce absenteeism and increase productivity. Workplace wellness programs, for instance, use apps, points systems, premium reductions, and other strategies to encourage employee physical fitness, healthy eating, and weight management, all with the goal of reducing employer-funded healthcare costs, although the effectiveness of such programs has not been clearly established.[13]

In the Canadian province of British Columbia, one such self-service initiative was the 2001 *BC Health Guide*, which was distributed by the government to every residence in the province.[14] This four-hundred-page guide offered step-by-step instructions for assessing injuries, ailments, and other conditions, as well as providing recommendations ranging from home remedies to emergency medical treatment. The handbook's ostensible goal was to empower individuals to take charge of their health, though it is not hard to see that it was intended at least equally to reduce publicly funded visits to healthcare providers. The *BC Health Guide* advocated a do-it-yourself approach to health care by shifting the authority to make medical decisions from health practitioners (especially doctors) to informed health consumers who assume responsibility for their own health and well-being. More recently, health agencies have relied on the web and telehealth programs to alleviate pressure on chronically underfunded health systems, although calls to help lines often result in exceptionally long wait times, potentially leaving individuals truly on their own to make medical decisions.

The public comments on the "Stop Bill C-51" petition demonstrate that Canadians have taken to heart the messaging of initiatives such as the *BC Health Guide*. The petitioners have so internalized personal responsibility as a condition of good health citizenship that they assert their right to use whatever products they choose to protect and promote their health and well-being. Throughout the dataset, commenters pledge their desire for unrestricted access to natural health products, citing past successes as evidence of the products' safety and efficacy. Commenter Lyse captures the essence of this position:

I feel that herbal products sold to the public should be regulated for content and strength only. Herbal remedies have been used for all time. There is no evidence that for chronic conditions, they are any less effective than most current pharmaceuticals. In fact, many drugs used frequently have been proven to be no more effective than placebos. Obviously in acute illness modern drugs are more effective. It is the individual's responsibility to learn about all medicinal products they use both modern and herbal. The government should not interfere except to monitor quality of commercial products.[15]

In this comment, Lyse evinces two key principles that undergird wellness as a form of self-management: that every person is *responsible* for their own self-care and, correspondingly, that every person has a fundamental *right* to self-care. For Lyse, the prospect of losing access to natural health products would constitute government overreach because she regards self-management as a sacred responsibility and right of citizenship.

Individual Responsibility for Self-Care

Those who commented on the "Stop Bill C-51" petition powerfully affirm that they as individuals, rather than doctors, healthcare agencies, or governments, hold primary responsibility for their health. Like the interview participants I discussed in chapter 1, the petition signatories demonstrate a profound commitment to their roles as citizen-consumers within an open marketplace of health products and services. For instance, a commenter named Mary Lynne argues that "I'm responsible for my own health care, and I have to ensure that all my options are open," whereas Denise explains that "as our former Premier of [the Canadian province of] Alberta said, 'It is time Albertans take control of our own health and not expect the health care system to take care of us.'" The petitioners maintain that everyone needs to step up to do their part to manage their own health and wellness. To fulfill that responsibility, the petitioners argue, they should be able to choose from the widest possible array of products and services in order to make the best choices they can as private wellness consumers.

The overall picture of the good health citizen that emerges from the petition comments is one who actively seeks to restore and enhance their wellness through a suite of behaviors that includes consuming natural health products as well as eating well, exercising regularly, and avoiding toxic consumer goods. The petition signatories argue that regulating natural health products would restrict their ability to perform their duties of citizenship, and they emphatically resist government and medical paternalism, asserting that they alone hold responsibility for learning about and deciding which health products and services they use:

> As a Canadian citizen I insist on the right to be responsible for my own health and to be able to continue to choose products that are beneficial in maintaining my good health. I do not need Big Brother—I am competent enough to do my own research.

> I am one of many disillusioned with the state of our current health care system; and believe that through self-education, research and taking responsibility for our own personal health; we as individuals, and as a country, can reduce the current stress on the health care system and enhance our quality of life for years to come. Follow the lead of a number of our European friends and include complimentary [sic] and alternative medicines to the roster instead of removing them and thus limiting the choices available to us—treat us as the educated, responsible Canadian citizens that we are.

> I am an intelligent individual who is quite capable of researching and deciding what products I put in my body and am against government interference.[16]

In these three examples, the commenters not only assume responsibility for learning about and deciding upon their health interventions; more importantly, they assume and assert that they have the requisite expertise to evaluate the safety and efficacy of these interventions on their own. One significant consequence of responsibilization discourse about health, then, is that it may give a false sense of expertise to individuals who lack specialized knowledge and training, leading them to overestimate their ability to decide on important matters of health and illness.[17]

The petition comments also reflect and embody the transformation of wellness into what Cederström and Spicer characterize as a "moral demand," with signatories not only embracing that demand but also rising to defend it in the face of Bill C-51.[18] The strong moral undercurrent within the comments parallels that same undercurrent of morality that shapes wellness discourse more generally, particularly regarding the individualization of responsibility for self-care. Philosopher Alexis Shotwell defines this moral impulse for self-care, following Robert Crawford, as *healthism*, or "the idea that we are each responsible for maintaining our own individual well-being, even in contexts of collective harm."[19] In a healthist worldview, Shotwell argues, there is a "tendency to think about individual health as a moral imperative—individuals are held responsible for their bodies, and obesity, diabetes, cancer, and other chronic conditions are rendered as moral failings."[20]

It is healthist, for instance, for my employer to tell me, during an unprecedented public health emergency that collapsed my home and work lives and closed my child's school, to make sure to take time out for myself to avoid burnout, while not meaningfully reducing my workload. It is healthist to tell would-be wellness seekers that feeling tired in the morning is a sign they need to take a supplement, while not discussing potential structural problems that might affect their sleep, mood, or energy. It is healthist to urge people living in insecure housing or lacking access to affordable food to practice mindfulness to quell anxiety or improve digestive problems. The moral imperative of wellness discourse tells each of us as individuals to do our part, regardless of larger structural factors that might ultimately determine how well we are.

The "Stop Bill C-51" signatories do not merely assume responsibility for making choices about their own self-care, however; they also assert their responsibility for making *appropriate* choices. Commenters perceive that there are right ways to restore and enhance wellness and wrong ways. Most pressingly, petitioners argue that natural health products are safer, gentler, and more effective than pharmaceuticals because they are "natural" and therefore the best choice for self-care. For example, Cindy explains that supplements allow people to go "back to nature," back to a time of pure wellness, whereas Jayne values supplements because they let people care for themselves "the way that nature intended." Signatories such as Anni cherish "the power of the nature gifts" to restore individuals to health, gifts that many commenters frame as divine in substance or origin, as Irene does here: "We all have a right to use the gifts that G-d has given us to take care of ourselves and our loved ones." In each of these cases, nature is cited as a pristine originary force, something that writer Eula Biss argues in her powerful book about vaccine hesitance, *On Immunity: An Inoculation*, is framed in public discourse as "pure and safe and benign."[21] Nature represents Eden before the Fall. In the eyes of those who oppose it, Bill C-51 therefore threatens to limit moral self-care through government restriction on products the signatories see as the most pure, most direct route to health and wellness.

The ideal form of moral, responsible self-care as imagined in the petition comments is to use natural health products to prevent illness before it can set in. According to the petitioners, there are two key components of prevention using supplements: proactively fostering a sense of multidimensional, holistic well-being and avoiding chemical harms in conventional medicine and in the environment. On the first component of prevention, those who oppose Bill C-51 echo the interview participants I discussed in the previous chapter by resisting atomistic understandings of health. Whereas an atomistic approach to health would view a single problem or symptom as treatable by a single drug, a process repeated with other drugs as needed for other problems or symptoms, the petitioners instead believe that true wellness is holistic. They view the body not as a collection of discrete physical parts and problems but as a whole entity that must be considered comprehensively:

> In the natural product industry (or at least in more traditional systems of medicine) synergy and wholeness are important aspects. There isn't really a reductionist approach to single (synthetic!) products; it's a wholistic approach to giving our bodies the best things they need so that they themselves can work for us to keep us healthy. Our bodies are really good at keeping us healthy. Nature has provided tons of help for us too.

> The whole herbs and nutrition market is a grass roots phenomenon evolving from people who know that good nutrition comes from good soil and care all along the way, from harvesting to bottling and transportation and has been successfully married to scientific knowledge to bring out formulations that do not treat disease but nurture health and vitality for the body which then itself overcomes unwanted conditions. Who can legislate away the body's inherent ability to heal itself when given the nutritional support and environment it requires?[22]

These commenters invoke holism as a central component of true healing because, in their view, it addresses underlying causes rather than merely masking problems by treating symptoms individually. Further, these commenters maintain that a holistic approach to health allows the body to heal itself by providing an appropriate nutritional environment. Natural health products therefore "nurture health and vitality," as the second commenter above, Andrew, puts it, not only by treating problems within the body but by creating optimal conditions for the body to both heal and thrive.

The petition comments also attribute duties of care not just to individual people with independent agency but also to the human body and to nature itself. That is, the commenters not only take up the terms of responsibilization for themselves but extend those terms to entities that cannot, in a strict sense, be "responsible." For example, both of the comments quoted in the previous paragraph figure the human body as itself responsible for and capable of self-healing. The first commenter argues that we need to use natural health products to support our bodies so "they themselves can work . . . to keep us healthy," whereas the second similarly suggests that natural health products will support "the body's inherent ability to heal itself." In these examples, the logics of restoration and enhancement are interbound: the body is always edging up against illness, requiring natural health products to restore it to good health, whereas those same products can also ignite within users a natural healing impulse that enhances health before one can become ill.

The petition comments also task nature with responsibility for health and wellness, imbuing it with the ability to engage in intentional, purposeful behaviors. For instance, the commenter who explained above that "our bodies are really good at keeping us healthy" added that "nature has provided tons of help for us too," aid that comes in the form of natural health products that help our bodies keep us healthy. Jayne goes even further by wondering whether her own children "will have the freedom of choice to take care of their bodies the way that nature intended or are they going to be forced into a medical communism where it's what someone else decides what they get for care?"[23] Jayne frames nature as having its own identifiable beliefs and desires ("nature *intended*"), which correspondingly situates human bodies as extensions of nature that draw on natural wisdom to self-regulate and self-repair, rather than requiring external, artificial interventions ("medical communism"). In this line of thinking, dietary supplements enhance the body through nutrition to create an environment in which it can fight off illness before it can set root, as commenter Penny explained: "Herbs and herbal products often allow us to treat the cause [of illness], not the symptom, which is all that our 'Doctors' do."[24]

The first step of preventing illness as a condition of responsible health citizenship in the "Stop Bill C-51" petition is to use natural health products to promote holistic well-being; the second step is to use natural health products to avoid and reduce harms from toxins and pharmaceuticals. Commenters worry that everyday life is steeped in hazardous chemicals, from polluted crops to contaminated air and water to home furnishings doused in flame retardants. Similarly, the commenters characterize pharmaceuticals as dangerous to health because they are "chemicals," "synthetic," and "toxic," characterizations that I discuss in detail in the next chapter. Here, I want only to highlight that the petitioners explicitly assume and accept responsibility for avoiding and reducing potential harms of toxins and pharmaceuticals. For instance, many of those who object to Bill C-51 believe that pharmaceuticals are inadequately tested and have dangerous side effects. However, rather than calling for expanded pharmaceutical regulations, the commenters instead cite these potential dangers as reasons for turning toward natural health products. Mary Catherine, for instance, argues that "many of the pharmaceutical drugs do not cure, but their side-effects actually do more harm than good," while an unnamed commenter says, "I am tired of the side effects related to prescription medications and the negative impact it has had on my families health."[25]

For many petition signatories, the apparent absence of side effects from supplements is a signal that they are safe and healthy to use. For example, Louise states that "the side effects from prescription drugs are many, and why would I want to subject myself to that, when there are natural remedies far healthier."[26] Louise implies that natural remedies are healthier at least in part because they do not have side effects. In these examples, the good wellness citizen discharges their wellness duties by making smart consumer decisions to avoid insidious toxic harms.

Of course, a crucial factor in the operation of wellness as an autopoietic discourse is precisely that it is difficult to dispute arguments that natural health products prevent illness. If a person taking a supplement for prevention does not fall ill, then the product seems effective regardless of whether it has any actual effect. If, instead, the person does fall ill, the supplement's failure to prevent illness could be explained in a variety of ways. One could argue, for example, that a given pathogen was particularly potent or that the natural health product was too gentle to fight it off. Or perhaps the person's own physical condition posed too much of a challenge—perhaps they were feeling especially run-down or had been living under greater stress than usual, so the supplement was not enough to counter it. As with public health measures such as vaccination or medical treatments such as cholesterol-lowering drugs, the success of natural health products for prevention can only be marked by a nonevent—by nothing happening at all. For vaccines, disease prevention can work against public enthusiasm and uptake, since the successful eradication of a pathogen such as the virus that causes polio can make preventive interventions seem redundant. For natural health products, the rhetorical situation is even more complex because wellness functions as a condition of good health citizenship that can be measured as much by the act of taking action, even if unsuccessful, as by the reduction of illness.

One further dimension of good health citizenship that emerges in the "Stop Bill C-51" petition comments may be unique to publicly funded health systems such as Canada's: the good wellness seeker, as figured in the petition, assumes responsibility for self-care at least partly to reduce burdens on the health system. Petitioners such as Andrew believe that dietary supplements alleviate demand on formal medical services in Canada: "People taking these products along with eating and growing their food consciously, exercising and not buying toxic products are keeping our health costs way down by needing less medical intervention."[27] Angela similarly explains that she is doing her part as a good health citizen: "I take herbs and vitamins to maintain excellent health and by doing so I help all Canadians by having to use the Canadian Health Care system quite a bit less often (perhaps only 3 times in 5 or 6 years)."[28]

Petitioners frequently cite the "broken" healthcare system as a reason for paying out-of-pocket for natural health products because wait times are excessive, doctors often cannot provide adequate care, patients often undergo unnecessary screenings and tests, and the whole system costs the public a lot of money. Additionally, commenters believe that taking natural alternatives whenever possible will mean that drugs are more effective when they are taken. As the commenter Ausra writes, "I want to be able to use cranberry, for example, to prevent bladder infection, so that I only need to use antibiotics when absolutely necessary. This reduces antibiotic resistance. We need both streams of health care to be able to flourish." It is not clear in Ausra's comments whether the primary concern in reducing antibiotic resistance is to preserve antibiotic efficacy across the whole population or in one's own body; in either case, her comment reveals her deep concern for the health system as a whole. Overall, the petition signatories assert that they require substantially less medical care as a result of taking supplements—which, in an age of managed care and limited resources, is itself an act of good citizenship.

In crediting natural health products for reducing the burden on formal medical care, those who signed the "Stop Bill C-51" petition illustrate the extent to which Canadians have internalized public health messaging about individual responsibility for health. They demonstrate a strong sense of personal and civic responsibility for both their own health and the health of their families, even at substantial personal expense. In debates about wellness and natural health that focus solely on whether a given intervention works, this account of supplement users as civic-minded, active, responsible health citizens is often lost. If we shift our attention instead toward what individuals expect to achieve by the decisions they make, their careful attention to fulfilling their obligations as responsible health citizens comes into sharper relief.

Individual Right to Self-Care

The corollary of the responsibilization of self-care is empowerment. According to the petition signatories, if individuals bear responsibility for managing both their own and their families' health, then they should have the right to access supplements without regulation or interference. Choice becomes a central value of empowered self-care, and choosing appropriately and responsibly thereby becomes another marker of good health citizenship.[29] Consider, for instance, petitioner Kathryn's objection to Bill C-51's perceived impact on consumer access to natural health products: "Our body is just that, 'OUR BODY', and how we choose to look after and care for our body should be 'OUR' decision alone, no one else's. It is outrageous that there are individuals who think they have some right to try to control that decision process regarding one's body."[30] Kathryn suggests that by potentially impeding people's right to choose what they put into their own bodies, the government is overstepping its legislative authority and infringing on citizens' freedom. Given that Bill C-51 did not propose any such broad power, the petition appears instead to have tapped into broader anxiety about health, healthcare, and the government's ability to make health-related decisions on the public's behalf. In this section, I illustrate how arguments about the right to self-care in the "Stop Bill C-51" petition reveal how wellness products and services reframe consumer choice for self-management as effectively a matter of life and death.

A prevailing argument about the right to self-care in the petition comments is that freedom of choice, including choice in healthcare, is a cornerstone of Canadian democracy and a central right of citizenship. Commenters view decisions about health as deeply personal, not to be made by governments or corporations. They argue that the ability to make one's own health decisions is a constitutionally assured right:

> It's not right to legislate what the individual chooses to put into their body. That's not the government's business.

> Another outrage by our Canadian government! How dare they remove my right (not privilege) to ingest what I feel is beneficial to my health.

> As a Canadian citizen I insist on the right to be responsible for my own health and to be able to continue to choose products that are beneficial in maintaining my good health. I do not need Big Brother—I am competent enough to do my own research.[31]

In the first two examples, the commenters invoke the body as a sovereign entity governed by individual citizens, who alone have the right to decide what does or does not cross its boundaries ("what the individual chooses to put into their body"; "my right . . . to ingest"). In the third example, the commenter aligns Bill C-51 with totalitarian models of governance by alluding to Big Brother, the surveilling ruler in George Orwell's novel *1984*. Similar references to totalitarian regimes are pervasive throughout the petition, including numerous other references to Big Brother, as well as to communism and dictatorship. Signatories frequently express surprise that a Conservative government that usually favors free-market activity would try to limit consumer choice through Bill C-51. Jeffrey, for instance, identifies as a longtime Conservative and wonders why the government does not "leave us as educated individuals in Canada to make up our own minds about what we consume." Sheryl, also a Conservative, explains her own consternation about Bill C-51: "I have been a Conservative all my adult life and am appalled that this bill would even be introduced." Sheryl wonders how this legislation will affect other choices down the road: "Are you thinking of banning food next??"

Virtually every petition commenter asserts in some form that caring for their own health with natural health products results in better and more lasting health than does relying solely on the publicly funded system. The petitioners argue that their right of access to these products must be preserved to reduce pressure on the public system and to alleviate their own frustrations with that system. The commenters decry medicine's emphasis on illness over health and wellness and on care of individual body parts rather than whole persons. Most importantly, however, the signatories argue that their right of access to natural health products should be preserved simply because these products work: in their view, the products achieve desired and noticeable effects. The commenter Maria exclaims, "Natural products have proven they work. Why is this a threat when the results are so positive . . . people are happier and healthier?"[32] In many cases, commenters choose natural health products when pharmaceuticals fail to help. Lorraine found success for a family member's psoriasis with an ointment made of essential oils after prescription steroids did not help. Other commenters prefer natural health products because they are more cost-effective than pharmaceuticals; for example, Sue uses vitamins and omega-3 capsules for osteoporosis because the drug alternatives "are very expensive" and Canada does not have universal pharmacare coverage. Similar comments throughout the petition regarding the relative affordability of supplements compared with pharmaceuticals illustrate that for the opponents of Bill C-51 the right to self-care encompasses affordability and financial prosperity as well as health.

Many signatories also indicate that not only are supplements effective but they provide critical, life-changing help. Boris, for example, comments that for him natural health products made the difference between life and death: "I would be dead or in a wheel chair if i listened to the medical industry.doctors have told me this themselves. Because of the supplemants i take i am pain and disease free." Tamara similarly, credits supplements with curing a range of chronic health conditions: "I am 53 years old and had an irregular heartbeat, goiter, hi blood pressure, vision deteriorating, brain fog,insomnia, bowell issues,and fatigue to the point of only being to able to work 4 hours per day. . . . I am now able to work a 10 hour day with an energy level I had in my 20's. This would not have been possible without these super food supplements."[33] Both Boris and Tamara argue that supplements have fundamentally altered the course of their lives. In Tamara's case, the curative potential of natural health products extends from health to work, economic stability, and the ability to engage meaningfully in everyday life activities.

Other commenters value supplements for reducing their overall medication load, which helps them optimize their own self-care. David, for instance, reports not needing to take any medication besides a daily dose of Lyrica since starting on supplements for pain. The supplements have been so effective, in fact, that David is now even "considering stopping this medication [Lyrica] because the 'natural' treatments are working so well." In all these examples, commenters describe supplements as providing important, natural options for self-treatment. Having options is important, as one signatory argues: "Natural health products have helped me at times that prescription drugs did not. The fact that I had a CHOICE to use either or meant a lot to me."[34]

Finally, the individual right to self-care, particularly as it concerns freedom of choice, is linked in the petition to wavering trust in science and medicine. The petition signatories maintain that Bill C-51 is motivated by greedy pharmaceutical companies seeking support from a corrupt government to accrue wealth at the expense of individual citizens as well as the public good. Jacqui argues, for instance, "I think that this Bill is just a way for pharmaceutical companies to fight back the natural care industry. Currently people are empowering themselves more and more when it comes to healthcare and are not as likely to believe in drugs and allopathic medicine."[35] Although there is no indication that Bill C-51 was indeed motivated by such a goal—nothing in my own research suggests as much—the prevalence of this argument within the dataset signals high public skepticism about the pharmaceutical industry, as well as its perceived embrace by government and the medical profession. More important, this comment that Bill C-51 is a machination of the pharmaceutical industry also reveals a deeper motivation for fighting the legislation: people who experience mainstream medicine as disempowering and view pharmaceuticals as unnatural find value in natural health products as alternatives for their own self-care. Taking those alternatives away would violate the petitioners' right to self-care as good health citizens.

Ultimately, by advocating for their individual rights to self-care by pushing back against legislation they believe will impede those rights, the signatories to the "Stop Bill C-51" petition do not oppose the responsibilization of health but, rather, carry that responsibilization to its logical conclusion: they so strongly fulfill their sense of personal and civic responsibility for health self-management that they seek interventions well beyond the bounds of conventional biomedicine, often at substantial personal expense. This particular account of supplement users as people who are motivated by deep concern about their responsibilities and rights as health citizens is often lost in debates that focus solely on whether a given health intervention works. Further, charging individual citizens with responsibility for self-management shifts the lines of influence in health and wellness by converting processes we might otherwise view as properties of medicine, such as diagnosis and treatment, into commodities in an open marketplace. The commodification of wellness has deep roots in the history of medicine, where self-management is not just a duty of citizenship but also an act of conspicuous consumption.

Wellness for Sale

The market for medical self-care is not a new phenomenon, as historian of medicine Roy Porter illustrates in *Quacks*, his sweeping account of shifts in the United Kingdom from the seventeenth-century medical market of "fakers and charlatans" to the emergence of professionalized medicine in the nineteenth century. During this period, Porter argues, "self-dosing" with proprietary medicines, culinary preparations, and lay procedures performed by wet nurses, maids, stablehands, and cooks was widespread, part of a culture of empowered medical consumption. Patients at this time were not passive supplicants to physicians; rather, they orchestrated their own care "much as they would hire a hairdresser or fire a cook," working with a range of practitioners as they pleased. The wide availability of populist health information such as home handbooks fed the demand for self-treatment, while the period's emergent commodity fetishism fueled the rise of new drugs as pills and ointments circulated as consumer items in the health marketplace. According to Porter, these shifts fostered the "reification of healing into commodity form," persuading the Georgian English public that "relief and health were things that money could buy."[36]

This consumerist view of health for sale—a phrase I take from the first edition of Porter's book of the same name—has only deepened today in the face of public health rhetorics of choice and responsibility accompanied by shrinking health funding in austerity budgets.[37] In the contemporary context, health is still sold as a product on an open market, whether in the form of pharmaceuticals advertised in the pages of *People* magazine, supplements sold at Whole Foods or naturopaths' offices, cosmetic procedures offered by dermatologists, or services provided at integrative health clinics. The marketization of health and wellness necessarily implies that the market will determine which interventions are more worthy (and by implication safer and more effective) than others. This model of determining the availability of supplements through market competition is fundamentally at odds with evidence-based medicine, wherein scientific evidence is the sole arbiter of a product's worth, but it is consonant with core Canadian and American values of freedom and consumer choice. In this section, I explain how wellness sells as a form of self-management by satisfying consumerist impulses that situate shopping as an act of good citizenship and a right of democratic engagement. I revisit some of the arguments I examined in the previous section because the responsibilities and rights of health citizenship overlap with those of consumer culture.

Shopping Your Way to Health

Within the comments on the "Stop Bill C-51" petition, arguments about the wellness citizen's obligations of self-care sit in tension with those about health as a consumer good because the consumer right to choose is rooted not in protected democratic rights of citizenship but in a market economy where sales figures are the ultimate arbiter of a product's worth. That is, within a consumer framework, the authority of science and government is displaced by the dictates of supply and demand. Accordingly, arguments within the petition that figure health and wellness as consumer goods illustrate the consequences of a neoliberal approach to health that frames the health seeker as a rational, "sovereign customer with a coherent shopping list and a fat wallet in a well-stocked market" rather than as a medical patient in need of expert help.[38] The market model of medicine pits medical expertise, which is based on a health provider's education, training, and experience, against patient empowerment, where individuals make autonomous health decisions based partly on expert advice but also on a range of other, often personal considerations such as life and illness experience, family history, financial resources, and values, beliefs, and feelings.

As sovereign customers in a wellness marketplace, those who signed the "Stop Bill C-51" petition seek to maintain their right to decide for themselves which products to take and how. They do not want to surrender their decision-making agency to doctors or the government, as Dianne argues here: "Everyone deserves the right to have alternatives (natural) vs. our non up to date advice from our Dr's. Our bodies = our own choices unless you would like to only receive advice from your GP. I think not for this body."[39] Many commenters argue that the popularity of natural health products is simply the natural outcome of market competition because consumers vote with their wallets. These individuals seek alternatives to what they perceive as deficiencies in mainstream medical care, such as a lack of access to doctors, inadequate care, overemphasis on pharmaceuticals, safety concerns, and failure to address root causes of illness rather than just focusing on symptoms. As one petition signatory exclaims, "If people are turning to alternative solutions it's because they are not satisfied with what they've been getting over the counter. If Pharma is losing money because of this they need to make better products."[40]

Within the argument that health self-management is a consumer choice, one dominant thread is that people should have multiple healthcare choices available to them, just as they would brands of apple juice or cell phone providers. The petition's commenters often consider biomedicine and natural health as equals in an open health marketplace. Accordingly, they figure the task of the health consumer as one of simply choosing their preferred option in a given situation:

[A]s a mother of a three and five year old I like having the options to pull from both of these important fields—medical and naturopathic.

I believe there is real value in pursuing a variety of options when it comes to one's health, and I fear that a single focus on "western" medicine leads society away from a holistic approach to health.

It's great that we have these options available to us. And there's no reason to dismiss either. If I've got a broken bone or something, I'm not going to the [health] food store to get some tea I'm going to the hospital to get pumped full of expensive synthetic drugs and get fixed up. If I've got chronic indigestion, I'm not going to the drugstore to get some strange synthetic concoction that happens to make me feel better temporarily, without fixing anything, that has a slew of really strange side effects. I'm going [to] the naturopath to find out what's wrong with my diet and see what natural remedies are available that can fix the problem. I don't need Zantac, I need a solution. There's a place in our society for all kinds of treatment options.[41]

In these examples, choice is an unqualified good that the petitioners want to protect. In the latter two examples in particular, the choice between natural health products and mainstream pharmaceuticals is marked by a difference not of degree but of kind, as they occupy distinct realms that for these commenters are defined by wellness and illness, respectively. While both commenters believe that mainstream medicine is appropriate for acute illness and injury, they prefer natural health products for improving their overall well-being through preventive care and addressing root causes of digestive and other problems. Especially given that natural health products are now shelved next to pharmaceuticals in major pharmacies and big-box stores, not tucked away in niche health food stores and organic co-ops, consumers have every reason to believe these products are distinct but equal.

Further, when health is marketized, the sheer volume and variety of natural health products available on store shelves alone imply that the products must be effective, or they would not sell as well as they do. Petitioners tasked with self-management argue for unrestricted access to natural health products by drawing on the classical Aristotelian topos of size, an orienting perspective that furnishes lines of argument about the relative greatness or smallness of something.[42] Many petitioners assert, for example, that supplements must be safe and effective because so many people use them:

> Natural supplements have been a benefit to *thousands and thousands of people*.

> Ridiculous law and will impact *many, many people* that currently enjoy the ability to treat themselves with natural alternatives to big pharma concoctions.

> If this bill were to get passed this country would have *more sick people*, more pressure on a crumbling health care system and an even lower GDP as *many people* are sustaining themselves on products from the natural health industry![43]

Commenters similarly cite the size of the natural product industry as evidence of the products' effectiveness. According to Jackie, "The very levels of profits from this industry should tell you what the people of this country support."[44] In all of these examples, people believe in the power of the market, rather than scientific evidence or doctors, to decide on the effectiveness of health interventions. If a product survives and thrives in an open marketplace, the logic goes, then it must be worth the money.

Another way the petition signatories argue from the topos of size to support the wide availability of natural health products is that the products have been used over long periods of time. Commenters such as Rose cite "ancient herbal wisdom" to argue that according to the dictates of market logic, supplements would have fallen out of use long ago if they did not work. Jayne similarly writes, "This bill . . . impedes my decision to use herbal remedies that have been around longer than pharmaceuticals for my own health." Denise figures competition and choice as cornerstones of an ideal health market, which draws on the best of contemporary science and traditional herbal remedies: "Living in Canada I should have the right to choose, just like I can choose who to vote for. . . . There is definitely a place for both our health care system and the natural way. The Natural way is how civilizations lived for thousands of years before penicillin."[45] The argument that natural health products are necessarily effective because they have been used for a long time is not logically sound, but it remains powerfully persuasive both among the petition's signatories and among the broader contemporary public.[46]

Natural health products' appearance of efficacy is further bolstered in Canada by the appearance on their packaging of a natural product number, or NPN, issued by Health Canada. The licensing of health products in Canada has undergone significant changes over the past decade, with all nonprescription pharmaceuticals and natural health products placed in a single category, along with disinfectants. But when Bill C-51 was proposed, in 2008, the NPN was an important marker of distinction for natural health products. The NPN distinguished natural products from pharmaceuticals, which were licensed in a separate category under a DIN, or drug identification number. Appearing on a natural health product's package, the NPN would have signaled endorsement from Health Canada, although the regulator did not necessarily verify claims of safety and effectiveness, and flaws in the approval process are well documented.[47] However, because regulatory processes are largely invisible to those who purchase and use natural health products, even the most savvy, cynical consumer could be forgiven for assuming that a Health Canada license number meant that a product was safe and effective. Indeed, for many consumers in 2008, NPNs and DINs likely seemed equivalent, if distinct, both endorsed by Health Canada. Although none of the petition signatories specifically cite the NPN as a reason for choosing natural health products, some do argue that the products must have already been approved as safe and effective since they have been commercially available for so long. Overall, for those who signed the "Stop Bill C-51" petition, the right to choose their own health interventions from a range of options is fundamental to their identities both as Canadians and as consumers.

Consuming Wellness as Agency

For those who signed the "Stop Bill C-51" petition, purchasing and consuming natural health products offers an opportunity to seek care, comfort, and cures they have otherwise been unable to access. The idea of health self-management is appealing partly because it invites people to take charge of their own health, appearing to free them of biomedicine's worst paternalist, "doctor knows best" tendencies. Further, as illustrated by comments from Tamara and Boris above, people living with chronic degenerative conditions or conditions that are difficult to diagnose and treat often view natural health products as vital additional options when mainstream pharmaceutical medicine is unable to help. Tamara credits supplements with successfully treating exhaustion and brain fog and giving her mid-fifties body the energy of a 20-year-old, whereas Boris argues that supplements were a cure for debilitating chronic pain. Similarly, as I discuss in upcoming chapters, those who seek wellness as a form of enhancement rather than restoration find in natural health products a powerful way to reshape their lives by optimizing their bodies, minds, and capacities. In each of these cases, agency over your own health becomes something you can buy in supplement form.

Agency is a central theme in the comments on the petition against Bill C-51: petitioners want to manage their own health, free of meddling governments, doctors, and pharmaceutical companies. For instance, a commenter named Lorraine argues that "Canadians are taking their health care into their own hands and looking for safer alternative medicine" made with "natural ingredients" rather than relying on "expensive and dangerous 'legal' drugs." Jayne, whom I cited earlier in this chapter, views supplements as a way of exercising agency against state-sponsored healthcare, or "medical communism." Other commenters similarly liken medical regulations to dictatorship and oppression and strongly affirm their ability to make their own health decisions, without government or medical mediation. Dominique, for instance, implores the government to "please realize that it is beneficial to all Canadians to be able to attend to their own health, especially at this time of crisis in the health care system. Give us the power to tend to our own bodies, our own needs. Trust that we know what is best for us."[48] For these petitioners, wellness as self-management means having the freedom and power to use interventions of their own choosing.

The petition signatories overwhelmingly express frustration with a disempowering, publicly funded health system as a reason for preserving their access to natural health products. They recount stories of doctor shortages, poor care, and feelings of powerlessness, whereas using supplements gives them a sense of control over their own care. Natascha, for instance, explains: "I have been sick for years following my regular doctor's advice and medications. Since I've been seeing a Naturopath, I am 95% better than ever and very frustrated with the health care system."[49] Many commenters credit natural health products with helping them avoid harsh treatments, such as pharmaceuticals or surgery, as well as bleak prognoses. One unnamed signatory writes:

> Herbs have helped me numerous times, especially this last year when the doctors were about to remove my thyroid, but then I took herbs and my health increased dramatically, and now the doctors say I can keep it!!!!!!! I just saved our health care system the $10,000 they said the surgery would cost by taking a few herbs for 6 months, which I payed for by myself! Why on earth would you not have wanted me to do that? For my own personal health, as well as the financial health of our health care system, please allow the continued use of plants for their health benefits.[50]

By arguing that herbal supplements preempted life-changing surgery, this commenter illustrates how wellness products offer individuals a sense of control over situations that threaten their autonomy. Further, paying for the supplements out-of-pocket seems only to confirm this commenter's agency to make decisions on their own, as well as their freedom from influence of medicine or government. Overall, the petition signatories assert their agency as consumers to decide how their money is spent, which in their view wrests control over health from doctors. Like many other petition signatories, Denise criticizes doctors for seeking profit from illness: "Doctors as a whole make their money off illness. [Bill C-51] is just another way to herd people into their twisted medical system."[51]

Opponents of Bill C-51 also find in natural supplements another form of agency: they feel more empowered in the face of illness, an experience that is disempowering at its core. Many commenters praise supplements for mitigating or curing conditions that in their view are not adequately treated or even diagnosed in mainstream medicine, including attention-deficit hyperactivity disorder, cancer, chronic fatigue syndrome, fibromyalgia, and chronic pain. Viviane, for example, describes becoming "very sick from taking conventional drugs" but, upon receiving diagnoses of chronic fatigue syndrome and fibromyalgia, finding hope of recovery in vitamins and supplements—"all the good of the earth, that can cure and help the helpless sick people like me." Lori too argues that natural health products are vital for her treatment: "I have been told by my doctor that there is no cure nor any therapies for my illnesses. Natural remedies have been sought and I am very thankful and hopeful of a full recovery."[52] In both examples, natural health products restore users' agency by resolving conditions that mainstream pharmaceuticals and practitioners did not, or could not, address.

Finally, for many of the petition signatories, agency also comes in the very fact of being able to choose nonpharmaceutical health interventions. Tara, for instance, is averse to conventional medicine, and so natural health products are a valuable alternative avenue for treatment: "I do not see a doctor and i don't use prescription medicine, neither do my children. The body can usually heal itself with the proper food, herbs etc. Drug companies do more harm than good." By choosing "herbs" over pharmaceuticals, Tara exercises agency as a wellness consumer. In other cases, petitioners assert that they cannot use pharmaceuticals because of "allergies and sensitivities to pharmaceutical drugs," as one commenter described; for these commenters, supplements become a necessity rather than a choice. Another petition signatory similarly explained, "Because of several severe health problems, I need natural products to cure and feed myself. I am allergic to the drugs that have been prescribed to me and natural products are my only alternative."[53] Bill C-51 threatens this person's agency in the most fundamental way: if they were unable to buy natural health products, they would have no agency at all.

In all of these examples, the "Stop Bill C-51" petition signatories value supplements as a means of restoring their agency to manage their own health, particularly since the government and doctors have not provided sufficient care or support. But leaving people to fend for themselves necessarily means leaving some to flourish and others, usually the most vulnerable, to starve.

Self-Management or Abandonment by the State?

One central principle underlying this book is that the state must not relinquish its responsibility for human health by repackaging abandonment of citizens as "self-care." Indeed, the very rise of wellness culture and natural health is fueled largely by government failures to provide for basic human needs through public health, adequately funded and allocated healthcare, housing and social welfare protections, education, and food security. As I have argued above, downloading responsibility for health onto individual citizen-consumers directly sponsors an individualist, market-oriented vision of health in which choosing health providers and interventions is analogous to choosing between supermarkets or product brands. It is for this reason that I have no tolerance for critiques of wellness culture that mock or ridicule people for choosing health products and services outside the realm of medical-pharmaceutical treatments. Wellness consumers are doing precisely what they have been told to do over decades of relentless public messaging, marketing campaigns, and government policies. The bootstrap mentality of late twentieth- and early twenty-first-century health policy and planning relies on rugged individualism; one need look no further than the global coronavirus pandemic that put at greatest risk of exposure those with the least social capital—low-wage earners, racialized people, people in low-income housing and neighborhoods—while people like me (and probably you) were able to work safely and financially secure at home.

An irony of shifting responsibility for health from the collective to the individual is that those who take on the moral weight of self-care often see the government not as *abandoning* its citizens by burdening them with the labor of self-management but as *caring for* its citizens by furnishing conditions that allow them to make individual choices as health consumers. For the signatories of the "Stop Bill C-51" petition, any limits on access to natural health products would therefore violate that principle of care by denying people the right and freedom to self-manage their health. Commenters argue that they should be able to choose natural health products for themselves without any government interference: "It is not necessary to regulate or control supplements," says Sandra, because, as a fellow commenter, Jeffrey, explains, "almost without exception products sold at . . . health stores are made from natural organic products and do no harm."[54] These commenters demonstrate a circular pattern of reasoning, arguing that the state is failing to care for its citizens by not allowing access to natural health products, when, as I argue in this final section, they largely seek access to natural health products precisely because they believe the state is failing to care for its citizens. The petition signatories demonstrate that the doctrine of self-management fuels demand for wellness products and services, while at the same time it arguably leaves citizens less well overall.

Most of the people who signed the "Stop Bill C-51" petition express deep mistrust in the government because, in their view, it refuses to properly care for its citizens. They regard the public healthcare system as critically underfunded, oversubscribed, and generally ill-equipped to deal with the basic health needs of those it ostensibly serves. Many of the commenters report using natural health products to treat chronic illness and disability, arguing that they have not been able to access the care they need because, in their experience, doctors are only interested in quick-fix solutions, usually in the form of pharmaceuticals, and not in alleviating their distress. Other commenters fear that the government is actively denying them the agency to care for themselves and their families. What is most important to understand about the petitioners' comments regarding wellness as a form of self-management, then, is that underneath arguments against supplement regulation is a persistent belief that the government has failed in its duty to care for its citizens.

A significant proportion of those who signed the "Stop Bill C-51" petition go a step further and argue that the government is not just negligent but also corrupt, actively seeking to capitalize on the population rather than to care for it. For these signatories, the ability to make choices about their health is a core right of both democratic governance and capitalist economies, and so losing the right to choose is a constitutional and economic violation. Some signatories, such as Cheryl, even argue that governments try to maintain control over citizens by deliberately delivering poor healthcare and restricting patient-consumer choice: "This is dictatorship . . . period. What is next. No more broccoli or asparagus as they may improve our overall health . . . is this the agenda . . . more sick people means better control of us and the bonus is supporting your bosses . . . the pharmaceutical industry. We all know your agenda . . . which is why you are trying to push this through quietly . . . in secret."[55] Like many others who signed the petition, Cheryl sees health regulations as a potential tool of oppression.

Other signatories characterize Canada as an emergent "police state," a "fascist state," a state that is "becoming more like a communist country rather that a free country that we are to be."[56] Here again the petition signatories link the right to choice in healthcare to their democratic rights as citizens. Some of the more extreme iterations of this argument are tinged with conspiracy theories about pharmaceutical kickbacks or foreign government influence on Canadian officials, but the petition's underlying position is clear: the government is oppressing the very people it was elected to serve by trying to limit or control their ability to seek the forms of healthcare they desire.

Greed also looms large in the petition comments more generally. Many of the signatories believe the goal of the legislation is to force consumers to choose pharmaceuticals over natural health products. A commenter named Paul, for example, argues that "the government is in it for the money but not for the people," while another, unnamed commenter cites the legislation as "yet another sign of the pull of the drug companies on our government." Many signatories also believe the government favors the pharmaceutical industry by hiding problems in conventional biomedicine to ensure its dominance in the healthcare sector. According to Jayne, "The government shades the truth on a lot of western medical practices in their greed for money and pass[es] it off as care and concern for their citizens!"[57] For these individuals, Bill C-51 constitutes a government intervention that protects the interests of the pharmaceutical industry over those of citizens by forcing people to use pharmaceuticals when they would prefer to use natural health products. Ultimately, the signatories believe that human health should be valued in its own right, not as an instrument of profit or political gain.

While some comments on the petition view Bill C-51 as a government conspiracy to increase pharmaceutical profits, others offer nuanced critiques of how current pharmaceutical industry practices erode public trust in both the industry itself and the government bodies that regulate it. For example, one unnamed commenter observes,

> The way I see this bill is a thinly veiled american style attempt to push through a bill that benefits the Pharma business. First, the minister of health has large investments in the business (which may very well be incidental). Also the argument concerning us being protected, especially in this particular business, is kinda ridiculous. When new drugs are introduced into the market it's the companies that manufacture them who perform the tests to see if the new product is safe; the company then submits this information to the regulatory body who decides if they can be sold. A sketchy process, with the prevailing interest likely to get the drugs on the market, safety second.[58]

In this example, the commenter lays out a reasonable basis for questioning the bill's integrity: well-documented problems in pharmaceutical research, approval, and marketing.[59] At the end of their comment, this petition signatory also suggests in a parenthetical aside that then prime minister Stephen Harper was in league with Big Pharma, "proposing other laws to make getting new drugs on the market even easier, by the way." Here, the commenter points to government conflict of interest and the clashing ideologies of universal healthcare and free-market capitalism as evidence that the government is corrupt in siding with the pharmaceutical industry over those it was elected to serve.

For the petition's signatories, the cost of government corruption is paid at the expense of human bodies and lives. Many commenters express deep discomfort with the tension between health as a public good and healthcare as a market commodity. Although many commenters defend their rights to purchase supplements as consumer products, at the same time they overwhelmingly resist the idea that health should be viewed as an opportunity for making money. They frequently figure supplement manufacturers as small-time good guys fighting evil corporate giants—the Davids of healthcare fighting Big Pharma's Goliath—often failing to recognize that supplement producers are themselves large, for-profit corporations that are often owned by pharmaceutical parent companies.[60] Penny argues, for instance: "I believe that natural health products need to be monitored only for quality purposes. The fillers etc. in the so called 'good prescription drugs' not to mention many of the actual ingredients are extremely unhealthy. In fact I am sure some only serve to keep people coming back to a Doctor repeatedly. . . . Herbs and herbal products often allow us to treat the cause, not the symptom, which is all that our 'Doctors' do." Here, Penny draws several key distinctions between supplements and pharmaceuticals, including their different contents (natural and pure versus "extremely unhealthy" fillers and ingredients) and their different purposes (treating underlying causes versus treating symptoms). Many petition signatories also argue that the supplement industry is more honest than pharmaceutical companies, particularly because they desire to heal rather than merely to make money. Barbara, for instance, writes, "I would not be alive today if it weren't for the natural health, alternative supplement industry. This industry has more self-governing integrity than most which exist today—please leave well enough alone!" Andrew similarly describes the natural health product industry as a "grass roots phenomenon" led by "people who know that good nutrition comes from good soil and care all along the way."[61]

Somewhat ironically, the petition's signatories often employ the logics of capitalism, such as the principles of market choice and individual responsibility, to critique Bill C-51 as an exercise in capitalist ideology. They charge then prime minister Stephen Harper and then minister of health Tony Clement with promoting profits for pharmaceutical companies without noticing or acknowledging that the natural health product industry was itself a profit-driven industry. Further, the petition signatories critique the government for eroding public, population-level investment in healthcare, while the commenters' own focus is trained solely on health at the level of individual consumption, each body responsible for itself. Kathryn's comment summarizes this position: "Our body is just that, 'our body', and how we choose to look after and care for our body should be 'our' decision alone, no one else's. It is outrageous that there are individuals who think they have some right to try to control that decision process regarding one's body."[62] Overall the petitioners frequently cite public good and public health as reasons for opposing the legislation, but they then argue for individual over collective solutions to problems of health. For those who signed the "Stop Bill C-51" petition, health self-management through wellness is ultimately a solo project.

As is true in wellness discourse more generally, the petition signatories seldom acknowledge systemic factors that negatively affect health, such as poverty, disparities of education and opportunity, inadequate housing, limited availability of healthy food and safe water, and racism and other forms of discrimination. Instead, they focus on individual acts of consumption, particularly of wellness products and services. Overall, the concept of health invoked in the petition is radically individualized; good health is seen not as a right of all citizens but, troublingly, as a choice for those wise and wealthy enough to make that choice. This model of wellness as an exercise in personal choice and consumption privileges only those who can afford it.

What is disturbing about wellness as a form of self-management, then, is that public health rhetorics of personal responsibility situate individual citizens as agents of their own health without ensuring that all citizens have the opportunity and means to assume that responsibility. Many signatories of the "Stop Bill C-51" petition believe that natural health products are vital to human health because they activate "the body's inherent ability to heal itself when given the nutritional support and environment it requires," as the commenter Andrew puts it.[63] If these products are accessible only to the wealthy, however, then they ultimately offer little opportunity to meaningfully shift the landscape of illness, health, and wellness. By privileging the perspectives of the already privileged, wellness culture therefore occludes the possibility of systemic change that would benefit everyone. If health is for sale, that is, then wellness becomes a consumer good traded on an open market that remains out of reach for many, particularly those who most need it. As the next chapter illustrates, the spoils of wellness culture are unequally distributed among the rich, whereas natural health products promise to reduce harms that disproportionately affect not the rich but the poor.

CHAPTER THREE

Wellness as Harm Reduction

When I began working on the project that would eventually become this book, I came across two cultural artifacts that unlocked for me the third vector of wellness discourse, that wellness constitutes a form of harm reduction. *Harm reduction* is a term from substance use treatment policy that describes the practice of proactively reducing exposure to or mitigating potential risks associated with substance use. The idea behind harm reduction is that when risk of harm cannot be avoided outright (e.g., through abstinence), the better policy is to do *something*, such as provide safe injection sites with clean needle kits and emergency overdose care, rather than nothing at all. In the realm of health and wellness, a similar idea of harm reduction is a key motivator of supplement use, with individuals relying on natural health products to replace or offset the harmful effects of pharmaceuticals and everyday exposure to potential health risks such as environmental contamination.[1] I argue in this chapter that the principle of harm reduction intensifies and expands discourse about wellness as people grapple with living in a world they view as increasingly harmful to their health.

The first artifact that shaped my thinking for this chapter on wellness as harm reduction was a banner poster that hung for years in the window of the health food store Sweet & Natural on busy Yonge Street in downtown Toronto. Situated on the ground floor of a tall, concrete building, the store offers a range of naturopathic and homeopathic remedies, nutritional supplements, and personal care products. In large pink and purple type, the poster exclaimed a warning to passers-by: "In Today's Toxic Environment CLEANSING is no longer an option. It's a NECESSITY!" In the middle of this text was an image of two product boxes in matching hues of pink and purple, packages for the supplements First Cleanse and CleanseSMART. Each box featured a stylized drawing of a sun and a logo for the products' parent company, Renew Life, set against a background color gradient suggesting bright midday light. On the bottom of the poster were five checkmark-bulleted reasons for "Why YOU should cleanse":

✓ Improves Overall Health
✓ Decreases Risk of Disease
✓ Increases Energy
✓ Improves Digestion
✓ Reduces Toxicity

Although the poster did not include specific product information, Renew Life's website explains that First Cleanse contains sixty capsules filled with "39 whole herbs to support the cleansing of all 7 channels of elimination"—liver, lungs, lymphatic system, kidneys, skin, blood, and bowels.[2] CleanseSMART, the other product depicted on the poster, is, according to the website, more powerful than First Cleanse because it includes an "added focus on the body's two main detoxification pathways, the liver and the colon," organs that together "reduce the toxic load in your body and relieve occasional constipation."[3] These promotional materials for Renew Life's cleanses are at once both vague and alarming: they do not explain how or why the products affect the listed organs and systems, but they do identify an urgent problem (toxicity) and offer a ready solution (a cleanse).

The second artifact that helped crystallize for me how wellness functions as a form of harm reduction was a gameshow-style segment from *The Dr. Oz Show* titled "Toxic Toss Out," which aired in 2010 (figs. 1 and 2). For the segment, Oz asked audience members to bring to the show the household items they believed to be most toxic. The items were placed on a steel table in front of the two competitors, Doris and Carla, who raced to find the three items Oz had chosen in advance as the worst offenders. As each woman made her selection, Oz praised her for being a wise consumer, for being "too smart" to buy toxin-containing products such as mothballs. He closed the segment by explaining why consumers should not buy the three products featured in the game.[4]

Together, Renew Life's cleanse poster and *Dr. Oz*'s "Toxic Toss Out" segment illustrate how toxins are figured in contemporary public discourse as weakly defined entities that lurk invisibly everywhere in our everyday lived environment. Rhetorician Phaedra Pezzullo explains in her book *Toxic Tourism: Rhetorics of Pollution, Travel, and Environmental Justice* that toxins "*by definition* . . . refer to those substances that pose environmental and human health hazards," including asthma, congenital disorders, memory loss, and perhaps above all, various forms of cancer.[5] In chemical terms, toxins can make us physically sick by disrupting how the body works. Toxins also serve as powerful social-semiotic

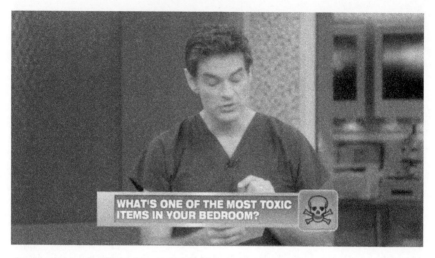

Figure 1. A video still of Dr. Oz presenting on "toxic" household items, *The Dr. Oz Show*, episode 80, "Toxic Home"

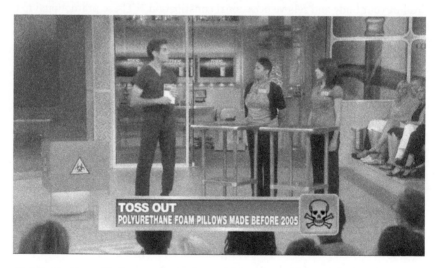

Figure 2. A video still of Dr. Oz quizzing competitors on "toxic" household items, *The Dr. Oz Show*, episode 80, "Toxic Home"

signifiers that, as Pezzullo points out, we use rhetorically to refer to substances, places, people, or relationships that we view as *figuratively* harmful.[6] For example, we often hear statements such as *She's a toxic person* or *They had a toxic marriage*. These expressions are obviously metaphors to describe personalities or situations negatively. But what about other common ways of talking about toxicity in contemporary culture? Is sugar toxic, for example? Or gluten? How about conventionally grown fruits and vegetables, which may or may not contain traces of herbicides, pesticides, or genetically modified materials? Headlines I have seen on magazines at supermarket checkouts suggest these foods are toxic, but whether they are literally or figuratively so is never clear.

Consumers may not always be certain about what toxins are, and yet they are well trained by marketing, media, and word of mouth to recognize their prevalence and to know that they, as good health citizens, can and should avoid them. As I outlined in chapter 2, neoliberal models of health establish self-care as an act of individual consumer responsibility by exhorting people to manage their own wellness through concrete efforts to restore and enhance their health. A key consequence of this shift toward individual health self-governance is that it personalizes risk, transforming collective potential problems into individual ones.[7] In the case of toxins, this shift transforms risk mitigation into a personal duty we fulfill for ourselves by buying organic fruits and vegetables, undertaking cleanses, and avoiding pharmaceuticals to reduce our toxic loads rather than by lobbying the state to regulate the chemicals we are exposed to in our food systems and healthcare. As I argue in the present chapter, in the vector of harm reduction the will to wellness therefore operates largely in the logic of restoration, serving as a defensive measure against invisible poisons. Nevertheless, the logic of enhancement also figures into people's efforts to proactively build up their defenses against toxin risk through the use of natural health products.

While the notion of risk saturates wellness discourse generally, I focus in this chapter on two forms of risk that undergird widespread use of natural health products: risk of pharmaceutical medicine as both morally and physically harmful and risk of exposure to ambient environmental toxins that enter our bodies invisibly. In the first section, I show how worry and doubt about whether we are healthy are amplified by the ways we talk about toxins in public discourse, creating the perfect environment for wellness to flourish as a form of harm reduction. In the remaining two sections, I explain the main strategies wellness seekers adopt to address the risks of harm they face, which include, first, avoiding perceived toxins by choosing natural health products over conventional "chemical" pharmaceuticals; and second, eliminating toxins through supplement-supported detoxification regimens such as cleanses. The toxins I discuss in this chapter are usually vague and nonspecific, which makes them more insidious. They are everywhere, all the time—in our food, in our furnishings, in our natural and constructed environments, in the water, and in the air. The detoxifier's work is therefore never done.

My analysis in what follows draws on the interview transcripts and "Stop Bill C-51" petition comments discussed in chapters 1 and 2. Together, these datasets offer some 320,000 words that reveal how people use natural health products to mitigate the various risks they face in their everyday lives. I have also woven throughout this chapter discussion of a pair of bestselling popular books by environmentalists Rick Smith and Bruce Lourie: *Slow Death by Rubber Duck: How the Toxic Chemistry of Everyday Life Affects Our Health* (2009) and *Toxin Toxout: Getting Harmful Chemicals Out of Our Bodies and Our World* (2013).[8] Smith holds a PhD in biology and is executive director of the Canadian Broadbent Institute, a socially and environmentally progressive think tank named for political scientist and former longtime leader of the New Democratic Party of Canada, Ed Broadbent. Lourie is an environmental policy analyst and speaker in Canada.

I selected these additional texts because of their broad reach and nuanced approach: both books are carefully researched and steeped in scholarly evidence, and they occupy what strikes me as a reasoned middle ground in debates about toxins in the environment and in our bodies. Although the books do paint an alarming picture of how deeply potentially dangerous chemicals have penetrated our everyday lives, they offer neither the simplistic cures promised by peddlers of detox-quick schemes nor reassuring pro-industry apologia. And yet, while *Slow Death by Rubber Duck* and *Toxin Toxout* are more robustly evidence-based than many public texts on toxins and detoxification, they nevertheless operate in accordance with the same self-driving tension between the logics of restoration and enhancement that are pervasive in the other texts I discuss in this chapter. Indeed, the books' more even-handed approach to toxic culture only seems to intensify the idea that risks are everywhere all the time and individuals must manage those risks themselves. What is particularly distinctive about these texts, then, is that even while they seem to tamp down the flames of wellness culture, they lock directly into the individual, consumerist impulses that drive that culture.

Before turning to my analysis, I want to note that although many of the claims about pharmaceutical harms or supplement safety and effectiveness that I discuss in this chapter are not necessarily grounded in scientific evidence, we must nevertheless take seriously the concerns they express about toxicity and drug side effects if we wish to understand why people use natural health products and services and to incorporate that understanding into health policy and practice. We can therefore set aside distinctions between true toxins—substances known or compellingly suspected to cause disease and morbidity—and their metaphorical cousins. We can also set aside the question whether detoxing cleanses "work": so long as people *believe* that toxins are a problem and that detoxing with natural health products is a solution, then what people *say* about natural health and wellness is our primary object of inquiry. For this reason, it is helpful to view arguments about wellness and toxins as instances of what communication scholar Robin Jensen identifies as *chemical rhetoric*. As Jensen explains, chemical rhetorics employ chemistry as a "public vocabulary" for nonexpert communication that invokes key terms, concepts, tropes, figures, appeals, and narratives from chemistry as "a shared communicative resource."[9] The language of chemistry provides a wealth of rhetorical resources for individuals and groups seeking to understand and explain the world around them, which for discourse about wellness and natural health includes employing technical concepts such as toxicity as conversational shorthands to signify impurity, moral ambiguity, and potential danger.

What I show in this chapter is that in aggregate terms the materials I analyze do not provide evidence of ignorant, uninformed rejection of medical science or unwarranted paranoia about toxic chemicals; rather, they demonstrate individuals' sincere efforts to grapple with well-documented problems in both science and medicine, as well as in health policy and administration. The individuals whose words I examine are skeptical about the extent to which doctors, regulators, and drug manufacturers have their best interests at heart—and many of those individuals cite specific evidence that they do not. Therefore, while we could read commentary on wellness and toxins through the lens of scientific fact, if we momentarily suspend concern about what is right or true, we gain the opportunity to understand what people themselves believe when they make decisions about their health. The perspectives I discuss in this chapter reveal a collective imagining not of how things *are* in contemporary healthcare but of how things *might be better*.

Two Kinds of Risk

Wellness culture is premised on the interleaving of (at least) two kinds of risk, which together situate the body as permeable and polluted, requiring constant vigilance and action. These two forms of risk—risk of pharmaceutical harm and risk of ambient, environmental contamination—are animated by medicalizing discourses that blur boundaries between illness prevention and incipient illness. As I discussed in chapter 1, active monitoring of health at the individual level may reduce illness by targeting and reducing illness risk, but as Peter Conrad explains, "the increased role surveillance medicine plays in the social context of behavior" also necessarily means that "in addition to focusing on those that are ill, the medical vision now includes an increasingly large number of people who are regarded as *potentially* ill."[10] The focus of wellness culture is trained on an idea of potential illness that appears to operate in the logic of enhancement by emphasizing positive, health-enhancing behaviors but is actually structured by its opposite, the logic of restoration. Joseph Dumit notes that within the landscape of contemporary pharmaceutical medicine there has emerged a "new grammar of illness, risk, experience, and treatment, one in which the body is inherently disordered." This new grammar creates "a new kind of health" that centers on risk reduction "in which to be normal is to have symptoms and risk factors you should be worrying about, and at the same time to not know whether you should be worrying about yet more things."[11]

In this new health landscape, being a responsible health citizen means seeking to know as much about your health and to do as much for it as you can. This breeds what Dumit calls a *double insecurity*: you can never be sure about your health because you are always at risk, and you can never be sure that you are effectively reducing that risk and thereby protecting your health. Unsurprisingly, symptoms and anxiety proliferate in a risk-preoccupied culture because when it comes to our health and health risks, "the more we know, the more we fear; and the more we fear, the more preventative actions and medications we need to take."[12] Rhetorics of risk similarly proliferate when we try to mitigate potential risks. As rhetorician J. Blake Scott explains, "Even reflexive efforts to contain or control risk often end up increasing it and causing it to spin further out of control."[13] Keränen similarly points out that the more we talk about risk, the more at risk we feel, and the more at risk we feel, the more we talk about it; this spiraling discourse about risk becomes the theater within which risk-mitigating industries grow.[14]

The double insecurity sponsored by heightened concern about health risks converts *uncertainty* (about the risks we face and whether we are doing enough to reduce them) into *worry*, according to Dumit: "Rather than illness punctuating ordinary life, the everyday conceals illness."[15] And so when health is redefined as a risk state, conditions of the body previously thought to be normal or harmless are refigured as potential threats: aches, pains, or fatigue are transformed into symptoms that constellate around a nameable state that merits attention or correction through an external intervention such as a pharmaceutical or natural health product. How, then, can we ever really know if we are healthy?

Worrying Our Way to Health

Bodies are stubbornly opaque. They do not simply reveal themselves to observers, nor do they surrender their secrets just any which way. I remember being starkly confronted by my own corporeal opacity while nursing my newborn baby, who was healthy but did not conform to the standard growth charts circulated by my local public health unit. What I thought would be a blissful bonding experience instead became an occasion for anxiety and concern because while she was a happy baby, she was small, and no one could tell just how much milk she was getting. I remember resenting my own body and hers—mine because breasts do not have gauges to say how much has been emptied, hers because babies' stomachs do not show when they are full. After anxiously weighing her and counting wet diapers, my midwife became worried enough that she advised me to take fenugreek capsules to stimulate milk production. (Her recommended dose: "Take them until you smell like maple syrup.")

My family doctor soon joined the team of worriers, prescribing me the galactagogue Domperidone, which swelled my breasts to alien proportions even while my daughter held tight to her low-slung growth curve. I nursed and pumped anxiously up to ten hours a day, thinking often about the legendary cow of my childhood, who lived on the nearby university farm with a plastic window along its flank so researchers could observe its stomach at work. If only my daughter had had such a window in her belly, or if I had had one in my breast, I would have been able to know with certainty that she was nursing well and so lighten the load of new motherhood, even just a little.

This story of my nursing experience is important because it is mundane: regardless of the cause of our worry, we remain an overwhelmingly health-anxious culture. My baby met all her important developmental milestones, had regular wet diapers, and was happy and playful. She showed no signs of illness or distress. Nevertheless, her failure to grow in accordance with epidemiological averages prompted two experienced healthcare providers with a combined sixty years of experience to risk overtreating a newborn and incapacitating a new mother with fear to allay the hypothetical risk identified by population-based estimates.

Of course, bodies themselves are part of the problem: because they are opaque, we can never be certain they are working as they should. For nursing infants, baby and breast work together behind a veil of tissue and skin. We can infer what they are up to by the way they move (jaw movement, breathing patterns) and by the traces they leave behind (spit-up, urine), but our bodies seldom tell their own stories. As literary and health humanities scholar Catherine Belling writes in her beautifully disturbing book about the meanings of hypochondria, "One reason that medicine is uncertain and interpretive is obvious yet worth restating: the body is not transparent. We do not, even with the help of biomedical science and technology, have real access to the inside of living bodies as they live."[16] Even if a diagnostic scan or test comes out clean, there is always a chance that an underlying pathology is just too small to visualize yet or is lurking somewhere else in the body. Health is thus always qualified, and fleeting: all of us will get ill sometime or another, and we will all certainly die. Anxiety about health is fueled by doubt that what we feel in our bodies can ever adequately convey what is really going on inside them. For me and my nursing daughter, for example, the opaqueness of our bodies did not conceal pathology but *potential* pathology. She seemed fine—but what if she wasn't?

My worry was not brought on by physical markers of illness but by statistical markers of not-health; my anxiety took hold, and expanded, in the space created by doubt about what was happening in our bodies, both hers and mine. Worry similarly drives wellness discourse because when it comes to our bodies, there is just so much we do not, and cannot, know about our health. The new configuration of health as risk avoidance thereby extends our realm of concern, propelled by the logics of restoration and enhancement. As risk awareness expands alongside a growing public preoccupation with wellness and optimization, we are increasingly encouraged to monitor and manage symptoms of wellness alongside symptoms of illness. This expanding scope of self-surveillance and management brings us back to toxins. Our bodies do not have built-in meters that can tell us our toxic load at any given moment. Without specialized testing, we simply do not know what courses through our bodies and whether it will hurt us.

Toxin Talk

In wellness discourse, the language of risk largely transposes rhetorics of *contagion*, centering on pathogens, with rhetorics of *contamination*, centering on toxins. Toxin talk shifts the grammar of how we understand and describe potential dangers to our health, shifting focus from a specific agentive force (such as a pathogen) acting within and against our bodies toward something more scenic or ambient that surrounds and permeates our bodies silently and unavoidably. Unlike pathogens, toxins do not move from body to body but from place to person. The everyday lived environment therefore becomes potentially dangerous, with threats lurking in household goods such as cleaners, plastics, and fire retardants; in the food chain from fertilizer to crops to livestock; and in land, water, and air. In wellness discourse, all we can do as individual consumers is try to reduce or mitigate our exposure to these potential toxic harms.

In *Slow Death by Rubber Duck* and *Toxin Toxout*, for instance, Lourie and Smith figure toxins rhetorically as both pervasive and insidious. They note that toxic exposure begins in the womb: "children are born pre-polluted."[17] Pregnant and nursing mothers are framed as sites of contamination that transmit "poisons" to their babies through umbilical cord blood and breast milk.[18] As Lourie and Smith explain it, human life is an endless barrage of toxins entering our bodies and potentially making us sick. Importantly, however, they do not use the term *toxin* in its precise scientific definition as a biologically produced poison;

instead they employ the term colloquially to mean something like "industrial by-products that are bad for you."[19] Drawing on this much broader understanding of toxins to emphasize their ubiquity, Lourie and Smith write, "At a very basic level it is frustrating for so many of us to realize that despite all of our best efforts to avoid toxins in our food, our homes and our personal-care products, we are still exposed to hundreds, if not thousands, of potentially harmful chemicals on a daily basis."[20] Lourie and Smith position their books as guides for navigating lives flooded in a toxic soup, helping us learn both to reduce our exposure and to repair damage that has already been done.

Regardless of whether we define toxins narrowly as biologically produced or more broadly to include industrial byproducts, toxins are ultimately risky because they can make human beings sick. Even so, where each of us draws the line for what counts as an appropriate and justified level of concern about toxins depends partly on where we stand in the world of wellness discourse. For wellness skeptics such as Timothy Caulfield, a professor of health law and host of the wellness-debunking Netflix show *A User's Guide to Cheating Death*, and Jennifer Gunter, an obstetrician-gynecologist who "wields the lasso of truth" in her science-based health advocacy, including the debunking podcast series *Body Stuff*, the threshold of concern is much higher than it is for the people that both Lourie and Smith and I interviewed. While Caulfield and Gunter rightfully expose misinformation and health fraud, their engagements with public interest in detoxification do not attend to the impact of personal experience and belief on people's perceptions of their health and well-being and how these experiences and beliefs in turn inform their decisions about the health practices they engage in and the products they buy.

In *Better Safe than Sorry: How Consumers Navigate Exposure to Everyday Toxics*, sociologist Norah MacKendrick chronicles how deregulation and reactive environmental policies in the United States, Canada, and elsewhere have resulted in widespread environmental contamination and caused significant illness and death, prompting justifiable public alarm. MacKendrick examines how everyday people, many of whom feel powerless to change regulations, scramble to stem the flow of potentially harmful chemicals into their own lives and homes by using the primary tool available to them: individual consumer choice.[21] By purchasing "green" variations of household products such as cleaners, laundry detergents, body-care products, food, and home furnishings, consumers try to do *something* to protect themselves and their families under chemical threat, even when they cannot know for sure whether those products will actually reduce their exposure to harmful toxins. I return later in the chapter to the principle of consumer choice in the realm of harm reduction, but for now I want to look more closely at the significance of toxin talk itself. How we talk about toxins and narrativize our scramble to avoid them can reveal important insights about how we, collectively, consider ourselves, our bodies, and our health in relation to the environments in which we live.

For instance, one dominant idea that circulates in toxin talk is that toxins cause all kinds of illness that manifest in unspecified, even mysterious ways. In *Toxin Toxout*, for instance, Lourie and Smith tell the story of the Californian "detox pioneer" Peter Sullivan, whose experience of food allergies and other undiagnosed health issues left him "irritable, stressed out, unhappy and feeling generally unwell." His two sons also experienced baffling symptoms that left one diagnosed with numerous neurological conditions and the other expelled from kindergarten for "antisocial behaviour."[22] In Lourie and Smith's telling, Sullivan saw toxins as the root cause of his family's unusual ailments, pinpointing mercury poisoning as the key culprit. When conventional doctors dismissed his theory, Sullivan consulted an integrative medicine specialist who subsequently found elevated mercury levels in the whole family. Having confirmed his hunch, Sullivan then set out to detoxify his life, removing his mercury-containing dental fillings and undergoing two and a half years of intravenous chelation therapy to strip metals from his bloodstream. He dabbled in colonic irrigation, initiated an intense supplement regimen that Lourie dubs "Peter's Purification Potions," and even installed a Faraday cage in his Palo Alto mansion in the belief that the enclosure's conductive material would reduce his exposure to dangerous electromagnetic frequency.[23]

Sullivan's story, along with the many similar stories in Lourie and Smith's books, illustrates how people concerned about toxins often associate toxic exposure with vague, nonspecific ailments that are dismissed by conventional doctors and only acknowledged by alternative practitioners such as naturopaths or integrative health providers. This diagnostic trajectory (marked first by rejection in mainstream medicine and then by recognition in the world of alternative health) is mirrored in my own datasets as well, with both interview participants and "Stop Bill C-51" petition commenters linking toxins to symptoms such as fatigue, brain fog, and chronic pain that are reportedly only relieved by natural health products. Lourie and Smith are more circumspect about the potential illness risks of toxic exposure than the people they interviewed, as the authors focus only on specific illnesses substantiated by scientific evidence. These toxin-induced illnesses include "several forms of cancer, reproductive problems and birth defects, respiratory illnesses such as asthma and neurodevelopmental disorders such as attention deficit hyperactivity disorder."[24] For Peter Sullivan and others with lived experience of nonspecific symptoms such as fatigue, distractibility, and confusion, however, identifying a cause for their symptoms can be tricky and often unsuccessful, so toxins offer a ready explanation. In toxin talk, the main emphasis is typically on the idea *that* toxins can make you sick, not on how, specifically, they do so.

In toxin talk, as I have argued, toxins are dangerous because they invisibly constitute part of the scene of our lived environments. But they are also dangerous because, in this language, they have agentive force, moving freely and invisibly through opaque bodies. In *Toxin Toxout*, for example, Lourie and Smith anthropomorphize toxins grammatically by warning readers that "pollutants are indiscriminately taking up residence in your body."[25] These pollutants can perform their own actions ("taking up") with affective intent ("indiscriminately") and purpose ("residence"—they are seeking a home). Other individuals who appear in Lourie and Smith's books use similar agentive phrasing, including researcher Philippa Darbre, who explained of her 2004 study that parabens that would normally be broken down by the liver "bypass the liver and remain intact" when applied to the skin.[26] In this example, parabens actively elude the body's defenses, moving stealthily through the body on their own power.

Further, in toxin talk, once toxins are in the body they are mobile. For example, Lourie and Smith describe the "propensity of toxic chemicals to move around" in the body, telling readers that "destructive chemicals don't remain stuck in one part of the body; they travel from organ to organ, finding a spot where they prefer to hang out. One of these chemicals might make its 'home' in a fat cell in your brain, or it may become embedded in cells in your small intestine—and it's impossible to know what kind of damage it may cause once lodged in those areas."[27] In this description, toxins are itinerant menaces that play hide-and-seek, afflicting our bodies differently depending on where they are. Figured in this manner, it is almost as if toxins operate according to their own drive or design, intending to overtake and reside invisibly in the body. Given the grammatical agency afforded to toxins in wellness discourse, it is no wonder that individuals have become concerned about the toxins that surround and occupy their bodies. That concern plants the seeds of wellness as a form of harm reduction wherein people strive first to avoid harm, such as by choosing natural health products over conventional pharmaceuticals, and then to reduce and eliminate harm through "detoxification" techniques.

Avoiding Harm

In *Toxin Toxout*, Lourie and Smith argue that "the first thing to do in order to get toxins out of your body is to avoid them in the first place." After all, as they note playfully in a later chapter, "if no toxins, we don't need toxouts!"[28] For Lourie and Smith, eating organic foods and using "green" cosmetics and cleaning products are excellent ways for people to reduce their toxic load at the gate, before toxins can enter the body. For wellness seekers, another primary strategy for avoiding toxins at the gate is to avoid pharmaceuticals. Nichter and Thompson identified this line of reasoning in their ethnographic study of individual supplement-related beliefs and behaviors in the United States, finding that their participants viewed natural health products as safe substitutes for toxic pharmaceuticals.[29] I consistently found the same arguments across all the materials I analyze in this book, including the interviews I conducted with wellness seekers and the petition comments against Bill C-51. In this section, I draw primarily on the interviews and petition comments to explain how wellness operates discursively as a means of avoiding pharmaceutical harm, although the findings I discuss here apply equally to other sources I have examined and are similarly prominent in both Canada and the US.

Three overarching statements of belief illustrate wellness seekers' chief reasons for choosing natural health products over drugs in the name of harm reduction:

- Pharmaceuticals are dangerous, whereas supplements are not.
- Pharmaceuticals are harsh, whereas supplements are gentle.
- Pharmaceuticals suppress symptoms of illness, whereas supplements address underlying causes.

All three of these beliefs were evident in my interview with Gene, a construction worker in his fifties, as he explained that in his view a supplement is "less toxic to the body and gets more to the root of the problem, I guess. Or improves your health overall. . . . It doesn't just treat symptoms. Pharmaceuticals are toxic and cover over symptoms."[30] I examine each of these three themes in turn, although as I discuss below, they are often entangled and overlapping in the interviews and petition comments. Further, individuals in both datasets similarly characterize natural health products positively as natural and fundamentally good and pharmaceuticals negatively as toxic and fundamentally bad, but the petition comments generally adopt more extreme positions on each end. Commenters frequently associate pharmaceuticals with a model of science gone wrong that results in toxicity, environmental devastation, human exploitation, and sickness and death. I suspect that the petition's more dramatically polarized account of supplements and pharmaceuticals is rooted partly in the comments' origin in an anonymous online forum and partly in the "spirit of protest" characteristic of the petition genre, whereas the interview participants' more measured and nuanced responses may stem from their origins in intimate, in-person interviews. Despite these differences, the individuals in both datasets maintain that natural health products are a direct output of nature itself, produced without distortion or impurity, whereas pharmaceuticals are products of corporate subterfuge, government corruption, and toxic, chemical processes that harm both human and environmental health. These beliefs, whether misguided or well founded, are a central driver of wellness discourse.

"Pharmaceuticals Are Dangerous"

Individuals in both datasets overwhelmingly characterize pharmaceuticals as toxic poisons produced in laboratories and natural supplements as plants grown in farmers' fields. These individuals believe that pharmaceuticals are dangerous to their health because they are chemical, synthetic, and toxic and therefore potentially harmful to human bodies. For example, when Mandy, an entrepreneur in her early fifties, was asked why she thought wellness and natural health had become so popular in recent years, she replied that "people want to be as close to natural as possible, they don't want to keep adding in more chemicals. And people want to get away from toxins."[31]

Terms from chemistry figure particularly prominently in each dataset, prompting high levels of concern among wellness seekers even though such terms refer, by definition, to value-neutral scientific objects and processes. One petition signatory argues, for example, that "prescription drugs don't exist withouth [sic] the synthetic chemical industry, which is about 100 years old, which is horribly polluting our enviromnent [sic] and bodies. And only a small percentage of the chemicals used in the manufacture of drugs have been tested themselves for safety, many of them over 50 years ago. And the synergistic effects of long term exposure to synthetic chemicals has virtually NEVER been explored."[32] Another signatory similarly contends that "most pharmaceutical drugs are chemicals the body cannot easily process. Subsequently, they cause toxins to build up in the body creating more health problems for the patient whose health is already compromised."[33] In these examples, the language of chemistry serves as a shared communicative resource, in Jensen's framing, in that terms such as *chemical*, *synthetic,* and *toxic* circulate in nonexpert contexts to impute a negative value to one set of substances (pharmaceuticals) but not another (supplements).[34] Pharmaceuticals are framed in both datasets as dangerous because they are products of chemical synthesis in a laboratory, which many people equate with pollution, toxicity, and illness.

Individuals in the interviews and the petition comments also argue that natural supplements are purer than pharmaceuticals because, in their view, supplements are produced without additives such as pesticides, preservatives, or fillers. For example, Andrea, a nonprofit administrator in her late forties, explained in her interview that natural health products are "just like herbs, you know, or like spices," whereas with pharmaceuticals "there's stuff in there that you don't need." She said she always tries preventive measures first and then natural products before trying medication: "The pharmaceutical stuff is like, it kind of scares me," she said with a laugh.[35] Mandy also worries about what is in pharmaceutical interventions and so "would rather use natural ones [because] they're less harmful, there's less extra additives and stuff like that."[36] Opponents to Bill C-51 similarly seek unhindered access to natural health products precisely because they believe natural health products come purely from nature. A commenter named Dawn argues, for example, that natural health products should not be regulated because they are natural, safe, and free of chemical and material interference, and therefore should be accessible to all: "Mother Earth provides us with the tools for finding balance and health, and it is our right to be able to accept these in their most natural state . . . unhindered!"[37]

Like Dawn, other wellness seekers frequently evoke botanical and culinary imagery such as seeds, gardens, farms, herbs, and spices to characterize natural health products as plants or foods rather than drugs. These images associate supplements with nature, earthiness, and purity and also with the homespun familiarity of a cottage industry comprising home gardens, hobby farms, farmers' markets, and agricultural cooperatives rather than with a sprawling, multibillion-dollar multinational corporate industry. One petition commenter explains that these products were "made from natural organic products and do no harm," a view shared by a commenter who describes supplements as "a kinder, safer method" for supporting their health. Another petition signatory, Lorraine, similarly argues that "Canadians are taking their health care into their own hands and looking for safer alternative medicine" made with "natural ingredients" rather than relying on "expensive and dangerous 'legal' drugs."[38] In all of these examples, claims about natural health product safety hinge on the fact that the products are *natural*—that they are made from plants ("herbs," "foods"), grown without chemicals ("organic"), and manufactured without artificial additives or fillers ("natural ingredients").

Supplement consumers find additional reassurance in natural health products simply because they are not pharmaceuticals. For instance, Nicki, a teacher in her forties, said in her interview, "I don't trust what's in the products from the pharmaceuticals. I just want to use more natural things where I can read the label and see what's exactly in it, things that I can pronounce."[39] People trust labels on supplement packaging even though numerous studies indicate that this information is not reliable and that many products contain unlisted contaminants or fillers.[40] Labeling conventions also contribute to consumer trust, as most supplement labels provide both scientific and common names for their ingredients and list their originating sources to accommodate untrained consumer-readers. For instance, the hangover supplement Over EZ lists ingredients first by more recognizable terms, such as vitamin B_6 and vitamin B_{12}, and then by their respective technical equivalents, pyridoxal hydrochloride and cyanocobalamin, in parentheses.[41] These labeling conventions fulfill consumer desires to recognize and understand what their products contain and foster trust in those who produce them.

One of the most revealing elements of both datasets from the perspective of wellness as a form of harm reduction is that people consistently point to problems of trust in the pharmaceutical industry as grounds for believing that drugs are potentially toxic and natural health products are therefore a safer choice. Interviewees and petition signatories alike cite well-documented problems of corporate involvement in pharmaceutical research as cause for concern about the reliability of data on drug safety and efficacy. For example, one person commenting on the "Stop Bill C-51" petition describes regulatory drug approval as a "sketchy process, with the prevailing interest likely to get the drugs on the market, safety second."[42] For this commenter as for others whose voices appear in this chapter, the true danger to public health is a pharmaceutical industry effectively left to govern itself.

Many of the petition signatories even argue that Bill C-51 was a pragmatic maneuver orchestrated by "a scared pharmaceautical [sic] industry," as a commenter named Anita put it, because companies "have discovered that people are choosing a kinder, safer method for their health." In the view of these wellness seekers, untrustworthy pharmaceutical companies are scrambling to rig the market in their favor. Here is how commenter Will summarizes this position: "The pharmaceutical industry is teeming with examples of unethical profiting and betrayal of trust. It is an outrage that our alternatives to this business would become more difficult to attain, most certainly for the sole purpose of funneling us into the purchase and use of drugs."[43] For these individuals, the pharmaceutical industry is dangerous and not to be trusted.

In some cases such fears are well founded. The history of pharmaceuticals is rife with examples of the very products intended to improve health sickening, injuring, or killing the individuals they were intended to help. In some cases, pharmaceutical-related injuries can be explained by treatment decisions based on poor research design and interpretation, as in the case of recommendations for hormone replacement therapy based on large observational studies.[44] Conversely, many other such injuries are caused by research misconduct, ethical violations, misleading marketing and advertising, industry sponsorship, and negligence.[45] Signatories to the "Stop Bill C-51" petition point to such cases as justification of their preference for natural health products over pharmaceuticals. For example, Marvin credits the Vioxx scandal that emerged in the late 1990s for his decision to choose natural health products, and Beverley similarly reasons that "thousands of people die every year from prescription drugs so this [legislation] can't possibly make things better."[46]

Beyond concerns about the pharmaceutical industry lie additional concerns among wellness consumers over doctor kickbacks, compromised regulatory mechanisms, and cuts to public health and healthcare delivery. Many who opposed Bill C-51 blamed the government for getting into bed with pharmaceutical companies and prioritizing profit over constituents. They also viewed doctors as complicit pharmaceutical gatekeepers who opposed natural health products to force public dependence on their own professional services, particularly their power to prescribe medications. For consumers who are suspicious of the entire mainstream health system, natural health products appear to provide a way to opt out of that system. Consider, for example, this unsigned comment on the "Stop Bill C-51" petition: "Man made pharmasuticals [sic] are poor attempts at copying natural substances and most often are toxic to the human body. I prefer to use natural substances whenever possible. This bill is one more attempt of the mega wealthy pharmacutical industry to dig deeper into citizens pockets and to stop the use [of] preventative treatments to keep people sick so they can keep selling their poison."[47] Commenters such as this believe the pharmaceutical industry should not be trusted because its goal is to make money, not to heal people. By contrast, natural health products appear to offer users a way to bypass pharmaceutical industry greed and government complicity, even if those products cost more than conventional pharmaceuticals.

On this last point, many individuals in both datasets interpret the high price point of natural health products as evidence that those products are the better choice, expensive only because they are produced in small batches with higher-quality materials and fewer impurities. Those who signed the petition against Bill C-51 in particular describe supplements as if they were produced in a cottage-type industry—farm to capsule, say—even though most Canadians access their supplements through major commercial distributors. This point is significant because it highlights the often wide gulf between what supplement users *believe* about the supplement industry and how that industry typically operates.[48] In both datasets, as in the other artifacts I analyze in this book, it is overwhelmingly clear that interest in natural health products is driven partly by falling public trust in mainstream pharmaceutical medicine; wellness rhetorics seem to offer consumers a way out.

"Pharmaceuticals Are Harsh"

Not only do the wellness seekers represented in the datasets believe that drugs are dangerous but they also see them as clumsy, poorly targeted interventions that are far too potent to address most health problems. For example, when I asked Clara, a former dance instructor in her late fifties, what she saw as the difference between natural health products and mainstream pharmaceuticals, such as Tylenol or cold and flu medication, she told me about a time when her doctor had prescribed antibiotics for an infection. She had accepted the prescription but worried about how the antibiotics would affect her gut microbiome so she sought out a gentler alternative. She tried taking garlic, herbal drops, and a homeopathic remedy for a few days, and her infection cleared up so quickly that her doctor was "shocked." She wondered aloud to herself, "Why would I ever choose to use something that's just going to be like a sledgehammer against the good bacteria as well as the bad when I can use something that doesn't have all those side effects?"[49]

Side effects serve as potent evidence for many wellness seekers that drugs are too harsh. One petition signatory notes, for example, that "many of the pharmaceutical drugs do not cure, but their side-effects actually do more harm than good," while another says, "I am tired of the side effects related to prescription medications and the negative impact it has had on my families [*sic*] health."[50] Steve, a retired businessperson in his early seventies, explicitly framed his supplement use as an effort to avoid the unintended consequences of taking a drug: "I try to go for natural in the sense that it's non-synthetic and non-pharmaceutical because more and more pharmaceuticals are known to have side effects."[51] The belief that supplements produce fewer side effects than pharmaceuticals signals to many wellness seekers that they are therefore safer and even healthier than pharmaceuticals. Louise, for example, explains in the petition that "the side effects from prescription drugs are many, and why would I want to subject myself to that, when there are natural remedies far healthier."[52] Of course, taking drugs is sometimes unavoidable, so many wellness seekers try to offset their side effects with natural health products. For example, Nicki loads up on probiotic supplements when she needs to take antibiotics in order to "balance the bacteria in the body, the good versus the bad."[53]

Many wellness seekers view pharmaceuticals as too strong for the problems they wish to treat, so they choose natural products as a gentler first line of treatment and only escalate to conventional products if needed. In the interviews, for example, participants frequently described trying different interventions in a progression from least invasive to most invasive. For example, for a headache, Coretta, a mid-fifties tourism employee, first tries essential oils or drinking more water "to try and release the headache" before moving to a "chemical-based" product such as Tylenol, and Suri, a graduate student in her mid-twenties, tries "natural cold and flu concoctions" before moving to more powerful over-the-counter products.[54] Similarly, Steve, the retired businessperson, explained that he often consults a pharmacist when deciding what strength of intervention he needs, asking, "Will this willow bark do the same as the Aspirin does, only in a less harsh manner?"[55] June, a call center worker in her late fifties, chooses natural products because they're more "subtle" than pharmaceuticals, which "hit hard" and "have a strong effect."[56] For all these individuals, natural health products are effective even if they are gentler than pharmaceuticals because, unlike their chemical counterparts, they are made of substances the body works with synergistically rather than against.

Marketing plays an unsurprisingly significant role in reinforcing the apparent synergy between natural health products and the body. Although supplements are widely available at regular pharmacies and big-box retailers such as Wal-Mart and Amazon, the wellness seekers in my datasets strongly associate them with natural health stores, organic markets, naturopaths, and home gardens. Many believe supplements are developed, produced, distributed, and consumed on a fundamentally different model than pharmaceuticals—a natural, grassroots model of wellness that works in sync with the body rather than an industrial, corporate model of illness that overpowers the body. The products' visual rhetoric reinforces their ties to nature with images such as suns, rainbows, leaves, and flowers incorporated into their logos and packaging. This imagery reinforces the widespread belief articulated by the petition commenter Jeffrey that "almost without exception products sold at . . . health stores are made from natural organic products and do no harm."[57]

At the same time, natural health product marketing also trades partly on the similarity of these products to pharmaceuticals: once relegated to specialty stores or small, visually distinct "natural health" sections in drugstores, supplements now are often mixed in with pharmaceuticals and nearly indistinguishable from them. For example, my local Shopper's Drug Market shelves the natural health product Helixia Sinus, a cold remedy that contains no regulated active ingredients, in between boxes of NyQuil and Advil Cold and Sinus. Nothing on the front of the package indicates that Helixia Sinus is an herbal product instead of a pharmaceutical aside from a small eucalyptus leaf in the bottom right corner next to text that reads "With Eucalyptus Oil Extract" (fig. 3). The package design is otherwise indistinguishable from its pharmaceutical counterparts, from the prominent bulleted list of cold and sinusitis symptoms the product purports to relieve to the reference in the bottom left corner to "liquid caps" accompanied by an illustration of two capsules that closely resemble capsules of NyQuil and Advil Cold and Sinus. Next to the product name, "Helixia Sinus," the package also lists a quantity, "200 mg," which presumably refers to the product's active ingredient even though no such ingredient is listed on the product face. Here, the Helixia Sinus box trades on the practice in pharmaceutical packaging to clearly identify the quantity of each active ingredient per dose, but without actually quantifying anything. The visual rhetoric of products such as this aims to establish sufficient continuity with pharmaceuticals to imply that the products are "real" medicine,

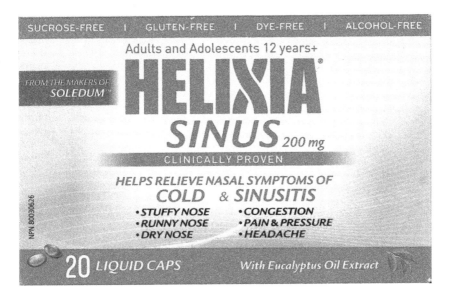

Figure 3. Helixia Sinus product package

yet they maintain enough discontinuity through their connections to nature that they are perceived as safer, less toxic alternatives.

This is not to say that supplement users are necessarily naive about the products they consume, however; even while they perceive natural health products as safer than pharmaceuticals, many individuals in the interview and petition datasets do recognize their potential dangers. For example, Steve, the retiree who described choosing between willow bark and Aspirin, noted that he worries about risks of bleeding ulcers associated with willow bark.[58] Owen, a schoolteacher in his thirties, similarly worries about the effects of ginseng on his liver.[59] As these examples show, most supplement users are passionate about their use of natural health products but do not take the products' effectiveness or safety as a necessary given. Participants in the interviews, for example, frequently reflected on the influence of marketing and media hype on their decision making. Many recognized that choosing supplements over pharmaceuticals can sometimes be dangerous, particularly for infections that can get out of hand if not addressed appropriately and promptly. Some interview participants also recognized that natural health products sometimes contain dangerous fillers or contaminants, as June notes: "I can't help but mention the recent articles in the newspaper about tests being done on natural health products in the health food stores and there being a big scare because they found all these really, for lack of a better word, bad ingredients in natural health products."[60]

Still, for many wellness seekers the bigger dangers are posed by pharmaceuticals, which they believe can produce dependence and overuse resistance. Some people try to head off such potential problems by choosing natural health products whenever they can. Ariel, a healthcare professional in her early thirties, explained that she tries "immune boosting herbs" and cranberry juice or Cran-Aid tea for bladder infections: "I don't want to have to go on a whole course of antibiotics . . . so I'll treat that naturally. Antibiotics sometimes aren't enough these days and I don't want to have too much resistance."[61] That drugs are becoming less effective because most people take too many of them was a frequent refrain in both the interviews and the Bill C-51 comments. These individuals have so strongly internalized public health messaging about their personal responsibility for health that they now believe not only that they should take medication when necessary but also that they are obligated to reduce risks posed by overuse by taking medication *judiciously*.

Notably, concerns in the interviews and petition comments about drug resistance are framed entirely in terms of individual health risks rather than public health risks. The chief worry among these wellness seekers is that taking too much medication now might reduce its effectiveness if they need it in the future. Only one participant alluded to potential problems of antibiotic resistance across whole populations—when overexposure to antibiotics allows bacteria to build up defenses that reduce antibiotics' effectiveness—but for that participant, Kayla, a tech worker in her thirties, the potential for public harm is overshadowed by her personal desire to avoid medication. She admitted that her practice of stopping antibiotics as soon as her symptoms clear rather than taking the full prescribed course may allow harmful bacteria to flourish and harm others, but she nevertheless chooses to prioritize her own wellness: "This is really bad . . . I'm probably, like, contributing to antibiotic resistance."[62] Similarly, Ariel tries natural remedies before antibiotics so that she will not develop "too much resistance" down the road, as does Ying, a 20-year-old student in the health sciences who chooses natural health products first because although they do not work quickly, "your body don't build, like, anti-resistant against it . . . and in the long run it works better for you."[63] For products such as Tylenol, Ying says, "you will see the result right away but your body becomes reliant on it so then, like, you're using more and it's less effective."[64] For wellness seekers, opting out of taking pharmaceuticals thus serves as a form of reducing the potential harm of drugs failing us when we need them most. This is particularly true when individuals hope to fix underlying issues rather than merely masking symptoms.

"Pharmaceuticals Suppress Symptoms"

The previous two subsections have examined wellness seekers' beliefs about pharmaceuticals as dangerous and too harsh for most health problems. Another key belief that motivates people to choose natural health products over pharmaceuticals is grounded in the idea of healing itself, as many individuals believe that natural products reduce exposure to pharmaceutical harms by correcting underlying pathologies rather than merely suppressing symptoms. Ariel, for example, stated that in her view taking a pharmaceutical "doesn't necessarily get to the root [cause of illness] and it's not going to help you prevent it from happening again. It's just going to suppress what's happening at the moment, so it's more of a bandaid solution, where natural health products are something that's going to help you build you from the inside out, can get rid of your symptoms and prevent you from having it again in the future."[65] Similarly, Nicki, a teacher in her forties, argues that pharmaceuticals "don't do anything to address the root problem and, in suppressing, they can cause a myriad of [negative side] effects. . . . They're not trying to build the system up, they're simply trying to suppress symptoms."[66] Arguments such as these run throughout the interview transcripts and the "Stop

Bill C-51" petition, figuring pharmaceuticals as harmful because they repress rather than resolve health problems. Whether this is actually true is irrelevant to what individual people believe and do about their health: if people do not believe pharmaceuticals will solve underlying issues, they will seek alternatives that they believe can.

One of the most prevalent arguments in both the interview and petition datasets is that the profit motive guiding pharmaceutical development, legislation, and marketing is directly at odds with the motive of curing people because people no longer require medication if they have been cured. Those who signed the "Stop Bill C-51" petition, in particular, made frequent reference to the deep contradictions between seeing medicine as a healing practice and seeing it as a business:

> Remember: THERE IS NO MONEY TO BE MADE IN HEALING PEOPLE!! THEY MAKE MONEY WHEN WE'RE SICK! [Bill C-51] IS NOTHING BUT ANOTHER STEP in their agenda to further solidify the insane POWER & domination that PHARMACEUTICAL COMPANIES & THE HEALTHCARE INDUSTRY now hold. . . . They WANT people sick, so they can siphon money not only from patients and insurance companies, but also from taxpayers.

> This bill is one more attempt of the mega wealthy pharmacutical [sic] industry to dig deeper into citizens pockets and to stop the use [of] preventative treatments to keep people sick so they can keep selling their poison.

> Pharma & medical companies, with lobbying pressure, stand to make money and that is the only concern. Chris Rock has said, medicine hasn't "cured" anything since Polio because the money is in the treatment not the cure. Natural supplements, herbs and vitamins aim, in large part, to prevent illness. Anyone who remains healthy their whole lives long is a missed financial opportunity for big Pharma.[67]

These examples illustrate the extent of public discomfort with the idea that health can and should be sold on an open market.

Further, concerns about the pharmaceutical industry prioritizing profit over health affects how people view medical practitioners as well. As one petition signatory explained, "Doctors as a whole make their money off illness. This is just another way to herd people into their twisted medical system."[68] One of the interview participants, Jana, a journalist in her early thirties, linked all these concerns together, noting with a wry laugh that "because we hear a lot about how the pharmaceutical companies are trying to run the world and make us hooked to

the drugs" and because "we know that [some] doctors are, you know, being motivated by the pharmaceutical companies," they "end up prescribing more than you
need or prescribing something that you don't need at all."[69] The individuals
represented in both datasets demonstrated acute awareness of the pharmaceutical industry's primary growth strategy, maximizing treatment (as Dumit terms
it),[70] a goal that, as I noted in the previous chapter, is resolutely contrary to the
values of health and healthcare.

The corollary to the argument that pharmaceuticals merely mask symptoms
is, of course, that natural health products address root causes. This belief is fur-
nished partly through marketing discourse that has long surrounded natural
health products, lifestyle advice gurus, and alternative health practitioners such
as naturopaths, all promising to solve underlying problems that have long been
neglected by conventional medicine. In his landmark 1995 book *The Yeast Connection and the Woman*, physician William G. Crook attributes a wide array of intractable health problems, such as premenstrual syndrome, chronic fatigue
syndrome, migraine, fibromyalgia, irritable bowel syndrome, and numerous
other conditions, to an overgrowth of yeast in the body. The way to cure these
conditions, according to Crook, is to fix the underlying yeast problem through a
specific diet and range of supplements to be taken under a physician's supervi-
sion. The central plank of Crook's argument is that natural health products stimulate the body to heal itself, a view that is echoed throughout both datasets; as
Jana put it in her interview, natural health products take effect by "using your
body's own immune system."[71]

Steve similarly noted in his interview that natural health products fix underlying problems by triggering the body's own healing response: "I had a bit of high
cholesterol for a while and I was told to take a statin but you can also buy an anti-
cholesterol herbal combination from Finlandia [a natural pharmacy] that they
say will do the same as the statin, only it's natural herbs and it does it in a different way which is not so much to suppress the build-up of cholesterol as to find
out what's causing the build-up of cholesterol, what's the imbalance in the body,
and curing the imbalance in the body."[72] As supplement users like Steve see it,
these products help them avoid risk of pharmaceutical harms by stimulating the
body to rebalance itself so that they do not have to rely on external aids such as
drugs. Seeking to restore and enhance their wellness, these individuals view the
use of natural health products instead of pharmaceuticals as a way to prevent certain toxins from entering their bodies in the first place. Once those toxins have
entered the body, however, the wellness seeker's task shifts to damage control.

Reducing and Eliminating Harm

Let us return to the two cultural artifacts I began with, Renew Life's poster warning that "In Today's Toxic Environment CLEANSING is . . . a NECESSITY!" and *Dr. Oz*'s "Toxic Toss Out" segment about common toxic items in our households. Both artifacts figure toxins as vague, omnipresent threats that we must vigilantly guard ourselves against, and purify ourselves of, in order to reduce our risks of harm. As I have illustrated thus far, wellness culture holds consumers ultimately responsible for avoiding these risks, whether the risks lie in the drugs we take, the goods we buy, or the food we eat. Tasked as we are with discovering what is in the products we interact with in our daily lives and deciding for ourselves which are safe and which are not, one strategy for avoiding risk is to buy products that seem more natural, whether that means choosing supplements rather than pharmaceuticals or organic fruits and vegetables rather than their conventionally grown counterparts. Part of what fuels wellness culture, then, is the scramble many of us experience as we try to steer clear of the dangers that invisibly surround us.

MacKendrick describes this scramble to avoid risk through careful shopping as "precautionary consumption."[73] It is labor-intensive and often gendered work that involves reading labels, looking for certification seals, checking "Dirty Dozen" lists for high-pesticide foods to avoid, searching product databases such as the Environmental Working Group's *Skin Deep* database for safe(r) cosmetics, and Googling ingredients and materials. Such vigilance can be exhausting, and as MacKendrick muses, "All of this reading and decision-making could prompt shoppers to drop their baskets in the middle of the aisle, walk out of the store, and vow never to read a label again."[74] Ultimately, no matter how much research we do, all the public messaging that surrounds us says we live in a world filled with invisible toxic chemicals—smog from traffic and factories; flame retardants on our couches and mattresses and in our kids' pajamas; pesticide and herbicide residues on our produce; dangerous fumes from cleaners, solvents, paint, and synthetic materials in our homes and workplaces; and preservatives, additives, and other harmful ingredients in our food, body care products, and pet supplies. Despite our best efforts, we cannot stop all toxins from sneaking in.

Enter at-home detoxification techniques such as cleanses, ionic foot baths, juice fasts, charcoal-infused foods, and recreational chelation therapy, which is an intravenous solution typically used to treat heavy metal poisoning but increasingly used in boutique alternative health settings to remove alleged contaminants from consumers' bodies. These detoxification techniques reassure consumers that they can reduce their own individual "chemical dose" or "body burden" of toxins.[75] As MacKendrick explains, marketing for detoxification products and services performs the simultaneous task of "stoking anxieties while promising to fix them" with supplements, infusions, and other toxin-fighting strategies.[76] Such marketing strategies echo rhetorics of "disease marketing," when pharmaceutical companies simultaneously promote both a health problem and its solution.[77] In a wellness-saturated world, argumentation surrounding this dual task practically completes itself.

Ambient Toxins

Concerns about toxic contamination are not new. MacKendrick, for instance, cites a 1928 text from scientist Karl Vogel that could have been written today: "The world we inhabit is permeated by this subtle poison so that the possibilities for its accidental absorption are countless. . . . It is an uncanny thought to realize that this lurking poison is everywhere about us, ready to gain unsuspected entrance to our bodies from the food we eat, the water we drink, and the other beverages we may take to cheer us, the clothes we wear, and even the air we breathe." Similarly, advice in the 1935 book *Eat, Drink, and Be Wary* to reject foods made with artificial ingredients, preservatives, and stabilizers would rival any contemporary "clean eating" manifesto.[78] Just as food entering the body constitutes one point of intervention for addressing potential toxic harms, its elimination has for millennia been another crucial site of preoccupation.[79] Constipation, for instance, is often seen as trapping toxins in the body, prompting a vast industry of treatments to promote colonic regularity, including laxatives, fortified foods, exercises, enemas, and devices, all believed to help the body expel the toxins harbored within. Fasting, leeching, soaking, and sweating also have long histories as detoxification strategies. Concerns about bodily purity and impurity are etched into the story of humankind itself.

Given this long historical context, we might wonder why toxins have assumed such renewed prominence in the cultural imagination over recent decades. Are contemporary consumers simply paranoid and gullible, convinced by marketing and sham gurus that they are under constant invisible threat? This is certainly what debunkers of celebrity health fads would have us believe. For many proscience advocates, giving people more and better facts (e.g., about how the liver works) will help them see they have been duped. But a richer and likely more accurate answer lies in understanding how public preoccupation with toxins and their removal is driven by broader tensions between the logics of restoration and enhancement, which in turn are influenced by the dynamic interplay of industry regulation, healthcare policy, pharmaceutical marketing, and a culture of personal individual responsibility. Consumers may be paranoid and gullible, but if they are, it is only because they have been trained to be so.

The twentieth century is rife with instances of regulatory failure to protect public health from toxic harm, whether through five decades of continued prescription of estrogen diethylstilbestrol (DES) to pregnant women even though it was long known to cause vaginal cancer, or industry suppression of research linking cigarettes with cancer, or policies allowing known carcinogens into the food stream because of industry pressure.[80] Even regulations explicitly designed to protect the public often fall short of their mandate; an example is the 1976 US Toxic Substances Control Act (TSCA), which, as MacKendrick notes, gave legacy approval to sixty-two thousand existing chemical substances, only 2 percent of which have subsequently been reviewed for safety.[81] The story in Canada follows similar contours on a smaller scale, with a nest of overlapping regulatory bodies that leaves plenty of gaps for potential health risks to escape notice. In both countries, in the absence of broader coordinated strategies for managing collective risk, the market has stepped in with ready solutions to help people manage their own individual risk.

Precautionary consumption with products such as natural health products, organic foods, and "green" cleaning supplies is ultimately inevitable: people see government inaction, worry about its risks, and want to find their own ways to act. As individuals, they have learned from public health messaging, governing agencies, and consumer culture that their primary form of agency is through consumer choice, so they work to become more responsible, knowledgeable consumers. As MacKendrick and others have carefully detailed, people widely believe they can insulate their families from ambient toxins by making better choices, whether that includes buying "clean" food and household products, investing in air filters and water purifiers, or even questioning vaccinations.[82] Of course, the corollary of this belief that you can shop your way to a toxin-free life is that if you or your family fail to remain safe and healthy, you have failed as an individual parent, partner, and health citizen.

Despite every precaution we take, our bodies are porous, their boundaries permeable. We are therefore affected by what surrounds us, and we are exposed every day to a litany of chemicals, some of which have been shown to be safe but many of which we cannot be certain about. Indeed, we do not even need to be in direct contact with toxic materials to be saturated with them. Consider, for example, that the breast milk of Inuit women contains high levels of PCBs, DDT, and flame retardants, which are brought by "global air and water currents" into the region, far from where they are produced and consumed, and then absorbed by local fauna that make up Inuit diets.[83] As living creatures, we, like fauna, absorb our surroundings through what we eat, drink, breathe, and touch. Kids and pets are affected by prescription hormone creams applied to adults' skin; families and roommates are colonized by one another's bacteria; cyclists and pedestrians breathe air that includes exhaust from cars, trucks, and factories. What is outside comes in.

Consumers are therefore left in a double bind: they know they have been exposed to a high chemical load over their lives, but they cannot always determine which chemicals matter or how to limit their exposure to them or reduce their effects. Left on their own, they end up practicing what Eula Biss calls "intuitive toxicology" by reading up online and in books, magazines, and newspapers; by talking with doctors, naturopaths, and friends; and by going with their gut instincts about what will be safe to put into their bodies.[84] However, even people who inform themselves and take precautions often cannot help which or how many toxins they are exposed to because individual body burdens are partly determined by race, class, and occupation.[85] Toxins disproportionately affect minoritized and immigrant workers, especially those in manufacturing, farming, and cosmetic salons, as well as lower-income neighborhoods located near freeways, industrial areas, and disposal sites. And yet, neoliberal environmental, health, and economic policies turn attention away from these social and environmental hazards by tasking each individual with personal responsibility for avoiding, reducing, and eliminating potential harms on their own. The wealthiest among us have therefore turned in staggering numbers to products and services that promise to eradicate toxins, and even those with less discretionary income are catching up.[86] Products such as Renew Life's First Cleanse promise to "gently stimulate the cleansing and detoxification process" to protect us from the toxins that lurk within by stimulating "the body's 7 channels of elimination: the liver, lungs, colon, kidneys, blood, skin, and lymphatic system."[87] The rhetoric of detoxification products is powerful because it provides a clear path forward to solving a problem that each of us, as individual consumers, otherwise cannot begin to touch.

Toxing Out

In *Toxin Toxout*, Lourie and Smith explain that because we cannot entirely avoid risk of toxic harm, we must reduce or eliminate the toxins that do enter our bodies. Their advice on how to do so comes with a warning, however: "Once you immerse yourself in the detox world, it's a hypochondriac's dream come true." The authors experiment with cleanses and intravenous chelation but dismiss these sorts of "wacky quick-fix detoxes" as doing little more than empty our pockets.[88] For Lourie and Smith, the real way to remove toxins from the body is through "a continuous lifestyle shift" that begins with the natural toxin-flushing processes of "breathing, sweating, peeing and pooing" and expands to eating more vegetables and less meat, exercising, drinking plenty of water, and protecting the environment by changing the ways we live, shop, and vote.[89]

Although Lourie and Smith dismiss detox products such as cleanses, they recognize the deep symbolic value they hold in contemporary American and Canadian culture. Just as toxins are loaded with metaphoric significance of "badness" or "impurity," detoxes signify redemption and purification, a chance to become clean without undertaking the difficult work of making the "continuous lifestyle shift" that Lourie and Smith prescribe.[90] Cleanses typically require only short-term dietary shifts that include abstaining from certain foods, fasting, consuming high levels of fiber and liquid, and consuming various supplements in capsules and teas. Whether a person does routine maintenance cleanses or engages in them only after periods of heavy eating or drinking, cleanses constitute the sort of harm reduction that Nichter and Thompson describe as counterbalancing the bad with the good.[91] MacKendrick similarly describes these practices as a strategy of "cancelling" risk.[92] Cleanses allow us to be good without requiring full-scale change.

Many of my interview participants described their use of natural health products in exactly these terms, as a means of counterbalancing busy work and family lives by helping the body clear itself of toxins accrued when they have not taken good care of their health. For instance, Coretta explained that she turns to another of Renew Life's products, Rapid Cleanse, when she feels "a little more bloated or . . . losing energy, feeling that there might have been a buildup in the toxins." Busy in her tourism job, she seeks the energy she gets from Rapid Cleanse "cleansing out toxins" by stimulating her colon. She finds evidence of her cleanse's success in the frequent and voluminous elimination from her body of what she euphemistically calls the "bad buildup." When she finishes the cleanse, Coretta simply resumes her usual everyday life, feeling "not physically lighter but . . . I just feel lighter and feel like I've gotten rid of, you know, just a lot of bad buildup."[93]

As in Coretta's case, poop—one of Lourie and Smith's primary toxin elimination strategies—is central to the rhetoric of detoxification: short of laboratory testing, changes in colonic output are often the only signs that a detox has or has not had an effect. Lourie and Smith explain in *Toxin Toxout* that while it is obvious whether a diet is working—you either lose weight or or you do not—"there's no such built-in quality control" for detox programs. We cannot tell by looking at our opaque bodies whether a cleanse has worked, and we cannot buy what Lourie and Smith cleverly call a "Tox-O-Meter" to read our bodies' toxic levels.[94] We can only guess on the basis of how we feel and what comes out of our bodies.

Many people report feeling energized and euphoric following a cleanse, though it is difficult to tell whether this feeling comes from reducing the body's toxic load or is instead an emotional or physical response to the difficult experience of eating very little for a sustained period of time.[95] As for what comes out of the body following a cleanse, the internet is, of course, flooded with images of what people believe is a toxic sludge eliminated through their colon, which they count as evidence of a successful treatment. The quantity and quality of poop that follows a cleanse is thus an important physical sign, and often the only one, that a cleanse has worked. As a material signifier that can be seen, smelled, and felt as it leaves the body, poop is easily persuasive. Rhetorically, this is the beauty of supplement-supported cleanses: cleanses provide enough evidence by proxy (e.g., increases in energy, euphoria, colonic output) to imply effectiveness without ever having to demonstrate unambiguously that they do eliminate toxins. This proxy evidence creates a mutually reinforcing cycle that strengthens and expands the realm of toxin talk because the poop produced during a cleanse becomes proof that the cleanse successfully removed toxins, which in turn proves that the body was full of toxins that needed to be removed. This cycle in turn both justifies the present cleanse and paves the way for future cleanses.

Lourie and Smith are themselves circumspect about cleanses, but they unwittingly perpetuate this mutually reinforcing cycle in both *Death By Rubber Duck* and *Toxin Toxout* by arguing so forcefully, first, that toxins are always all around us, and second, that the liver is one of the body's best routes for toxin elimination. Because the liver processes toxins and produces bile that winds up in the colon and comes out of the body in our poop, an increase or change in poop during a cleanse seems like a compelling indication that the cleanse has indeed worked. Any consumer therefore might understandably be persuaded of the product's effect, particularly given that all three of the Renew Life cleanses I have discussed (First Cleanse, Rapid Cleanse, and CleanseSMART) also contain laxatives. To put it more simply, undertaking a cleanse has a particularly physical persuasive force for the person who experiences it.

This mutually reinforcing cycle of toxin worry and detoxification brings us back to how the logics of restoration and enhancement drive wellness as an autopoietic rhetoric: we can avoid toxins, but there will always be more lurking, invisibly, around us; we can use cleanses to eliminate the toxins we could not avoid and to build up our bodies' defenses, but the effects are only ever temporary. There is no ceiling in the world of harm reduction. Supplement producers such as Renew Life capitalize on this cycle of avoiding and eliminating toxins by keeping open a wide window to further treatment. Indeed, on the product description webpage for the seven-day Rapid Cleanse, Renew Life advises consumers: "It is recommended that you cleanse 2–4 times per year as we live in a toxic world with chemicals from factories, trucks, and pesticides. Since we are constantly inhaling and ingesting toxins, it is better to remove them regularly, rather than to have them build up and lead to health problems."[96] A consumer following these guidelines exactly would spend between two weeks and a month each year on a cleanse. Worse, those seeking a "deeper, more advanced cleanse" with Renew Life's thirty-day CleanseSMART, which has the same recommended frequency of two to four times a year, would instead spend a staggering 120 days in treatment a year, or one out of every three days.[97] For all its antipharmaceutical posturing, the natural health industry thus operates virtually in tandem with pharmaceutical manufacturers by creating products that simultaneously identify problems and promise to fix them—but only if the products are used regularly. Surrounded by messaging about toxins fueled simultaneously by the logics of restoration and enhancement, the wellness consumer is caught in an eternal loop.

Importantly, however, not all wellness consumers have equal access to detoxification regimens that promise to restore our bodies to a pretoxic state and enhance our defenses against future toxins. Only the very wealthy—someone such as Peter Sullivan, the millionaire Californian "detox pioneer" I discussed earlier in this chapter—would have the ability to remove all their fillings, undergo years of chelation therapy and colonic irrigation, consume untold numbers of supplements, and renovate their homes in a bid to avoid contamination. Even maintaining a more modest wellness regimen requires considerable time and financial resources to read labels, research and buy specialty products, visit practitioners who specialize in detoxification, monitor symptoms, take supplements, follow cleanses, and cook from scratch, whereas minoritized people and those in lower economic brackets disproportionately bear the most toxic body burdens of contemporary life.[98] In wellness culture, harm reduction therefore belongs almost exclusively to the wealthy.

Social Contamination and Individual Action

When we conceive of wellness as a form of reducing or avoiding harm, we can see more clearly how contemporary neoliberal environmental and health politics have put us in a situation where we as individual citizens cannot win. The detoxi-fication practices described in this chapter are premised on the idea that each of us can and must purify ourselves of the invisible threats lurking in our bodies and in our environment, but those threats are produced not by individuals but by collectives, by whole populations, by industries, governments, and nations. These threats are produced in boardrooms, factories, advertisements, and legislation and cannot meaningfully be traced back to individual acts by individual consum-ers. MacKendrick says of precautionary consumption that "this approach, in so much as it hinges on suggesting that better label reading at the supermarket will address and mitigate chemical pollution, obscures the larger systemic context that has resulted in a marketplace awash in untested chemicals. By focusing on consumer practices, individualized precautionary consumption directs attention from the responsibility of government and chemical companies to enforce and enact responsible testing and manufacturing protocols."[99] In other words, precau-tionary consumption provides an individual solution to a collective problem and reframes the problem as if it had been an individual one all along.

Facing down a wall of cleaning products that may be toxic, for instance, con-sumers are put on the defensive, forced to decide between different products rather than ask why so many products are full of dangerous chemicals in the first place. The principle of consumer choice thus leaves many individuals wondering if they are bad people if they choose not to buy the "green" bathroom cleaner or if they have failed as parents if they cannot afford it. Just as expanding the ideal of health citizenship has downloaded responsibility onto individuals to care for their own and their families' health, the principle of harm reduction that under-lies wellness culture shifts attention away from broad, systemic action, the very place we are most likely to effect change, by reframing concerns about toxic con-tamination as matters of individual consumer choice.

In *Fear of Food: A History of Why We Worry about What We Eat*, Harvey Lev-enstein points out that "American capitalism had a remarkable ability to defang opposition by co-opting it—that is, by adopting the rhetoric of radicals' programs while gutting their content."[100] If what drives people to wellness culture is the desire to bypass corporate interests and return to a state of purity, then the irony is that neither is actually even possible in the current American and Canadian political-economic climate, where industries simply tap into and then neutralize activists' and consumers' desire for more equitable, safer, and more effective products through initiatives such as "eco," "green," and "natural" labeling.[101] And so while toxins may be invisibly everywhere, beyond our control, our available forms of remediation center primarily on individual consumption. This problem is compounded because, as McKendrick points out, when people "cocoon themselves from toxic threats, they are less likely to demand regulatory action to prevent toxic materials from being released into the environment and retail landscape."[102] There is little space within toxin talk for systemic or collective action, such as enhanced industrial and commercial regulations. It is instead about purification of individual bodies, a pharmaceutically motivated solution to social and environmental problems.

The final point in this chapter, then, belongs to those who took part in my interviews and in the "Stop Bill C-51" petition. While all those whose words I have analyzed in this chapter assert their rights to use natural health products to protect themselves from toxins, nearly all of them explicitly noted that problems they seek to solve with supplements are not of their own making. They instead lay the fault with government inaction, lax regulations, pollution, poor-quality food, overwork, economic anxiety, and chronic illness, none of which, in their view, been sufficiently addressed by health authorities. In the petition, for example, the commenter Mary Catherine reported being forced to buy supplements at personal expense because "the ground that our toxic crops are grown in [is] depleted in many of the natural nutrients that God had placed in the first place and man has destroyed."[103] In the interviews, many participants described feeling pressure to use cleanses even though they feel skeptical about them because they know that as good health citizens they are expected to protect their health from harm. There is thus a prominent moral dimension within wellness as a form of harm reduction because we know we are supposed to care about, and act on, the potential dangers lurking among and within us. As Alexis Shotwell reminds us, "We are made responsible for our own bodily impurity."[104]

Shotwell advises that rather than simply assuming responsibility for our impurity by shopping for more natural or purer products, we should instead engage collectively in "practices of perceiving interdependence [to] nourish an ethical relation to complex ecologies in which we are implicated and through which we are formed."[105] By recognizing our interdependence, she says, we can embrace our vulnerability and fight back against models of health and illness that exhort us each to act as individual islands of one. I agree with Shotwell's argument in principle, but then I think back to all the individuals I cited in this chapter who explain that they turn to wellness particularly when they are overworked, sleep-deprived, and too busy to eat well, exercise, and relax. How can we engage in collective action if we are exhausted, barely hanging on? This is the topic of the next chapter.

CHAPTER FOUR

Wellness as Survival Strategy

The motivating situation of the fourth vector of wellness, and the keyword of this chapter, is *exhaustion*. I begin from Lauren Berlant's provocation to consider how we might view so-called unhealthy behaviors—consuming junk food and alcohol, playing videogames, or even smoking—not as disregard for life but as attachment to it. In Berlant's view, these behaviors resist rhetorics of self-discipline and medicalization that define the body as a tool of capitalist production that requires constant observation and management—of what we eat, how we sleep, and how we feel. Berlant invites us to view behaviors commonly considered unhealthy as survival strategies, as ways for people to find *life* within moralistic logics of self-surveillance and self-improvement. As the previous chapters have shown, these are logics that exhort us constantly to be our best selves, to be the smartest, most efficient, strongest, most attractive, and most self-actualized versions of ourselves. In Berlant's view, so-called unhealthy behaviors instead offer "vitalizing pleasure," a kind of respite for the exhausted self.[1] This vitalizing pleasure is a space where the body becomes a refuge, through sensory relief, from the labors of the day.

In this chapter I explain how the concept of wellness similarly operates as a survival strategy, the flip side of a tub of Haagen-Dazs at night. Wellness-oriented products such as supplements offer a sense of agency, a means of reducing the burdens of everyday life when nothing else seems possible. For example, if we are feeling tired or beaten down, we might try one supplement to boost our energy, another to boost our thinking, and a third to boost our mood. If we are hung over, we can get vitamins infused intravenously so we can continue working. We have collectively become so exhausted, in fact, that in 2019 the World Health Organization officially recognized burnout in its *International Classification of Diseases* (ICD) as an "occupational phenomenon" that stems from "chronic workplace stress that has not been successfully managed."[2] While the ICD emphasizes the role of individual stress management for addressing burnout, a better way to address the problem is to understand burnout in the broader contexts of human life, to explore how exhaustion figures into our personal, political, economic, and health decisions. Viewed from this perspective, wellness discourse constitutes an optimistic rhetoric: it promises improvement in lives increasingly lived in permanent states of temporary crisis as individual rights, worker protections, housing security, economic stability, and environmental stewardship erode under global capitalism and as human bodies reach their limits under physical and mental stress.

In what follows, I argue that although public discourse surrounding wellness and natural health products is steeped in pathologizing medical-pharmaceutical rhetorics of bodily imbalance and dysfunction, users of these products nevertheless find within them resources for resilience—and therefore for political possibility. That is, if, as Sara Ahmed argues, "exhaustion [functions] as a management technique: you tire people out so they are too tired to address what makes them too tired," then rhetorics of wellness provide hope of change by promising to reinvigorate those who seek it.[3] At the same time, however, wellness seekers may ultimately be caught in a relation of what Berlant calls "cruel optimism" with respect to the object they seek because their drive to wellness may actually impede their odds of ever reaching it: with no ceiling, wellness is discursively constituted to remain ever just out of reach.[4] Drawing on recent scholarship on rhetorics of resilience, I argue that reliance on wellness-oriented products such as supplements does not optimize our health as much as it props us up just enough that we can keep going.[5]

I must admit at the outset that thinking about the ideas of this chapter makes me tired—and if I have done it right, it should make you tired too. But the chapter's topic alone does not precipitate my fatigue. Rather, what makes me tired is that for all the problems I address in this chapter, as for many I discuss over the course of this book, there is almost nothing any one of us alone can do to fix them because they are not individual problems of living but collective problems of social structures, of systems. We can buy all the organic produce we want, we can meditate and do therapy and get twelve hours of sleep at night, and we can "vote with our wallets" to try to change the status quo, but none of these individual actions will move the needle on our collective exhaustion. One of the ways wellness operates in contemporary culture is as a promise—a promise that if we can get through the labors of the moment by giving ourselves a little boost, we will be ready for what comes next; a promise that we will not always feel so tired, so powerless, so overwhelmed; a promise that we can and will feel better. Wellness culture is in large part about surviving life in a state of exhaustion.

I know this on a vital, visceral level because I have experienced it myself. When I began planning this book, it was going to be a cynical takedown of wellness culture, but as the project progressed, I started to see things differently. I began to experience the shifts we all go through at some point: I started to get older, my body registering the cumulative effects of a busy professional and family life, the stresses of graduate school, the academic job market, and the tenure track. I experienced the losses and griefs of aging and sick relatives, including my own mother's death from cancer. Life happened while I kept working at the pace I had been habituated to in my early career, and I got totally burnt out. Then, as I started writing this book in earnest, I went on sabbatical. It was the first time I paused to catch my breath, indeed the first time I felt I *could* pause to breathe, since graduate school. Without really thinking about it, I started taking more time to take care of myself. I did yoga, Pilates, and therapy. I slept. I cooked leisurely meals and read for pleasure. I ignored email. And I hired an academic coach to help me restructure my working life so I could have more clearly demarcated working hours and more unambiguous time off. Normally tense from head to toe, with chronic neck and jaw pain, headaches, and all the other hallmarks of stress and anxiety, I began to unfurl during my sabbatical as my shoulders moved away from my ears down my back and the crease between my eyes softened. As this happened, I started to see wellness a little differently. While I remain largely cynical about wellness culture, I came to see for myself that one of the things wellness does is give us a break, a moment of rest when we really need it. My experience is echoed throughout the materials I discuss in this chapter, where people find in wellness small ways to survive the overwhelming present.

Over the course of this chapter, I examine wellness as a survival strategy, a key driver of wellness discourse. I return to the interviews I conducted with wellness consumers and analyze the marketing of a range of natural health products that differently address our prevalent collective exhaustion. My discussion unfolds over two parts. I begin by illustrating how exhaustion is often at the center of discourse about natural health and natural health products, operating primarily in the logic of restoration: individuals use supplements as a source of support or rest when they feel depleted so they can return to what they see as their normal functional self. I then show how wellness activities can also work as vitalizing pleasures, serving not merely as a stopgap for fatigue and frustration but sometimes as a source of nourishment, of joy. I situate wellness as a survival strategy within the broader context of what can be achieved through individual action, as well as whether (and how) wellness and natural health may ultimately reduce the odds that we will ever actually become *well*. In this argument, I am motivated by Berlant's orienting observation that "we must begin thinking about how to survive and thrive not by imagining people in the tableau of their greatest self-conscious control but by seeing the patterns of activity that at once advance and contradict survival in light of the pressures of contemporary everyday life. Then we need to rethink everyday life."[6] Short of a fundamental remaking of who we are collectively and how we live, I suggest in this chapter that sometimes all we can do is make sure we are each comfortable as we sail sinking into the sea. And that alone is significant. Sometimes the best we can do is simply draw attention to things that need attention.

Maintaining the Exhausted Self

Several months prior to the global coronavirus outbreak in 2020, I needed to change an airline ticket, which meant calling the company and speaking to an actual person. I put off the task for weeks because I knew what it would entail: my call would be greeted by the now-familiar message "Due to unusually high call volume, wait times to speak with an agent will be longer than usual," and then I would sit on hold for upwards of an hour before it was my turn. I knew this because I have heard this same message and held for the same length of time every time I have called this airline for as long as I can remember. I have also heard a similar version of the message when calling my bank. And my cell phone provider. And my city's 311 service. And chances are that you have heard it too.

This time, though, instead of the airline's usual message of feigned surprise that so many people would try to reach its call center simultaneously, a different recording alerted me that the queue to speak to an agent was in fact full and I would need to try again later. Undaunted, I called right back and this time was placed in the queue, annoyed but grateful for making the cut. Calls like these are such a widely shared experience that the internet is filled with memes about them. My favorite, a comic from syndicated cartoonist Randy Glasbergen, features a businessman on a call at his desk, listening to a recording that says, "Due to unusually high call volume, this conversation will be really loud."[7] Playing on slippage in the meaning of *volume* from a quantity to a property of sound, the comic finds a sliver of humor in an otherwise mundane and frustrating shared experience; the joke lies in the fact that we all know what the recording really means. Another of these memes features a tight shot of Keanu Reeves as the slacker character Ted from the 1989 film *Bill and Ted's Excellent Adventure*, overlaid with the question we have all certainly asked ourselves: "What if an unusually high call volume is really the usual call volume?"[8] (The comedic effect is more impressive if you hear it in Ted's characteristic "Whoa, dude!" voice.) These memes together highlight how well trained we are as citizens and consumers to accept that this is just how things are now when we try to reach large institutions and corporations. We have learned that exceptional circumstances eventually become the norm and that we can only shrug and wait our turn.

This normalized "abnormal" state is akin, in miniature, to what is known in politico-legal terms as a *state of exception*. A state of exception arises during a period of crisis when governments suspend normal juridical order and place legal limits on certain human geopolitical and biological rights in response to a perceived emergency. This is an interim state that can then effectively become the new normal as temporary restrictions harden into established practice and policy.[9] What I have in mind here is far broader and more diffuse than the state of exception as it is enshrined in law. Instead, I want to pick up specifically on how the concept is generative for thinking through how human beings live under and respond to ever-increasing physical, psychological, social, economic, and environmental pressure in the contemporary age. Whether we are thinking of telephone hold times, lineups at government offices for passports or driver's licenses, invoice processing delays, or diagnostic and surgical wait times, we have become habituated to perpetual states of crisis in every aspect of our lives. Consider, for example, our collective (but unevenly distributed) experiences with cuts to education, healthcare, and social supports; crumbling civic infrastructure; increased bureaucracy and decreased services; and loss of permanent employment with benefits in a new gig economy of insecure, short-term, low-paid work. The state of exception in which we currently find ourselves, in which most of us live exhausted lives under conditions of austerity, has become the new normal.

Unmoored in this sea of normalized low-level panic is the human body, the most elemental part of our existence, the thing that constitutes *us*. Even under ideal circumstances, the body eventually breaks down, gets sick, tires out, and ultimately stops living. But for bodies trying to live within and respond to a system of labor and capital that is, in an important sense, inhospitable to life, the effects are particularly "wrenching," to use anthropologist Emily Martin's term. She notes that as "people stretch and are stretched to adjust to . . . fit their circumstances" under trying conditions, bodies become sites of struggle where survival does not necessarily mean triumph but simply adapting successfully enough to continue for another day.[10] Martin's focus on the body's ability to survive trying conditions brings us back to Berlant's consideration of so-called unhealthy acts such as eating junk food, drinking alcohol, or playing video games as "a kind of rest for the exhausted self."[11] All-consuming sensory experiences allow people to escape momentarily their stressful lives through the experience of pleasure and feelings of engagement and resilience. Wellness discourse therefore shapes and is shaped by exhaustion, as well as by its seeming antidote, resilience, while focusing primarily on the (re)insertion of human bodies into spaces of work.

The Rhetorical Work of Resilience

If you look past the veneer of energetic self-empowerment in wellness culture, you do not need to look far to find exhaustion lurking in its shadow. Indeed, if illness is the "night side" of life, as Susan Sontag once famously said,[12] then we might say that exhaustion, in all its forms, is the night side of wellness. Whether we are exhausted physically, psychologically, spiritually, or financially, wellness appears to provide replenishment in one form or another. For example, the writer Charlotte Bayes, who dubs herself on Twitter as "Femme Fatigue," experimented with rejuvenating supplement infusions in a 2019 *VICE* exposé of posh London wellness clinics. She found temporary relief from an anti-aging treatment, but as with the other injections and intravenous solutions she sampled, before long she was right "back to feeling like the same tired, dried-out slug as always."[13]

Similarly, Brigid Delaney writes in her popular nonfiction book *Wellmania: Extreme Misadventures in the Search for Wellness* about her efforts to transform her life through cleanses, yoga, and various forms of healing and self-discovery such as mindfulness and meditation. Her goal was to alleviate "the sensation I carry in my body [that] is an almost ever-present discomfort" from too much food and drink and long days of sitting at the office: "This is the discomfort of a person who has a lot on her mind and worries for the future, her work, her family, waking sometimes at 4am and having a hard time getting back to sleep. This is the discomfort of a person for whom exhaustion—or at least a low-level version, with its minor aches and pains, a bit of brain fog and forgetting names, the *hmpruff* sound when bending to put on her shoes—is the new normal."[14] This new normal eventually becomes old as our frame of reference for what is physically tolerable shifts ever further from what we might call "healthy" to a place where our collective imaginings of what people can and should endure become ever more unrealistic. For example, if we can function with only six hours of sleep, it is not long before six hours becomes five; if we can make do while short-staffed by one person, one soon becomes two.

The experience of exhaustion that both Bayes and Delaney recount shares roots with nineteenth-century rhetorics of hypochondria and neurasthenia, or nervous exhaustion, the range of cures for which varied from total rest to vigorous physical exertion, punctuated by regimens that included medication, massage, and other treatments.[15] Exhaustion then, as now, was often attributed to overexertion and the demands of a sped-up culture in combination with the struggle to become and stay happy; in this respect, the phenomenon I am discussing here is not entirely new. What does seem to be new is how much closer we are, collectively, to the edge of our ability to withstand physical, mental, social, financial, and environmental crises.

A precarious form of exhaustion loomed large in the interviews I conducted for this book, particularly in relation to stress and work. Initially, the participants praised wellness culture for shifting public attention from strictly physical understandings of health to multidimensional models of human flourishing that encompass not just bodies but minds, souls, and social relations. In these moments, the participants explained wellness in the logic of enhancement. However, when they explained what wellness means in their own lives, the participants' focus often slipped quickly into the logic of restoration, a logic not of flourishing but of just getting through another day. As I explain over the following pages, wellness serves as an important source of resilience in contemporary culture, a strategy for maintaining the exhausted self by helping individuals to weather and recover from difficult circumstances.

The concept of resilience currently organizes much activity in journalism, environmental and community organizations, educational and research institutions, and government policy. As communication scholar Bridie McGreavy argues, *resilience* does not refer merely to an individual capacity to cope with, bounce back from, regain control over, and reduce vulnerability to difficult or undesirable circumstances. Rather, as McGreavy explains, resilience is also importantly discursive: what resilience is at a given time is determined by how it is performed in a given context by a given set of actors. McGreavy illustrates how we can track these performances to understand how resilience operates both materially and ideologically in the contexts within which it is invoked. She cautions that our collective definitions and understandings of resilience directly "influence how we become resilient" in ways "that foreclose other ways we might respond" to difficult or harmful circumstances.[16] Examining the rhetorical performance of resilience in wellness culture reveals that although natural health products may provide short-term relief to those who seek it, they advance a medicalized, individual-psychological approach that does little to address the root causes of problems for which people seek natural health products in the first place. Ultimately, natural health products do nothing to alleviate the penetrating exhaustion that characterizes much of contemporary life.

For example, the participants I interviewed defined being well primarily in terms of having enough energy to endure the stresses of demanding jobs and busy lives. Gene, a construction worker in his fifties, explained that he understands wellness as being able to "get through a day and have lots of energy, . . . to be able to endure stresses physically or mentally." For him, illness is the reverse, characterized by "aches and pains [in your] body, your joints. Fatigue, tired—tiredness, fatigue."[17] Productivity thus serves for Gene as a benchmark of wellness, whereas feeling tired means one is ill. Similarly, Coretta, a tourism professional in her early fifties, defines wellness as the ability to get things done, to be able to go to work, run errands, and engage in physical activities. For her, being ill is "where you're physically not able to, or just too tired, too exhausted, don't have time or don't have the energy."[18] Exhaustion is a defining reason why these and other participants seek wellness products and services.

When asked how they can tell whether they are themselves well, numerous participants likewise framed their answers in terms of productivity and function, of being able to get things done. Steve, a retired engineer, explained: "I can tell if I'm sufficiently well if I get up in the morning and I'm full of energy or I'm tired, and if I'm tired I say the body's not in balance."[19] For Steve, wellness is not a place you inhabit but a transient state that shifts from morning to morning, moment to moment. Knowing whether you are well means reading your body at a given point in time; it is like reading a thermometer or a barometer. Clara, a retired dance teacher, also tracks her body internally to determine whether "the energy is there, the clarity, the mood, a feeling of comfort and peace and freedom in the body." Her sense of wellness at any given moment depends on how she perceives her present "ability to do things without any reservation [so] I don't worry, 'Oh my god that's too tiring or too heavy or too this or too that.'"[20] With regard to wellness as a survival strategy, the interview participants almost universally expressed the belief that wellness has become a massive industry specifically because it responds to people's unmet needs for rest, care, and vitality in their everyday lives. For Steph, a 40-year-old office administrator, exhaustion is pervasive, and it negatively affects all aspects of her life: "I'm always tired and sluggish and I just feel like because that affects my general well-being, I'm not a happy person . . . because I'm tired all the time. So how do I fix that? How do I make myself better?" In her view, wellness and natural health appeal to people who "want to know more about how to make ourselves better, [who] want more resources." Steph's quest for restored energy and vitality leads her, like so many others, beyond the mainstream health system to the world of natural health products and practitioners: "I'm asking a wider range of resources to get more information."[21]

Mandy, an entrepreneur in her early fifties, offered an even franker explanation of why people are interested in wellness: "Because they're not happy. They're sick. They're sick and tired of being sick and tired. They feel like crap, everybody else feels like crap. . . . And people want to feel better, you know? Everybody wants just to be healthy, happy . . . but it's very hard to do." Mandy, like Steph, feels she has to seek care for herself because she is not getting what she needs from her regular health providers: "If you go to the doctor's office and it's one thing at a time . . . so you can come back twelve times. Again."[22] In Mandy's view, wellness offers her a way to fight for her health because everyday life makes her feel sick and tired. Similarly, Vanessa, a graduate student in her early thirties, views wellness as a response to "stress in everyday life. Everything's messed up. Our culture is so opposed to actually being well [that] exhaustion is kind of seen as a status symbol." Like Steph and Mandy, Vanessa is not surprised that people are taking their health into their own hands by choosing natural health products because "wellness is something that's a kind of counterpoint to acknowledge how messed up our everyday life has become."[23]

Vanessa's characterization of wellness as a counterpoint to stress and exhaustion echoes the main reasons her fellow participants also gave for using specific natural health products to enhance their energy, immunity, mood, and sleep. For instance, Erin, a nutritionist in her mid-twenties, said that when she is tired she seeks "that extra boost" she gets from supplements containing so-called superfood greens such as kale, wheatgrass, kelp, beets, and algaes such as spirulina and chlorella so that she "can have more energy and feel well."[24] Andrea, a nonprofit administrator in her mid-forties, similarly described taking multiple vitamins daily "for energy to stay healthy," with a special focus on B vitamins because "I feel much less stressed if I take a B vitamin, I feel that that really helps with my stress."[25] Jasmine, a public policy professional in her early thirties, takes vitamin supplements for the same reasons, complementing them with teas that have "healing properties."[26] Each of these women sees natural health products as an important source of extra support when she needs it.

One element of Jasmine's interview that stands out is her mention of using a homeopathic remedy recommended by her naturopath for "adrenal fatigue." Jasmine explained that the theory behind adrenal fatigue, as she understood it, is that living through "a period of chronic stress" places extra pressure on the adrenal glands, which then require support through supplementation while the body recovers from overexertion. She expressed some hesitation about the diagnosis because she had learned that adrenal fatigue is not recognized by biomedical health professionals, but she ended up trying the remedy "because it wasn't too cost prohibitive and I was at a point where I was willing to kind of take any advice." The most important thing, she explained, is not whether a health intervention actually works on a physiological level but whether she experiences positive effects from trying it, even if those effects are imagined rather than real. In particular, she values the increased sense of agency she feels when she tries natural health products: "I think they give me a sense . . . of control that kind of goes into it. Like, I have this issue, I'm feeling this way, I'm doing something that . . . I'm proactively doing." She said she is not as concerned about whether the product "actually makes a difference: I don't know if it's placebo or not, or if it puts me at ease that I'm doing something."[27] As this example from Jasmine shows, whatever else wellness and natural health products do (or do not do), they offer people ways to claim some agency for themselves when they feel overwhelmed by exhaustion and stress.

The interview participants also frequently pointed to anxiety prompted by exhaustion and stress as a main driver of their use of natural health products. Gene, who earlier defined wellness as being able to "get through a day and have lots of energy," correspondingly associated the degree of anxiety he feels at a given moment with his ability to get things done.[28] Similarly, Tania, who is in her late forties and on sick leave, described her anxiety in inverse relation to her fatigue: "When my anxiety gets really high I find it hard to control my mind and then I don't feel like doing much of anything. You know, my anxiety kind of has been in line with my energy lately and my energy's been very low and anxiety makes you not want to necessarily go out and socialize and do things in public."[29] Both Gene and Tania seek natural health products on an episodic basis to treat their anxiety in much the same way that a person might take a benzodiazepine such as Lorazepam. Operating in the logic of restoration, for relief of symptoms they choose natural health remedies such as Bach's Rescue Remedy, an herbal preparation advertised as "the world's traditional anxiety remedy."[30]

Products such as Rescue Remedy offer an alternative to the distressing experience of anxiety for others I interviewed as well, such as Nicki, a teacher in her forties: "I take the Bach Flower Remedy Rescue drops . . . if I feel stressed out or full of anxiety, you know if I'm travelling or something." Nicki takes comfort in knowing that if she feels overwhelmed, liquid relief is close at hand in a small amber bottle administered with a dropper directly onto her tongue.[31] For each of these individuals, wellness and natural health products function as purchasable solutions that give them the ability to withstand and bounce back from the pressures they face, to feel more at ease, and to restore their energy.

Retail Resilience

The marketing of products intended to treat stress, anxiety, and fatigue illustrates the rhetorical work of resilience within wellness culture because marketing lays bare the ideological currents that animate the retail landscape. The Rescue Remedy product line from Bach Original Flower Remedies taps into the persistent exhaustion and stress that we all experience at various points in our lives, establishing itself as a ready solution in the form of quick-acting drops, sprays, melts, candies, and chewing gums. Rescue Remedy was formulated in the 1930s by Edward Bach, an English physician who closed his Harley Street practice in London to practice homeopathy and herbal medicine. Rescue Remedy is the jewel accompanying Bach's line of thirty-eight individual "flower essences," which contain homeopathic dilutions of flowers that ostensibly correspond to each of thirty-eight negative emotional states organized into seven "emotional groups."[32] After cultivation, each flower variety is diluted in a solution of water and brandy until all that remains is its "vibrations or energy";[33] users are intended to ingest these solutions alone or in combination to remedy their negative emotional state. Nearly a century later, Bach's Original Flower Remedies are widely available in mainstream pharmacies and natural health stores and on wellness websites worldwide. My own midwife, who held hospital admitting privileges and taught in the local university's accredited midwifery program, enthusiastically recommended Bach's Rescue Remedy when I was overwhelmed after my daughter's birth. (I declined.)

Marketing discourse surrounding Rescue Remedy moves fluidly between clearly defined medical-diagnostic categories such as depression and anxiety and more ordinary problems of living such as frustration and nervousness. For example, on Rescue Remedy's website, its product overview explains, "The RESCUE family of products combines the original flower essences discovered by Dr Bach in the 1930's to provide support *in times of emotional demand*."[34] The nature and limits of what constitutes "emotional demand" remain fuzzy, edging around but never fully invoking diagnostic categories such as anxiety or depression: "Whatever the day throws at you, a challenging agenda at work, school exams, or balancing the demands of a busy family life, keep on top of things and get the most out of your busy day with RESCUE Remedy® by your side."[35] None of these problems of living are medical in nature, but according to Rescue Remedy's website, they are nevertheless treatable conditions that people need not suffer when "rescue" is available. By expanding the realm of problems that natural health products are advertised to treat, companies such as Rescue Remedy end up mimicking the pharmaceutical industry marketing strategy of selling "an ill for every pill" rather than the other way around.[36]

The traffic between pharmaceutical and natural modes of healing is clear throughout Rescue Remedy's website, vacillating between the logics of restoration and enhancement. While the impetus to use the remedy is reactive—one seeks restoration ("rescue") in response to stressful situations—the remedy itself is framed as proactive, using positive terms of enhancement rather than negative terms of restoration. For example, according to the "Bach & RESCUE Remedy®" page, Rescue Remedy comprises "five individual flower essences" from Bach's original line, "which were specifically chosen for a sense of calm and emotional balance, especially in times of difficulty." These five essences possess "positive potential" to help consumers "stay courageous," with Rock Rose essence (which, according to the website, promotes fearlessness); "stay patient," with Impatiens essence ("to think and act less hastily, and deal easily and diplomatically with all problems"); "stay engaged," with Clematis essence (for focus); "stay strong," with Star of Bethlehem essence (for comfort); and "stay in control," with Cherry Plum essence (for composure). The use of *stay* in each of these descriptions suggests that Rescue Remedy users already possess these qualities (fearlessness, patience, focus, strength, and composure) and that Rescue Remedy merely helps them remain so "in emergencies."[37] Enhancement terms are used to similar effect in the individual product descriptions on the "Our Range" page (see table 1), where Rescue Remedy is said to help people "keep on top of" their busy days rather than

TABLE 1
Web copy from Rescue Remedy, "RESCUE Remedy®—Our Every Day Essentials," accessed May 10, 2020, https://www.rescueremedy.com/en-au/rescue -range/rescue-remedy

RESCUE PLUS® Lozenge
"On busy days we all need to maintain our concentration and reasoning whatever the day holds."

RESCUE Remedy® Dropper
"Whether it's a frustrating commute, approaching exams, a difficult day at the office, or the demands of a busy family life, keep on top of your busy day with RESCUE."

RESCUE Remedy® Pastilles
"Keep RESCUE Pastilles nearby with our handy, on-the-go tin for your handbag or in your car."

RESCUE Remedy® Spray
"Today people across the world take comfort that RESCUE is by their side when they need to get the most out of their busy day."

get on top of them. Ultimately, however, the dominant logic of wellness employed on both web pages is the logic of restoration: Rescue Remedy is a plant-based cure for problems that are not quite medical but nevertheless warrant "rescue."

Rescue Remedy similarly promotes resilience as a consumer product in a series of four interlinked commercials on its YouTube channel, which feature women struggling to cope in stressful everyday situations.[38] Like the product's website copy, these commercials invoke both logics of wellness at once: Rescue Remedy restores its users to prior states of wellness by enhancing their capacity to respond to crisis. These commercials are filmed in black and white except for the product itself, which appears in its characteristic bright yellow, and feature various combinations of the same four characters, including a mother in a luxurious home preparing a meal when her child races into the room waving a sword that knocks a glass of red wine onto a light-colored carpet; a teenager in a school uniform looking panicked as she begins to take a final exam; a young woman nervously waiting in a line of applicants for a job interview; and a bride preparing for her big moment when her necklace snaps, sending pearls flying everywhere. All the women are white, conventionally beautiful, and judging from their grooming and setting, they enjoy a certain measure of wealth.

Each commercial features a different combination of the four characters, but the narrative structure of each woman's "story" is the same: facing situational pressure such as trying to balance caring for home and child (the mother) or applying for a job (the interviewee), she reaches a point of crisis (spilled wine, pre-interview nerves) with visible distress (yelling, grimacing; see fig. 4, top images). Each character then administers Rescue Remedy in a dropper, spray, or candy and immediately responds with a look of clear relief (breathing in deeply with closed eyes, giving a small smile; see fig. 4, bottom images) while a woman's voice says in a voiceover, "The world's traditional anxiety remedy."[39] The character then returns to her task, looking refreshed, as the voiceover names the product, "Rescue Remedy." The final shot in each commercial features images of the full product range while the voiceover clinches the overall message: "Rescue Remedy: for natural stress relief." The message of these commercials is that Rescue Remedy is like a pharmaceutical in its efficacy—it works quickly, in tangibly recognizable ways—but because it is "traditional" and "natural," it is safe and gentle. Rescue Remedy thus positions itself as a treatment for ordinary stress and fatigue by marketing resilience as something you can get from a lozenge or a few liquid drops on your tongue.

I am of two minds about how the concept of resilience works in these examples and in wellness discourse more generally. In one mind, the louder part,

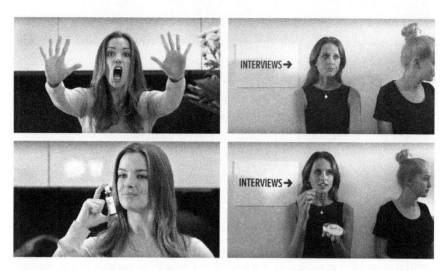

Figure 4. Video stills of Rescue Remedy commercial, *Rescue Remedy Mother and Interview*: "before" (*top*) and "after" (*bottom*). In the commercial, the product bottle (*bottom left*) and the product tin (*bottom right*) are highlighted as bright yellow within a black and white scene.

I know that resilience is not an unproblematic good. Resilience as it is currently invoked in discourse in public health, public policy, education, economics, and psychology favors individualist models of building a person's capacity to respond to stress, which does little to address the sources of that stress.[40] Addressing our collective burdens—tight finances, housing and food insecurity, long working hours, poor job security, hypercompetitive educational environments, lack of affordable childcare, insufficient time for exercise and leisure, little access to mental health and social supports, social expectations, and increased duties of care for ourselves and our families that have been downloaded onto us from the state—would require broad, population-based efforts, not drops or lozenges or lessons in mindfulness or meditation. Further, as I emphasize later in this chapter, the valorization of wellness as a form of individual resilience may ultimately make all of us less resilient and therefore more vulnerable to self-generating rhetorics of wellness.

At the same time, the idea of wellness as resilience for sale may also have positive effects we can learn from. It is easy to be cynical about wellness culture. It is easy to look at fad diets, treatments, or rituals as superficial self-indulgence or desperate, gullible consumerism. It is easy to mock Gwyneth Paltrow's wellness empire and the often implausible treatments she promotes. It is much harder but I think more valuable to focus not on the products or those who produce and sell them but on the people who buy and use them. When we shift our perspective from the *what* of products such as Rescue Remedy to the *how* and the *why*, we can see something different about wellness—that for many of its adherents wellness may not be a panacea but simply a way to survive, to restore their exhausted selves just long enough to endure another day.

Marketing does not invent markets from scratch. As much as promotional activities such as advertising play a role in selling illnesses and treatments, marketing must nevertheless tap into an existing public need or desire to gain traction.[41] Products such as Rescue Remedy thus may serve mostly as a reprieve, a moment of rest in relentless lives, as Berlant might put it.[42] In the interviews, for example, participants valued the "boost" they get from the various supplements they consume, knowing that the supplements will not fix their problems but might give them a bit more *oomph* to face them. Similarly, Rescue Remedy does not promise that its products will fix commute times, demanding jobs, or busy families. Rather, it offers temporary respite, "a moment to relax with refreshing, sugar free RESCUE chewing gum," for instance, or a little extra support to get through a "frustrating commute, approaching exams, a difficult day at the office, or the demands of a busy family life."[43] In other words, what Rescue Remedy promises most is a brief break.

Let us return to the commercials. On the one hand, they seem to be a clear-cut case of medicalization in that they first redefine normal stressful situations as "anxiety" and then position Rescue Remedy, "the world's traditional anxiety remedy," as its treatment. On the other hand, if we think carefully about the pressure experienced by the women in the commercials, the freight of the remedy itself becomes clearer: the situations depicted are banal—a wedding, an exam, an interview, a day at home with kids—but they place particular, and particularly gendered, pressures on the women who experience them. For example, in an age in which lifestyle gurus such as Marie Kondo set the cultural tone, mothers are under extraordinary pressure to care for their children, prepare nutritious and delicious meals, and keep immaculate homes, all while keeping themselves fit and fashionable, so it is no wonder the mother loses her cool when her child knocks red wine onto the carpet. The same goes for the bride: the gendered and heterosexist cultural codes baked into contemporary weddings can compel even the most easygoing women to panic about having the perfect day. That panic is both reflected in and reproduced by the face of presumably the bride's mother, who with a resigned expression of forced patience appears holding a bottle of Rescue Remedy. In both cases, the women are responding to situational pressure that is nevertheless shaped by more than situation: weddings and mothering are both fraught with sociocultural significance that can negatively affect even the most resilient among us.

For the other two characters, the student taking an exam and the young woman waiting for an interview, the pressures they face are marked both by gender and particularly by age. Math has been historically coded as masculine, whereas the workplace has historically favored male candidates and employees with higher pay, greater opportunity for advancement, and more explicit recognition. Because both women are young, they also face uncertain futures that depend on the outcome of the events that are about to unfold. For the student, the stakes of the final exam she is taking are particularly high, as the commercials were shot in Australia, where graduating high school students take exit exams such as the one depicted in the commercial. Because these exams determine students' eligibility for university and other future career paths, when the student appears to freeze up, the potential consequences are even greater than North American viewers might expect.[44] For the interviewee, the results of her interview might shape her entry into the workforce and the course of her career and earning potential.

For all the characters in these commercials, Rescue Remedy provides a moment of much-needed relief from exhausting and overwhelming situations. The narrative arc renders visible this relief in distinct stages: each woman begins in a situation that prompts a frantic, frustrated, or worried response; then she uses the remedy and subsequently looks reassured, calm, and focused, signaling immediate relief. While it is tempting to ask whether Rescue Remedy really does work in this way, if we instead focus on what it works *for*, we gain different knowledge about wellness—that wellness is in part a response to the unrelenting demands of contemporary life. Although public discourse about wellness and natural health products is generally steeped in pathologizing medical-pharmaceutical rhetorics of bodily imbalance and dysfunction, users of these products may nevertheless find within them resources for resilience, and therefore for political possibility. Before we consider these possibilities, however, let us return very briefly to exhaustion and to one of its primary sources, work.

Restoring the Exhausted Worker

The rhetorics of exhaustion that permeate wellness culture—from quelling the anxiety of busy lives to getting a better night's sleep to powering up with smoothies and supplements—frequently center on facilitating one's active participation in the workplace. The pivotal role of work in this discourse was clear in the interviews. For example, Gene, the construction worker in his fifties, defined wellness specifically as "being able to get up and take on a day's work without feeling exhaustion, without feeling fatigue. So much fatigue."[45] Similarly, Steph, the 40-something office administrator who sees multiple practitioners to try to address her long-standing fatigue, spent much of her interview focusing on work. She described feeling pressure from her employers to be productive as well as friendly and sociable. The additional burden of affective labor weighs on her because even if she gets her work done quickly and well, she feels she has to hide her true, tired self at the office: "So I'm like, 'Okay, put on my game face [and say] good morning' when I'm just like, 'Ugh! I hate the world today, I'm tired.'" She fears that her job could be at risk if she does not play along because "nobody likes Debbie downer."[46] Steph is caught in a cycle of exhaustion that she is trying desperately to escape, and she sees wellness as her most viable means of exit.

Steph's exhausting days at work lead to exhausting evenings at home. Too tired to eat a healthy dinner, she ends up settling in with a bag of chips "and then I pass out on the couch and then it's like, 'Oh great, now another night of bad sleep.'" The cumulative effects of poor sleep followed by early mornings of snoozing through her wakeup alarm mean that she spends her days alternating between coffee and nodding off at her desk, and then another difficult sleep at home at night. Steph describes this as a "domino effect" cycle in which "it's really hard to get back on the good foot" of sleeping well enough to eat well and exercise, which would in turn allow her to sleep well.[47] This cyclic story of exhaustion is repeated over and over throughout wellness culture, where natural health products and services draw exhausted workers looking to stay afloat as they manage the demands of their jobs and make the most of their time off.

Marketing strategies for natural remedies for fatigue closely resemble those of Rescue Remedy because they package up extra energy and better sleep as solutions you can also buy in a handy little box or bottle. The company EZ Lifestyle, for instance, produces three related natural health products that it advertises with the tagline "Recover. Energize. Sleep."[48] These products include EZ Lifestyle's signature product, the hangover remedy Over EZ, as well as the energy booster Fuel EZ and the sleep aid Dream EZ. Over EZ promises to improve hangovers with a "scientifically engineered" blend of vitamins, minerals, and herbs that "detoxify your liver while you drink," while also boosting nutrients and immunity that according to its website are depleted by alcohol consumption.[49] Fuel EZ appears to consist primarily of stimulants, including extracts of the caffeine-containing guarana seed and green coffee bean, as well as numerous vitamins and minerals that the product website tells us will "boost" users' brains, energy, and metabolism. Dream EZ contains "science-backed ingredients—sourced ethically from the Amazon Rainforest," including the sleep-regulating hormone melatonin, the sleep supplement valerian root, and the amino acid tryptophan to increase serotonin levels.[50]

EZ Lifestyle's "About Us" webpage urges potential customers, "Forget compromise. Get more out of life." The world is speeding up, the website says, and so "we exhaust ourselves" simply to keep up: "Think sluggishness, brain fog and anxiety. You know, the usual suspects. Add in the fact we're only human—and well, that's the biggest part of the problem."[51] I want to highlight that according to this supplement company, the biggest problem we collectively face is that we are "only human." Rather than being urged to slow down to live within our biological capabilities or fight for more humane living, working, and economic conditions, we as consumers are exhorted to turn to supplements from companies such as EZ Lifestyle, which boast that they have "found the answer" and will sell it to us in quantities of up to 120 "servings" per order.

EZ Lifestyle thus promotes its products as quick fixes for busy, tired people who need to get things done. The webpage for Fuel EZ promises customers "hours of sustained focus, mental clarity, and energy" that will allow them to become more productive, to complete big projects, to work for long periods, and to manage the demands of busy work and personal lives. Three of the four images provided on this page depict places of work: two people in work attire in a meeting with laptops, smartphones, and coffee on the table, a person writing out tasks "in progress" on a glass board covered in sticky notes while numerous smiling colleagues look on, and a younger-looking person wearing glasses seated at a table covered with what appear to be pens and markers, working on a computer (fig. 5). Work is also central to the remaining image insofar is it depicts a smiling man giving a thumbs-up with a small child, presumably his own, looking happy while

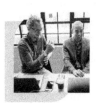

Increase work productivity   **Juggle your family, social and work life**   **Follow through with projects**   **Power through long study sessions**

Figure 5. Fuel EZ webpage image

seated on his dad's shoulders; the accompanying text reads, "Juggle your family, social and work life." In this image, we see that the father has struck the elusive balance between parenting and workplace success, which we are invited to attribute to Fuel EZ.

The supplement company Natrol similarly commodifies sleep explicitly by promoting melatonin products under the tagline "Sleep. Owned."[52] In a video hosted on its website and on YouTube, Natrol outlines the benefits of sleep, including improved memory, mood, productivity, immunity, looks, and overall health, but it draws sharp lines around what counts as "healthy" sleep and what does not. According to Natrol, unless you fall asleep in twenty minutes, sleep uninterrupted every night for seven to nine hours in ninety-minute cycles, *and* wake up "refreshed and ready to own your day," your sleep is unhealthy and warrants treatment.[53] This tightly circumscribed definition of healthy sleep pathologizes the sleep patterns of nearly everyone I know. So, either we are all sick or none of us are. Or, alternately, maybe there is good reason why we are having difficulty sleeping. Maybe our exhaustion is not the cause of problems but a consequence of a different set of problems? Perhaps trouble sleeping is a trade-off for busy personal and professional lives or an artifact of living with economic, job, housing, and food insecurity, systemic inequity, care responsibilities, social isolation, debt, and more. For participants in my interview study such as Steph, for example, getting a better night's sleep is not as much about having healthy sleep and feeling multidimensionally "well" as it is a tool for recovering enough from job-induced exhaustion to return to work.

Foucault indirectly predicted the exhaustion that characterizes early twentieth-century North American life in his explanation of biopower in the first volume of *The History of Sexuality*. As Foucault explains, capitalism depends on "the controlled insertion of bodies into the machinery of production and the adjustment of the phenomena of population to economic processes," which means that people become resources to be managed, and part of that management involves making sure their bodies are working efficiently.[54] Sick bodies and tired bodies are not productive bodies. This is the central motivation behind workplace wellness programs that promote health checkups, exercise, mindfulness, smoking cessation, and team-building exercises. These programs are not provided to employees because employers truly care about them; they are provided because employers want to reduce absenteeism and insurance costs and increase productivity.[55] Viewed in this light, my own university's "Recharge" plan during the COVID-19 pandemic, discussed in my introductory chapter, offered a veneer of care, but given how little institutional expectations of faculty changed even while the campus was closed, it strikes me instead as intended to reduce attrition and prevent faculty revolt.[56] In workplaces more generally, employees bear the weight of maximized profits with their bodies, whether through the wear and tear of physical labor or intellectual, affective, and psychological labor that manifests in bodies through chronic pain symptoms (headaches, backaches, jaw and neck problems), digestive disorders, insomnia, and situationally induced or exacerbated mental illness such as anxiety and depression.

If sleep is "one of the last barriers to capitalist production and consumption," as Cederström and Spicer observe, then it is no wonder that people like Steph take supplements to counteract the stresses of work and to sleep well enough to return the next day.[57] Human beings are only productive as long as they are energetically awake. If they are too worn out to get by on their own but are also worried about long-term effects of pharmaceutical sleeping pills, products such as Natrol stand ready as wellness-oriented alternatives. (Note even how the brand name, Natrol, lines up its flagship product, a melatonin supplement, with the well-known antihistamine marketed as a sleep aid, Nytol.) When it comes to exhaustion and sleep, then, the holistic images we conjure about wellness as a multidimensional model of health and well-being slip easily and imperceptibly into an instrumental view of sleep as a mathematical equation of energy in, labor out. Despite all the other good things that sleep does for us, such as improving diet and symptoms of depression, wellness discourse largely frames sleep as above all a tool for working better and harder. If we look again at products such as Rescue Remedy and Natrol, this time from the perspective not of what the products contain or whether they are effective but of why their users seek them, we can understand more deeply the hold that wellness culture has on us.

The "Vitalizing Pleasures" of Wellness

Viewing wellness through the prism of exhaustion makes it easier to see that one of the things natural health products offer is hope—hope that things can get better, that life will become easier, that we are not just spinning out of control. In the first half of this chapter, I showed that wellness functions as a survival strategy in that it provides people with ways of coping with persistent, low-level exhaustion. By promising moments of escape (Rescue Remedy) or a better night's sleep (Natrol), natural health products offer a cushion against the grind of everyday life. But wellness does more than allay fatigue and frustration: it also creates space for pleasure, for enjoyment of the body, for nurturing, and for experiencing the positive feelings that come with feeling good.

Consider again Berlant's discussion of moments of indulgence in "bad" or "unhealthy" behaviors. For Berlant, such moments "are not just symptoms of something off in individuals. These moments also point to social problems in maintaining equilibrium and optimism in everyday life." Berlant reminds us that despite the widespread prevalence of disciplining neoliberal discourses that emphasize personal responsibility over health, neither exhaustion nor the desire for sensory relief from "the pressures of contemporary everyday life" are necessarily personal failings. Instead, they might best be understood as appropriate responses to conditions of living that are hostile to life.[58] When people are exhausted, for instance, they may seek the restorative pleasure of curling up on the couch with a bag of chips, like the wellness-conscious Steph of my interviews, who seeks sensory relief in television, salt, fat, and carbs at the end of her workday.

Wellness-seeking behaviors may seem like the opposite of spacing out with salty snacks, but wellness often works in the same way, operating as a form of vitalizing pleasure whose comfort comes not in the pleasures of taste but in the pleasures of being "good." Activities such as eating superfoods and using natural health products give us pleasure partly because there is pleasure in striving to feel good, strong, and healthy. In my own case, for example, I feel better after working out, of course, but even those times when I dress in gym clothes at the start of the day, intending to exercise at some point but then not managing to, I still end up feeling a bit more fit and a bit more virtuous than if I had worn my regular attire. The workout clothes change my posture (I feel more limber, my limbs more organized), my mindset ("I am going to do something good for myself today"), and my affect (I feel good about caring for myself even when I am, at that moment, technically not).

Feeling as if we are taking care of ourselves can be an antidote to fatigue and frustration, particularly because self-care is something directly within our control, unlike so many other things in our lives. Recall Jasmine's desire for the "sense of control" she gets from trying natural health products because she chooses for herself when and how to take them.[59] Rather than worrying about whether the products really do have a physiological effect, she appreciates simply that she feels good about doing something good for herself. Working within prevalent definitions of wellness, which hold that one can be physically sick and still emotionally, socially, and spiritually well, even people who live with chronic or acute illness can find a form of pleasure in self-care. When we set aside the question whether natural health products actually do boost energy, sleep, or mood, we can examine how these products can restore life even by simply restoring one's sense of comfort and control. In this final half of the chapter, I illustrate how wellness helps us feel good and explain why feeing good is so desperately important to so many of us. The vitalizing pleasures of wellness are no mere add-on; they constitute a crucial form of survival by promising what Berlant calls "a kind of rest for the exhausted self."[60]

Feeling Good, Being Good

Wellness provides vitalizing pleasure in at least two distinct but overlapping ways, both of which draw on and feed into the twin logics of wellness. Tapping into the logic of restoration is the pleasure that comes from feeding the "appetites" through indulgence in alcohol, drugs, or junk food, say, and then offsetting those indulgences with supplements, injections, and intravenous solutions. Tapping into the logic of enhancement is the pleasure that comes from taking the same sorts of products to optimize energy, productivity, or nutrition. Feeling good in this way can be as much about virtue as it is about physical sensation: maybe you do feel stronger or more energetic, or maybe you feel good about trying to do something good for yourself. For many wellness seekers, cycling between these mutually reinforcing forms of pleasure—the pleasure of restoration and the pleasure of enhancement—creates a positive feedback loop wherein the ceiling of wellness once again retreats ever further.

We can see both forms of vitalizing pleasure, and indeed both logics of wellness, at work in marketing for a suite of intravenous treatments by a company called REVIV, which is headquartered in Manchester, United Kingdom, with global branches that include eight locations in the United States and two in Canada. Visitors to the main "IV Therapies" page of the website are invited to select "the right IV therapy" for their needs by clicking one of two links that generate different decision trees. Clicking the link labeled "RECOVERY" takes users to a further set of links for health problems that include "ILLNESS & HANGOVERS" and "ALLERGIES"; clicking on one of those opens a further set of links suggesting relevant IV treatments to restore customers to health. By contrast, clicking the "PRODUCTIVITY" link takes users instead to enhancement-oriented topics such as "BEAUTY & REJUVENATION" and "WELLNESS BOOST," which then further link to a range of suggested treatments. Regardless of whether a visitor begins their visit by choosing a therapy for recovery or for productivity, REVIV's website promises that its products "will help you work hard and play harder."[61]

The two logics of wellness are invoked independently of each other on REVIV's main IV webpage, with the binary structure funneling visitors toward its IV treatments for recovery or for productivity. Other pages on the website draw on the logics more fluidly, often simultaneously. The product page for the Royal Flush treatment, for example, describes Royal Flush as "a single therapy that is designed to supercharge recovery and maximize your wellness."[62] In this one sentence, website visitors are invited to view Royal Flush as both a form of restoration, a way to "supercharge recovery," and a form of enhancement, a way to "maximize your wellness." Similarly, the page blends together both forms of pleasure, the pleasure of indulgence and the pleasure of good health citizenship. The text never mentions alcohol or drugs explicitly, but both are implicit in nearly every sentence, veiled in the wink-nudge language of marketing. For example, Royal Flush allows users to "push your boundaries and experience a life beyond limits," especially if "you need a pick me up following a party," because the product will help you "supercharge recovery" by allowing you to "rehydrate" and "detoxify your body," "cleanse vital organs," and "relieve pain and nausea." Further, at the same time that the Royal Flush page hints at the pleasures of (over)indulgence, it also calls upon the pleasure of good health citizenship in its description of Royal Flush as a tool for achieving "maximum wellness" by boosting a user's energy, cleansing them of toxins, and allowing them to become better than well by pushing beyond their present limits.

Another product page on REVIV's website is less coy about the treatment's goal of restoring rather than enhancing health: "Give your body the helping hand it needs to aid recovery from ailments such as common colds, seasonal allergies, the flu or even a hangover with the help of the Ultraviv IV therapy." Unlike the page for Royal Flush, the Ultraviv page forges much tighter links to the logic of restoration, particularly by carefully framing the product's development and use in close association with doctors, illness, and medicine. The product description notes that the "clinician devised" therapy Ultraviv was "developed by an experienced team of physicians" and contains supplements such as antioxidants, minerals, and vitamins as well as "medications."[63] These references to doctors and medications seamlessly trade on both logics of wellness at once, creating space for wellness-minded consumers who want "a wellness boost" alongside those who may feel uneasy about receiving an intravenous treatment outside a medical setting such as a clinic or a hospital.

The images on this same page stand in sharp contrast to the text because they are entirely devoid of medical imagery. The page features a young woman of color with stylish natural hair and large silver hoop earrings reclining on a white-sand beach wearing a beach cover-up, surrounded by palm leaves (fig. 6). Like the other images on the website, this image seems better suited for a fashion spread than

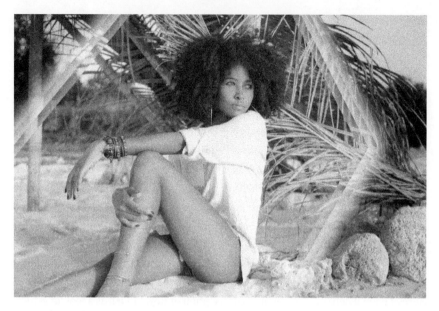

Figure 6. Detail of REVIV IV Ultraviv product page

for an intravenous treatment. The top of the page features an image of water in a rectangular shape that evokes an IV drip bag, with two large drips at the bottom suggesting an IV line (fig. 7).

The current version of REVIV's website deemphasizes the product line's association with biomedical processes and devices, but an earlier version preserved at the Internet Archive on July 2019 features unambiguous medical signifiers throughout the website, including intravenous catheters, needles, and medical personnel. In one archived image, for example, a young, white, seemingly heterosexual couple stand smiling into the camera while hooked up to IV drips and flashing peace signs (fig. 8).[64] The woman has the inside of her right elbow open to the front so that the IV line is visible at its insertion point, the catheter attached to her skin with transparent medical tape, while the man holds an IV pole the same way ambulatory patients do in a hospital. While these elements undeniably signify illness and medicine, both individuals are dressed not in medical gowns but in street clothes. He is wearing a collared button-up shirt, baggy jeans, and brown boots and has close-cropped hair and a short beard, whereas she is wearing a stylish blue tank top, distressed skinny jeans, and heeled boots, and her hair dyed in a "grown-in" style of dark roots and blonde ends that was the peak of fashion in 2018. These individuals radiate balance in a twenty-first-century idiom: they are confident and self-assured, reasonably wealthy, physically fit, and happy.

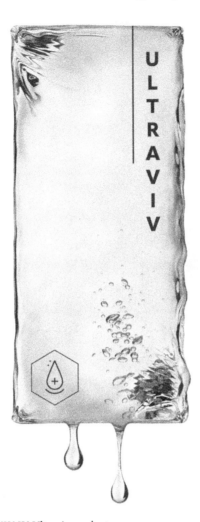

Figure 7. Detail of REVIV IV Ultraviv product page

Other images on REVIV's archived website repeat the pattern. One features the same woman, still smiling and making a peace sign and wearing a similar outfit, though this time she is receiving an injection in her shoulder from another young woman, a nurse or doctor of South Asian descent wearing light blue latex gloves and dark blue scrubs with an embossed REVIV logo. Both are smiling directly into the camera. In another image, the man, who has also undergone a change of clothes, is receiving his own shot, though this time both he and the nurse are looking off into the distance. In all these images, the couple's looks and Instagram-ready poses minimize the potential ick factor of intravenous

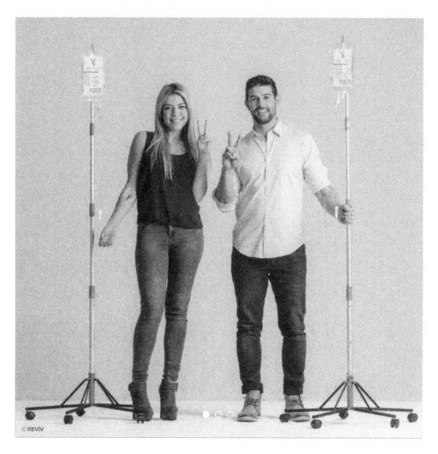

Figure 8. "Balanced" REVIV IV customers

therapy by packaging such treatments as a new, sleek, and utterly mainstream way of life.

EZ Lifestyle, maker of the energy supplement Fuel EZ, discussed above, similarly invokes both forms of pleasure associated with wellness seeking. Promoting its hangover remedy Over EZ, for example, EZ Lifestyle links its product directly to the vitalizing pleasure of indulgence: "Over EZ stops you from feeling sick after a night of drinking—so you can make the most of your day. No more waking up with headaches, cold sweats, and nausea. Our battle-tested formula is designed to target, and neutralize hangover-causing toxins left over from drinking." The product's sole purpose is to restore the body to a state of prior health by alleviating hangover symptoms: if you take it with your first drink, website visitors are told, "you won't need to cancel your next-day plans."[65] However, much like the images on REVIV's website, the images accompanying the text on the Over EZ product page tell a story not of restoration but of enhancement (fig. 9). Four side-by-side photos each depict an idealized life above text that implicitly claims that using Over EZ will transform people into optimal versions of themselves. The first photo on the left, for instance, features three thin, smiling white women in an exercise class above text that reads, "Get in your morning workout," and the second photo from the right pictures a young African American man putting headphones on while walking in an urban environment in bright morning light above the caption "Go to work refreshed." The other two images feature equally happy people who, thanks to Over EZ, can do all they want to do without being sidetracked by a hangover. The Over EZ product page suggests that those who use it can have a big night of drinking and still engage in positive, wellness-promoting behaviors the next day, even early in the morning.

But how often do any of us go to work feeling refreshed—even *without* going on a bender the night before? And how often, on average, do we get in our morning workouts? Certainly the more disciplined among us do, but when we add to the mix family and caregiving responsibilities, long commutes, and even longer to-do lists, the post-bender morning exercise class may become a little more difficult to manage. I would argue that the claim that underlies Over EZ's product page is subtler than it seems at first because while the page may be selling a product, it is also selling absolution of the sins of overindulgence. There are two elements of pleasure at work here, then: first, the pleasure of feeling good by having a good time; and second, the pleasure of absolving yourself of that indulgence through harm-reducing measures to minimize the duration and intensity of the aftermath.

Popular culture is full of references to just this sort of strategy for surviving stress and exhaustion. An episode from season 2 of *Grey's Anatomy*, for instance, features the title character, surgeon Meredith Grey, stress-drinking near the hospital when she is called back to respond to a multicasualty accident. Unable to

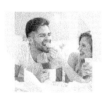

Figure 9. Detail of OverEZ hangover pill webpage. *Left to right*: "Get in your morning workout," "Enjoy your day with your family," "Go to work refreshed," "Enjoy your vacation."

practice until her blood alcohol level returns to normal, she hooks herself up to a "banana bag," an IV containing a vitamin and electrolyte solution, as ordered by her supervisor.[66] Similarly, the hedge-fund drama *Billions* included a storyline in which a character known to be a heavy drinker describes to a colleague his trick of using IVs to recover from a night of partying before work the next day. That colleague, a trained nurse, subsequently brings IV drips to the office to sell to coworkers who want to unwind from their stressful jobs at night and still get back to work in the morning.[67] Other popular shows such as *Scrubs*, *House MD*, and *How I Met Your Mother* have featured similar storylines, showing just how prevalent this narrative of "sin" and absolution has become. Collectively, stories like these figure wellness as a zero-sum game: as long as you offset your indulgence with a ritual of detoxification and rehydration, you are advancing on the path to wellness.

Further, progressing along the path to wellness is a vital component of contemporary health citizenship, and this fact alone constitutes a vitalizing form of pleasure that we cannot discount. As the interviewee Jasmine explained, it feels good to do something you perceive as good for yourself, even if it has no physiological effect.[68] The positive feelings associated with taking natural health products can kindle the pleasure of being a good health citizen—of *being* good. These positive feelings can also produce the pleasure of *feeling* good, physically. Jasmine illustrates this positive feedback loop when she describes how taking natural health products enhances her sense of agency and self-care: "I think they give me a sense . . . of control, [something] I'm proactively doing. Whether it actually makes a difference, I don't know, if it's placebo or not, or if it puts me at ease that I'm doing something."[69] Ultimately, taking steps to improve her wellness makes Jasmine feel well. Although wellness debunkers are right to critique those who produce and sell natural health products for capitalizing on collective exhaustion, the products themselves may serve as lifelines for people who feel they are out of options, out of energy, and out of health. When someone has no choice but to get up for work in the morning and do it all over again even when they are completely spent, a quick fix that may or may not work probably seems a better option than doing nothing at all.

The marketing of products such as REVIV's IV treatments and EZ Lifestyle's supplements makes wellness seem fun and fashionable, as well as empowering. But underlying this marketing is the disturbing fact that we have become so collectively disempowered that we want or need these products to patch ourselves up so we can head back out into the ring and battle another day. Like advertising for Rescue Remedy, the websites for REVIV and EZ Lifestyle construct wellness primarily as the ability to work. In this construction, the marketing of these products is in lockstep with pharmaceutical advertising: supplements are sold alongside migraine medications, antidepressants, and anxiolytics primarily as tools for maintaining and enhancing productivity rather than as methods of reducing suffering or improving human experience.[70] The ideal self in the materials examined in this chapter is thus the one who works out before going to the office, has the resources and leisure time to go on vacation, *and* spends their time smiling widely (and wildly) wherever they go. This ideal self in wellness culture is therefore the medicated self—or, more precisely in this case, the supplemented self.

The connections between supplement marketing and pharmaceutical advertising bring us back to Berlant. The products discussed in this chapter are sold under a fun, glossy sheen of marketing, but when we really think about the products themselves—what they are, what they purport to do, and what drives the people who use them—the reality is distressing. We are so exhausted, and face so many demands, that we are collectively compelled to maintain our active participation in lives that hurt us rather than withdrawing for rest and repair. This process is circular because, as Ahmed points out, when we are exhausted, we are too tired to fix what makes us tired; all we can do is whatever it takes to just keep going.[71] To break this cycle, what we need to fix most is our mistaken belief that we are machines, capable of running 24/7. We are not. We are biological creatures who need rest and who need care.

We Are Creatures That Need to Be Nourished

In this contemporary moment, the search for wellness is caught up at least partly in hashtag-driven consumerist culture, but under the gloss of celebrity endorsements, coaches, and clinics and the arsenal of products we can buy to put on or in our bodies lies the fact that people are searching for something they desperately need. What they seek is another way of living, a way to feel better, a way to rest and recover. This could come about in many ways, including large-scale social-systemic change, but as ever, solutions found in the market seem the most manageable, the most accessible, and the most realistic. For example, someone under mounting pressure to perform at work or experiencing the fatigue of managing multiple responsibilities seems likely to prefer the idea of buying a supplement or two over remaking their life and fighting the very system that threatens to break them. The quest for wellness is no mere whimsy. Even if wellness does not do what its proponents want or need it to do, it does offer a way to imagine another way of living. And yet, advocates and skeptics of wellness both miss the important point that wellness neither starts nor ends with individuals. We need to grapple with this fact if we want to understand what wellness is and how it affects us.

In *Biocultural Creatures: Toward a New Theory of the Human*, feminist political scientist Samantha Frost points out that of all the ways the human body has been conceptualized—whether culturally, socially, as a locus of power and subjectivity, or as an abstract idea or theory—we have not fully reckoned with "our biological, organismic, living animality" as "living bodies persisting with and because of biological functions and processes." Although we primarily consider human beings as self-mastering agents, Frost reminds us that we are all connected to and dependent on one another, our social frameworks, and our lived environments. Like all living creatures, we live (or not) and thrive (or not) in and because of the habitats within which we are embedded. And so, Frost argues, to say "You are a living body (you are alive)" is therefore to say that you are a living creature who needs to be nourished, who grows, lives, and dies in the very habitat that enables your existence.[72] This defining element of our existence is easy to forget in the speed and complexity of everyday life.

For the study of wellness, Frost brings into sharp relief the reality that many people who seek natural health products in the name of wellness are exhausted bodies trying to stay alive within physical, psychic, medical, and economic structures that threaten their existence. It is in this way that wellness can constitute not merely an act of resilience but an act of resistance: wellness offers a way to carve out space for self-care, problematic though that idea is, so that we, as biological creatures, can keep on living. In some respects, wellness therefore resembles what French literature scholar Richard Klein describes as an Epicurean model of well-being, which asks us not to avoid temptations such as alcohol, sweets, carbs, and cigarettes but to seek out those things that bring us pleasure, which in turn can bring about a different sort of health. Adopting the rhetorical strategy of what he calls "contrarian hyperbole," Klein urges us to recognize the value of behaviors framed as unhealthy so we can critique the moralization at the heart of contemporary approaches to health.[73] The vector of wellness analyzed in this chapter, in which wellness serves as a survival strategy, can usefully be seen as Epicurean because it can be a way of engaging in bad behaviors (overwork, stress, poor sleep, late nights of drinking) and maintaining your wellness too. Because many of those so-called bad behaviors arise not from poor self-control but from systemic factors such as increasingly demanding jobs, increasingly unaffordable housing, and increasing expectations for family and personal care, the path to wellness may indeed result in a zero-sum game of survival.

So how can we get out of this game? The performance artist, activist, and theologian Tricia Hersey offers one potential solution through her organization The Nap Ministry, which operates under the tagline "REST IS RESISTANCE." According to its website, The Nap Ministry draws on Black liberation theology, Afrofuturism, and related feminist and African American initiatives in performance art, site-specific installations, and community projects to create "sacred and safe spaces for the community to rest together" as a matter of racial and social justice.[74] These projects include collective napping sessions that invite viewers into welcoming public spaces to rest together, to take up space in celebration of the restorative power of sleep in a culture that valorizes overwork. The Nap Ministry's social media accounts feature directives from the "Nap Bishop" to "LAY YO ASS DOWN," reminding people that "you are not a machine. Stop grinding."[75] Hersey explained her mission to reclaim sleep as active, not passive, in her appearance on the *Social Distance* podcast from the American magazine *The Atlantic*: "When you're sleeping, you are actually doing something. You're honoring your body. You're giving your brain a moment to download new information. You're disrupting toxic systems by reclaiming rest."[76] Hersey's project provokes public reconsideration of how we might find ways to truly flourish, to speak back to systems that fail to recognize that we, as biological creatures, need to be nourished.

As a cultural signifier, wellness as it currently manifests in Western culture ultimately does not live up to its promise of improving lives increasingly lived with ever-rising stakes and scarcer resources. Part of the problem, as Sara Ahmed illustrates in her essay "Selfcare as Warfare," is that this promise is more readily realized for some (specifically, those who are white, wealthy, straight, cisgender, abled) than for others.[77] Looking back at the Rescue Remedy commercials I discussed earlier in this chapter, for instance, the women are all in stressful situations, sure, but each situation signifies a certain degree of wealth and privilege that suggests that even if they were not "rescued" by the product, they would eventually be just fine. As far as we can tell, none are facing problems such as mass incarceration, immigration denial, housing and food insecurity, substance dependence, abuse, or other problems that disproportionately affect those with less privilege. As writer Adebe Derango-Adem argues in the Canadian magazine *Flare*, "What happens when the very stresses of life make self-care solutions inaccessible? What if we can't afford pedicures or ultimately are too busy to #mealprep or #eatclean?"[78] Similarly, *Vice* staff writer Shayla Love writes, "If we lived in a world in which we were being properly taken care of, would self-care have the same appeal? Is self-care a symbol of a generation that wants to take care of itself, or does it reveal how our society has failed to take care of us?"[79] While wellness constitutes a survival strategy, this strategy will never be more than a stopgap so long as we do not recognize and reckon with what people are trying to survive.

There is an important contradiction built into the idea of wellness as a survival strategy, then. On the one hand, it serves as a source of vitalizing pleasure in the ways I have described in the foregoing pages. We can only absorb the shock and the stress of everyday life for so long before we hunt for ways of reducing that shock and stress, even just a little. But on the other hand, wellness may at the same time constitute a form of what Berlant calls "cruel optimism" because our efforts to become well may impede our ability to truly *be* well. As an autopoietic, self-generating rhetoric, wellness has no ceiling: it is discursively constituted as always just out of reach, a place where we may be going but never where we are. As Cederström and Spicer put so pointedly, "Where does our preoccupation with our own wellness leave the rest of the population, who have an acute shortage of organic smoothies, diet apps and yoga instructors? Withdrawing into yourself and treating the signals of your body as a good-enough ersatz for universal truth has become an increasingly appealing alternative to thinking soberly about the world."[80] The wildly individualist, neoliberal flavor of contemporary wellness culture, centered on productivity and self-actualization, occludes what is really at stake and what we can do about it.

As critiques of resilience rhetoric have shown, simplistic models of resilience as the individual capacity to bounce back from or manage the stresses of hardship obscure the collective, systemic nature of problems we face, problems that can only be addressed by collective, systemic solutions.[81] Thus, wellness-oriented products such as supplements may indeed enhance our health and wellness, but likely only by propping us up just enough that we can keep going. Wellness may not constitute giving up or giving in but simply getting on, getting through the day. Ultimately, when we view wellness as a survival strategy, products such as Rescue Remedy, Dream EZ, Over EZ, and REVIV IVs function as a Band-Aid applied to a gaping wound, a topical antibiotic given for a pervasive infection. Our ability to live, get by, and maybe even prosper in everyday life is dangerously compromised, and workplace wellness programs, mindfulness, meditation, puppy rooms, and resilience training are not going to fix it. It is like trying to fix a cracked foundation with a bucket of putty and hoping for the best.

CHAPTER FIVE

Wellness as Optimization

This chapter picks up where chapter 4 leaves off: if exhaustion is one of the core vectors of wellness, optimization is its inverse, more ambitious twin, focused less on keeping up than on getting ahead. In what follows, I consider wellness as a form of multidimensional self-actualization, an aspirational state driven by the logic of enhancement toward becoming "better than well."[1] Focusing on the use of supplements to enhance functioning and performance beyond one's usual capacity, I examine how wellness seekers are groomed not only as consumers taking charge of their health but as patients dependent on an expanding array of supplements. Consider, for example, Suzanne Somers, the former star of *Three's Company*, whose ThighMaster exercise device launched her second career as a celebrity wellness guru in the 1990s, well before Gwyneth Paltrow or Dr. Oz launched their own wellness empires. Today, Somers runs a sprawling lifestyle and health enterprise that includes her own line of supplements, called RestoreLife, along with weight loss products, cleaning supplies, skincare, makeup, hair products, jewelry, and clothing, and she has written more than a dozen books about health and wellness on topics ranging from menopause and aging to toxins to natural cures for cancer.

In January 2009, Somers appeared on the *Oprah Winfrey Show* to discuss bioidentical hormone replacement therapy (BHRT) alongside celebrity doctor Christiane Northrup, an obstetrician-gynecologist. BHRT is widely promoted in wellness culture as a natural, safe alternative to allegedly harmful pharmaceutical hormone replacement therapy (HRT). Proponents of BHRT such as Somers and Northrup argue that BHRT is more "natural" because it is derived from plant-based sources such as soy and wild yams, rather than from the urine of pregnant mares (the primary source of HRT), and therefore its molecular structure is more compatible with women's bodies.[2] Both Somers and Northrup urge women to track their hormone levels through urine and blood tests so that their BHRT levels can be adjusted precisely for their own bodies. Several years earlier, in 2005, Somers published *The Sexy Years: Discover the Hormone Connection; The Secret to Fabulous Sex, Great Health, and Vitality, for Women and Men*, where she asserted that BHRT is precision medicine at its best: "Instead of a doctor prescribing for me a synthetic 'one pill fits all' type of regimen, my hormones are tracked through blood tests to see exactly where my levels are; and because of this, an endocrinologist can prescribe combinations of the real bioidentical hormones to replace what has been lost."[3] Importantly, bioidenticals are largely unregulated and in some cases molecularly identical to conventional prescription hormones. The Mayo Clinic's website for patients cautions potential users that BHRT has not been shown to be safer or more effective and that urine tests cannot appropriately measure blood hormone levels for hormone replacement.[4] In Somers's view, however, optimizing when and how she uses hormones and other natural health products allows her to enhance her experience of menopause and aging.

In an *Oprah* segment filmed at her home, Somers walked viewers through her daily wellness routine. Every morning, she rubs what she describes as a natural estrogen cream into one arm, and for half the month, she rubs a progesterone cream into the other. She then injects estrogen compounds vaginally with a syringe (she did this off-camera) and finishes up by taking some forty dietary supplements. In the evening, she takes another twenty supplements to cap off a routine that she says "tricks" her body into thinking she is a woman of 30 rather than her then 62 years.[5] In addition to all the pills and creams, Somers also regularly injects human growth hormone and undergoes blood and urine tests to monitor her hormone levels. At the end of the *Oprah* segment, Somers sat in her kitchen with her sixty daily supplement capsules lined up neatly in front of her, the line stretching almost the length of her kitchen table, and explained directly to the camera: "You don't have to take all this. Although the deeper you get into [this regimen], the more you're apt to want to keep adding to it."[6] For Somers, the project of optimizing her body in the face of age is like pulling a loose thread on an old sweater: once you start tugging, it has the potential to just keep going.

Although the cultural moment of bioidentical hormone replacement therapy peaked early in the first years of this century, it is still very much alive twenty years later, animated by the same principles of optimization, surveillance, and intervention that drive public interest in wellness more broadly. To set the scene for this chapter on wellness as a form of optimization, here is Somers's advice to readers in her 2006 book *Ageless: The Naked Truth about Bioidentical Hormones*:

Being ageless takes a little work. There is no free lunch, but the rewards of this outweigh all the money in the world. . . . I embrace bioidentical hormone replacement and antiaging medicine. I gladly take my supplements, vitamins, herbs, hormones, human growth hormone injections, and vitamin B injections, and follow a healthy lifestyle and diet. I embrace my exercise and yoga programs. . . . I have never felt better or been happier in my life. I love my age. I don't dread my next birthday, because I feel great on the outside and inside. Good health brings joy, balanced hormones brings joy, a well-running body brings joy, and emotional health brings joy.[7]

What is so striking in this passage, and indeed in all of Somers's books and others like them, is that taking charge of one's health involves mounting an intense, defensive response to ordinary bodily states, which in this case include menopause and aging. For Somers, the empowerment she experiences from self-optimization means running through a vigilant (and expensive) daily regimen of supplementation and surveillance that involves ingesting more than four hundred capsules a week while routinely sending blood and urine samples for laboratory analysis. The logic of enhancement comes to mirror the logic of restoration.

The example of bioidentical hormone supplementation is useful for framing my discussion of wellness as a form of optimization because it illustrates how public discourse about wellness "direct[s] the attention" in ways that can make other perspectives harder to see.[8] For example, Somers, Northrup, and other advocates of so-called natural menopause frame the practice of using bioidentical hormones alongside a wide range of supplements and regular laboratory testing as a way to free women of harmful commercial interference in their wellness, even while urging expensive and labor-intensive regimens that may be ineffective or even potentially more dangerous. Wellness routines such as Somers's may, for example, result in polyherbacy, a situation in which individuals take potentially harmful combinations of pharmaceuticals and supplements, perhaps in the belief that if some wellness is good, more is even better.[9] In the vector of optimization, the ceiling of wellness does not just recede out of grasp; there is effectively no ceiling at all.

I begin this chapter by situating wellness within overlapping cultural frameworks oriented to optimization that transform self-improvement into a moral and social obligation. I then examine the two key elements of wellness optimization: surveillance and intervention. I first discuss wellness surveillance through self-tracking and testing as a means of generating data to support strategic and precise enhancement strategies. I then examine wellness intervention through self-hacking, which involves the targeted use of supplements to optimize how the body works. I close the chapter by showing that although the logic of enhancement propels rhetorics of optimization within the realm of wellness, those rhetorics necessarily feed back into the logic of restoration, where optimization may be as much a means of gaining or maintaining an edge in a cut-throat capitalist economy as it is a way of taking charge of our health. Optimizing wellness may, in the end, not help us move forward as much as keep us right where we are.

Optimizing the Body

Public interest in wellness and natural health has flourished within the wider culture of optimization that increasingly dominates Western capitalist life. To *optimize* is to make something as good as possible, to make it the best or most effective it can be, to make it optimal. Contemporary culture is saturated with quests for optimization, from reality shows about fitness, weight loss, surgical transformation, home decluttering, business deals, and baking competitions to celebrity gurus dispensing advice about health, wealth, technology, or life, whether on TV, online, or in books, magazines, videos, or even live tours and expos. As individuals, we can enhance ourselves nutritionally, pharmacologically, cosmetically, surgically, and spiritually. We can surround ourselves with "smart" machines—smart phones, cars, thermostats, baby monitors, coffee makers, and home assistants. And we can track, streamline, and improve our performance in nearly every aspect of our lives, including exercise, relationships, jobs, finances, hobbies, and our bodies, minds, and perhaps even souls. Western culture's overwhelming preoccupation with optimization has been broadly memorialized in popular culture, from Holly Theisen-Jones's parody essay in *McSweeny's*, "My Fully Optimized Life Allows Me Ample Time to Optimize Yours," to well-known songs such as Radiohead's "Fitter Happier" and Daft Punk's "Harder, Better, Faster, Stronger." Wellness discourse is both a part and a product of this more general and radically consumer-oriented culture of self-improvement.

Our everyday lives are saturated with messaging that frames optimization as a moral and civic duty, framed as if we *of course* want to improve everything we do, in every part of our lives. When I visited the website of the Canadian national newspaper the *Globe and Mail* one day back in 2012, these were the top stories: "How to build a healthier, smarter student"; "How to pick a healthy snack"; "How to make the perfect pancake"; "4 Tips to Get your BBQ Ready for the Season."[10] These headlines are significant only because they are so mundane: a decade later, you can still find virtually the same headlines all over the web, in new iterations of the same sorts of stories. Googling the last headline alone yielded 72 million results, the narratives so alike they could have been written by a bot. These stories' particulars do not matter; they could be about almost any topic at all, from making pancakes and barbecuing to cardio workouts, investment strategies, skincare routines, or happiness. What matters is the general message underlying stories such as these, which, by the mere fact of their existence, constitutes a kind of command: improve yourself (or else).

The obligation to self-improve is not new, and neither is scholarly criticism of that obligation, so I will not repeat that criticism in detail here.[11] However, some basic outlines are worth sketching as they illuminate wellness as a form of optimization. As I illustrated in the previous chapter, the human body has been transformed under global capitalism into an instrument of production that must be managed and maintained through practices of surveillance and intervention, such as workplace wellness programs, to ensure the continued functioning of the body-machine. An ill worker or a tired worker is not a productive worker. For people who are exhausted or stressed by their jobs, or who are facing precarity in a belt-tightening economy, products such as Fuel EZ, Natrol, and Rescue Remedy offer the boost, rest, and respite they need. However, under capitalism, keeping up is only one part of the equation because there is always room for greater productivity and efficiency. Capital therefore requires not only the ability to manage people as resources (what Foucault calls *biopower*) but also the ability to grow those resources by developing "methods of power capable of optimizing forces, aptitudes, and life in general."[12] In other words, managing human bodies as resources means not only restoring those bodies sufficiently so they can keep working, as I discussed in the previous chapter, but also enhancing them to optimize their ability to produce. Within this growth-oriented framework, people become infinitely improvable.

This formulation of the human body as an instrument of labor to be optimized deeply informs how we presently understand our health, wellness, and lives. As anthropologist Emily Martin argues in *Flexible Bodies* and elsewhere, the United States (and, I would add, comparable nations) experienced a significant transformation in perceptions and practices of the body toward the end of the twentieth century, which can be keyed to a similar transformation in prevalent economic models that began in the 1970s. This period was marked by a shift from a model of Fordist mass production to late capitalism, or what geographer David Harvey termed *flexible accumulation*. As Martin explains, the hallmarks of flexible accumulation include "technological innovation, specificity, and rapid, flexible change."[13] Martin's examination of how people understand and describe the human body in settings such as university research labs, urban neighbor-hoods, community organizations, and healthcare facilities revealed shifts in im-agery and language from terms of mass production, where bodies are perceived as "organized around principles of centralized control and factory-based produc-tion," to the view that bodies are "flexible," able to adapt seamlessly and effi-ciently to highly specific, ever-shifting contexts.[14] Flexible bodies must innovate constantly to deal nimbly with any number of external threats through careful, needs-based regulation and production, paralleling the just-in-time models of production and distribution characteristic of late capitalism.

We can usefully extend Martin's analysis of the flexible body to wellness cul-ture, as consumers similarly seek the latest fat-busting, mood-boosting, energy-giving, cancer-fighting products available in the health marketplace. In Brigid Delaney's memoir *Wellmania*, for example, the author describes undertaking a 101-day cleanse to address her long-standing exhaustion. The cleanse began with fourteen days of no food at all, only water, black tea, and a tincture of traditional Chinese medical herbs taken three times per day, and then graduated to an alternating-day cycle of minute quantities of cucumber, chicken, or egg. Delaney describes the first week and a half as pure agony: she was haunted by headaches, low mood, and chest pain. But on the eleventh day, she awakened transformed into a highly efficient machine: "My concentration and energy levels are through the roof! I don't think I've ever felt so sharp. My brain is a Rolls Royce, purring and preening, just out of the factory, in mint condition." As her body shifts from burn-ing carbs to fat stores—a state of ketosis, the founding principle of the low-carb, high-fat Keto diet—she exclaims, incredulously, "I have gone from being barely able to lift a teaspoon to super-productive. I throw myself into job hunting. . . . I write stories, I answer emails." Ultimately, Delaney credits her cleanse with opti-mizing her brain, leaving it feeling as if it "has been thoroughly rinsed, tuned and given extra component parts."[15] Despite Delaney's own stated misgivings about wellness culture, the narrative of her cleanse is fairly standard in wellness dis-course: a given practice such as a cleanse, elimination or superfood diet, medita-tion, or supplementation is credited with supercharging the body, the mind, and the self.

Within moralizing frameworks that task individuals with responsibility for self-improvement, the quest to become better than well is not necessarily a self-indulgent or narcissistic project.[16] For those such as Delaney, optimizing their bodies, minds, and energy for peak performance may feel critical for career growth or keeping pace with the culture at large. In this respect, whether someone uses supplements to manage exhaustion or to maximize energy and performance, they are motivated by the same desire to cope with the demands of every-day life. Self-improvement is also tied to individualistic notions of good citizen-ship, which in turn casts the failure to optimize as a personal failure. As sociologist Deborah Lupton observes, "Individuals can be regarded as fulfilling their obli-gations as citizens if they devote attention to optimising their own lives. . . . In the discourses that champion the ideal of the rational neoliberal citizen, social structural factors that influence people's living conditions and life chances—such as social class, gender, geographical location, race and ethnicity—are dis-counted in favour of the notion that people are self-made."[17] By obscuring the social-structural factors that determine collective health and well-being, self-optimization thus seems to be reducible to a clear set of steps that any individ-ual with the right knowledge and the right tools can simply follow. In nearly every aspect of our lives—public discourse and policy, advertising, employment prac-tices, and other frameworks that govern how we live—we are exhorted to become the best version of ourselves we can be by systematically observing and enhanc-ing our performance.

Over the remainder of this chapter, I pull apart and explain how the two over-lapping steps of wellness optimization fuel wellness culture both separately and together. In the realm of optimization, practices of wellness surveillance crystal-lize here as *tracking*, which includes measuring, recording, and monitoring wellness through various, often technological means. Practices of wellness inter-vention likewise manifest as *hacking*, which is the strategic and highly specific use of natural health and related products and services to enhance wellness. I draw both terms, *tracking* and *hacking*, from Silicon Valley startup culture, which has given rise to a massively profitable self-optimization industry. As communi-cation and digital culture scholar Joseph Reagle explains in *Hacking Life: System-atized Living and Its Discontents*, a *hack* is "a novel solution or fix" aimed at optimizing anything from how a computer runs to the length and quality of your sleep to how much time you spend working in a day.[18] For hackers, Reagle notes, "most everything is conceived as a system: it is modular, composed of parts, which can be decomposed and recomposed; it is governed by algorithmic rules, which can be understood, optimized, and subverted."[19] If we follow Reagle, the way to make a perfect pancake and the best way to get your barbecue ready for summer are both hacks: once you figure out the right formula, you simply need to apply it.

Wellness is harder to optimize than a pancake or a barbecue, however, because it is a multidimensional concept, an aggregate of different domains that resist clear categorization and tug continuously against one another. It is also difficult to know what the markers of wellness are or to determine when wellness has been maximized. Consider the rhetorical situation of wellness itself: it exhorts individuals without specific illness symptoms to monitor bodily states such as digestion, mobility, energy, cognition, and mood and then to intervene in states they perceive as suboptimal by using dietary supplements and other regimens.[20] However, without clear symptoms that resolve when an intervention has been successful, the wellness seeker lacks concrete ways to mark their progress or to know when they have reached their goal. By reducing wellness to a system, people can more easily track where they currently are and then identify solutions, or hacks, for optimizing their performance.

Tracking Wellness

Many methods of assessing wellness have emerged over recent years. One of the most common is the genre of the wellness "quiz," available widely on the web and in high-circulation magazines and newspapers. Many such quizzes can be found in the magazine *Dr. Oz: The Good Life*, which ran monthly from 2014 to 2017 and subsequently as annual themed issues under the same banner. One such quiz, in the 2020 theme issue of Oz's magazine, includes an eight-item assessment tool that allows readers to test their memory, balancing ability, aerobic fitness, and core strength and to evaluate their weight, relationships, fruit and vegetable intake, and sugar dependence.[21] Users assign themselves scores for their performance in each domain, which together form a metric that determines how well they are. Some wellness seekers may be satisfied with such a general measure of wellness, but for those who crave more precision regarding how to enhance their individual wellness, standing by is an array of tracking tools, such as apps, wearable devices, and laboratory tests.

In this section, I examine how individuals track their wellness through at-home hormone and gut health tests, which analyze urine and stool samples to recommend specific supplement regimens for optimizing users' health. I focus on a virtual nutrition coaching practice and supplement dispensary, Composed Nutrition, which is run by Chicago-area nutritionist Krista King, and a microbiome testing company, Viome, whose website invites prospective customers to "measure your health right now and get precise food and supplement recommendations to help you live a healthy lifestyle."[22] Wellness testing services such as these constitute a form of what Judy Segal calls "recreational diagnostics," a category that includes direct-to-consumer laboratory and imaging services that cater to people who want to learn as much as possible about their health.[23] Users of these services can buy tests and scans for themselves or gift them to others with no medical referral required, secure in the belief that if something harmful lurks invisibly inside the body, the tests will find it.

At-home wellness tests such as Composed Nutrition and Viome promise to reveal and treat users' unseen deficiencies, dysfunctions, sensitivities, and inefficiencies, while defining their services in legal terms as information and entertainment, not medical diagnosis or treatment.[24] For both tests, customers collect their own urine or stool samples at home and then send them for laboratory analysis. When the analysis is complete, users receive detailed reports of their results along with comprehensive recommendations based on those results. These sorts of testing services constitute the ultimate form of wellness tracking because their painstakingly detailed data are derived directly from users' bodies and their recommendations are based on those data, tailored for each user to improve their wellness. Wellness tracking emerges out of digital life-optimization and laboratory diagnostics, which together establish a ready, wide consumer base for at-home wellness testing services.

Digital Life Optimization

Just as my Nest thermostat can learn my home heating preferences and make my HVAC system run more efficiently, a FitBit's biosensors can track and help me improve my daily activity levels, heart rate, and sleep duration and quality. I can download iPhone apps to track my investment portfolio, to-do list, fertility, and mood and then use the tracked data to illuminate patterns that help maximize my efforts to improve in each of those areas. I can use apps such as Strava to map my cycling and running routes, calculate and improve my speed, and share my data with others. If I want to lose weight, I can record my current weight, body shape, "vitality," hormonal cycle, and more with the "Female Transformation Tracker" spreadsheet from the company Metabolic Renewal, which according to its website is "the first doctor-designed lifestyle program that optimizes your female metabolism by turning your natural hormonal rhythms into a fat-burning, body-sculpting, health-rejuvenating advantage."[25] The human body is figured in this description as a high-performance machine that with fine-tuning can be supercharged into a state of ultra-efficiency along the lines of how the formerly intimidating android played by Arnold Schwarzenegger in the *Terminator* movie franchise is outpaced by the nimble new shape-shifting T-1000 model first played by Robert Patrick in *Terminator 2*.

Smart devices and tracking apps give users a sense of empowerment by promising them special knowledge about their bodies that they can use to improve their health and well-being. These apps and devices emerged out of the Quantified

Self movement pioneered by Silicon Valley tech enthusiasts under the motto "Self-knowledge through numbers."[26] Self-tracking makes visible minute, often invisible details about our lives, giving us opportunities to intervene with an eye toward greater efficiency and impact. For example, Gary Wolf, one of the movement's cofounders and a *Wired* magazine writer, reported his daily numbers in the lede of his 2009 article introducing quantified living:

> I got up at 6:20 this morning, after going to bed at 12:40 am. I woke up twice during the night. My heart rate was 61 beats per minute, and my blood pressure, averaged over three measurements, was 127/74. My mood was a 4 on a scale of 5. My exercise time in the last 24 hours was 0 minutes, and my maximum heart rate during exercise was not calculated. I consumed 400 milligrams of caffeine and 0 ounces of alcohol. And in case you were wondering, my narcissism score is 0.31.[27]

This is a lot of information. Some of those numbers were gleaned through sensors such as accelerometers, GPS locators, gyroscopes, and optical monitors, while others have been calculated using data entered through in-app questionnaires and rating scales. These numbers provide a sense of certainty and control, a way to see global patterns in the vast webs of information we can produce through the minutiae of our everyday lives. As Kevin Kelly, Gary Wolf's former *Wired* coworker and cofounder of the Quantified Self, quipped in a 2007 blog post, "Unless something can be measured, it cannot be improved."[28] Self-tracking is rhetorically powerful because the special knowledge it confers appears to unlock our ability to become our best selves. That is, if I know what time I fell asleep or how many times I woke up, I have a benchmark for measuring my sleep improvement. If my mood was a 4 out of 5 today, I can aim for a higher score tomorrow. If I want to sharpen my mind by cutting out alcohol, I can count the number of consecutive days when I have none.

There are two other key reasons why tracking apps and devices are so compelling from the perspective of wellness as a form of optimization. First, these apps and devices are vitally personal. They hold vast reams of individualized data along with private biographical information such as a user's birthdate, weight, height, and gender. These apps live in our phones next to other apps that contain personal photos, text messages, social media accounts, and banking information. When certain settings are enabled, these apps know what we are doing, when, and where; they can even learn from our previous patterns to anticipate our next steps. (I was startled when I got in my car one Saturday morning, for example, to discover that my iPhone's Maps app had learned that I coach skating on weekends when, unbidden, it suggested a route to the arena.) We share intimate details of our lives with mood logs, period and fertility trackers, and symptom diaries, and then these apps, in turn, synthesize those details as datapoints in elaborate charts and statistics to make sense of our lives as data. Some of these apps even greet us by name when we open them. Tracking apps and devices seem sometimes to know us better than we know ourselves.

The second reason why tracking is so compelling for wellness consumers is that it shifts expertise from experts to consumers, allowing individuals more agency in managing their lives. For health in particular, tracking can provide information to individuals living with chronic conditions or conditions that are difficult to diagnose or treat, which can help those individuals measure their progress, uncover symptom triggers, and aid in caregiver conversations and diagnosis.[29] The numbers produced by these apps and devices transform users' idiosyncratic experiences into data assemblages that seem more objective than a narrative account of symptoms or illness ever could be.[30] Despite the potential advantages of tracking, however, the very availability of such devices and apps has a broader effect on all of us, collectively, not just those who use them. As sociologist Deborah Lupton warns, self-tracking practices lend credence to "the notion that the ideal self is productive and efficient and makes use of time wisely and well."[31] Technological self-surveillance provides an avenue for fulfilling our duty to improve ourselves, through self-knowledge, to become fully optimized health citizens.

Laboratory Diagnostics

At-home wellness tests also emerge out of laboratory diagnostic practices employed both in mainstream medicine and in alternative health modalities such as naturopathy. In medicine, patient reports of subjective experience are typically augmented with objective data obtained in the clinic. Healthcare providers such as doctors and nurse practitioners examine patients' bodies by sight, sound, and feel, sometimes with assistance from instruments such as otoscopes and stethoscopes. When they need further insight into what is happening inside an opaque body, they order tests: imaging, analysis of biological samples such as fluid and tissue, and monitoring devices. The results of these clinical and laboratory tests help guide further investigation and care and point to diagnoses.

Such tests serve important authorizing functions because they provide ostensibly objective assessments of a person's health status.[32] In my own life, for example, I remember times when I have felt unwell and found myself hoping, somewhat perversely, that something would turn up in a blood test or scan as proof that there really was something wrong with me, validating my subjective lived experience with external proof. Diagnostic technologies transform us, whether for better (by confirming our experience, leading to effective treatment, or alleviating concern) or for worse (by confirming illness, confirming nothing, or turning us from persons into patients).

Much has been written on the sociology, culture, and rhetoric of diagnostic laboratory testing, but perhaps the most contentious issue is the diagnosis of conditions for which there are no specific lab tests.[33] Without laboratory evidence validating their experience, many people turn to complementary and alternative health for help with health conditions that are not easily diagnosed or treated in biomedicine. As I argued in my previous book, *Bounding Biomedicine*, one of the strongest rhetorical appeals of practices such as naturopathy, traditional Chinese medicine, and chiropractic is that they focus primarily on chronic, nonspecific conditions such as pain, digestive troubles, and fatigue. Clinical examinations in complementary and alternative medicine are typically much more intensive than those in conventional family practice, with longer appointment times, more in-depth discussion, sometimes more physical touch, and frequently the use of specific diagnostic practices not typically employed in medical clinics or hospitals. These diagnostics include readings of the pulse and tongue in traditional Chinese medicine, the use of various electronic scanners and sensors, and an array of laboratory tests. Alternative health diagnostics often claim the ability to identify conditions that slip under the radar of conventional Western doctors.

Consider naturopathy, for instance, which my interview participants referred to frequently. Most participants pointed to a diagnosis from a naturopath as a significant factor in their decision to use natural health products, and nearly half mentioned that they had seen a naturopath in the months immediately preceding their interviews. As clinical practitioners, naturopaths typically follow the same diagnostic arc as family doctors, moving patients from intake through diagnosis to treatment, although there are some significant differences in how the stages unfold. For example, according to the Canadian Association of Naturopathic Doctors, the average intake appointment with a new patient is 90 to 120 minutes, compared with the average appointment of 15 minutes in Canadian medicine.[34] The detailed intake process includes a comprehensive assessment of the patient's personal health history, family history, stressors, accidents and injuries, diet, and digestion, as well as a physical exam and laboratory tests.[35]

In Canada, where I live, naturopaths in several provinces can order a range of standard medical laboratory tests that family physicians order, but they also use a range of other lab tests through specialty testing services not used in mainstream medicine. For example, many naturopaths offer immunoglobulin G

(IgG) testing through companies such as Rocky Mountain Analytical, using a sample of a patient's blood to determine a person's sensitivity to more than two hundred different foods, according to the company's website.[36] These tests produce comprehensive reports that list specific foods a naturopathic patient ostensibly should avoid, as well as a range of remedies and supplements for the practitioner to prescribe. While the costs of physician visits and laboratory tests are fully covered by Canada's provincially funded health system in most cases, naturopath visits and naturopathic laboratory testing can cost hundreds of dollars out of pocket, depending on whether a client has employer-provided extended health benefits, which might cover some or all of the costs.

Food sensitivity tests such as those offered by naturopaths are closely related to at-home wellness laboratory tests because they promise individualized, targeted interventions keyed to each client's particular biochemical composition. As a form of tracking, laboratory and other highly specific diagnostic tests such as those from Rocky Mountain Analytical thus embrace the principles of "technological innovation, specificity, and rapid, flexible change," which are characteristic of rhetorics of optimization in wellness culture.[37] Indeed, the Canadian Association of Naturopathic Doctors explicitly differentiates naturopathy from conventional medical practice on its website because its aim is not merely to restore the human body but, rather, to optimize it: "Today's stressed, fast paced lifestyle . . . makes people seek alternative ways to realize optimum health. They want high level energy, immunity and overall health by incorporating a more natural approach and natural remedies."[38] Lab tests such as the IgG test provide naturopathic patients with the opportunity to track their overall health and wellness not only by finding underlying pathologies that require restoration but, more importantly, by uncovering opportunities for enhancement.

Of course, laboratory diagnostics are not limited to clinical settings. With a simple saliva sample, anyone can sign up for genetic testing through services such as 23andMe and AncestryDNA (an arm of the genealogy website Ancestry.com) and receive comprehensive, detailed results without leaving their homes. While AncestryDNA is limited to identifying a user's potential ethnic makeup, geographic origins, and living relatives, 23andMe's "Health + Ancestry Service" additionally tests for a comprehensive range of genetic markers that include genetic predispositions to conditions such as type 2 diabetes, breast cancer, celiac disease, dementia, Parkinson's disease, and vision loss and carrier status of inherited conditions such as cystic fibrosis, sickle-cell anemia, and Tay-Sachs disease. This same service also includes a range of "wellness reports" that inform consumers "how your genes play a role in your well-being and lifestyle choices," including alcohol flush reaction, caffeine consumption, quality of sleep, lactose tolerance, and genetic predispositions for weight and muscle composition.[39] The detailed reports that 23andMe's customers receive include the genetic result, their odds of developing certain conditions, mitigating risk factors, information about illness symptoms and treatment, and links for additional resources. One key difference between these at-home laboratory diagnostics and those administered in clinical settings, of course, is that users are on their own when it comes to interpreting and applying the results. People who want a greater sense of agency over their own health may feel empowered by do-it-yourself genetic testing, but such tests also leave wide open the door to increased anxiety, pathologization, and unnecessary surveillance and treatment.

At-Home Wellness Testing: Composed Nutrition

Digital life optimization and laboratory diagnostics converge in at-home wellness tests of biological samples such as saliva, urine, and stool. These testing services are powered by the same impulses that drive people to learn everything they can about how efficiently and well their homes, lives, and bodies are running. These services distill wellness optimization to its purest form because they center on surgically precise self-improvement: by tracking a user's hormone levels and gut microbiota, they pinpoint specific targets for intervention, recommend strategies for intervening with certain diets and supplements, and, for an additional fee, supply those supplements. At-home wellness testing animates life hacker Kevin Kelly's belief that "unless something can be measured, it cannot be improved," as people seek a clear picture of their current health and wellness through their own, personalized lab-measured results.[40] The numeric results they receive become benchmarks for tracking their progress as they work to restore and enhance their health. Consider, too, the rhetorical weight of undergoing lab-based wellness testing over, say, filling out a magazine quiz: the experience of taking and drying a urine sample to send to a laboratory and then receiving a detailed report with graphical data displays, charts that measure dozens of specific hormones in nanograms, micrograms, and milligrams, and comparisons of your results with those of others is a fundamentally different experience than seeing if you can hold a plank for more than a minute. For people who want to maximize their health and well-being, lab-based tests are likely far more compelling.

A wide range of US-based nutrition consulting businesses offer such tests, including Composed Nutrition, from registered dietitian and health coach Krista King. Like similar web-based services such as The Women's Dietitian and Lindsay O'Reilly Nutrition, Composed Nutrition combines the scientific cachet of laboratory testing with the aesthetics of Instagram, the promise of precision medicine, and the breathless enthusiasm of wellness culture.[41] Through the Composed Nutrition website, King offers a range of nutrition services that constellate around hormone and gut health tests and supplement sales. Drawing simultaneously on the logics of restoration and enhancement, her website's homepage greets visitors who "are ready to truly thrive and are over just not feeling well." King describes her own role as part scientist and part guru: "I equip you with the tools + support you need to feel vibrant, energized, and confident in your body. I use a functional + integrative approach, which means that together we are going to get to the root of any body imbalances as opposed to simply addressing symptoms. I look at the whole picture of you to see what is causing you to feel less than your best + use an individualized approach to create a path to reclaim your health."[42] From that main page, customers who want to get "the whole picture" of how their body is doing can sign up for various packages by clicking on links that correspond to what they want to do, including "have a normal period," "improve my digestion," and "boost my fertility." Composed Nutrition customers can choose to take an at-home hormone or gut health test, or both, along with one or more nutritional consulting sessions to follow up on the test result by learning how they can adapt their diet and use supplements to improve their test results.

Like similar websites, Composed Nutrition uses the DUTCH hormone test from Precision Analytical, which also sells kits directly to the public on its own website. DUTCH is an acronym for Dried Urine Test for Comprehensive Hormones; this is the test recommended by gynecologist Christiane Northrup for menopausal women seeking bioidentical hormone replacement therapy. To use the test, Composed Nutrition customers who have menstrual periods must first calculate where they are in their cycle and complete the test between days nineteen and twenty-two, whereas others can take their samples any time of the month. All users take five samples over a two-day period, each time soaking a test strip with urine and allowing it to dry for twenty-four hours before closing the collection device. Once all five samples have been completed, users send the samples back to the laboratory and receive their results in five to ten days.[43]

Although I did not try the test myself, Precision Analytical's website includes a sample report on its website. This report is fifteen pages long and contains a single-page visual summary of the test's sex hormone and adrenal hormone results (fig. 10), followed by detailed charts with numeric values of specific hormone levels, graphical representations of the user's hormones at different times of day, an extensive reference list (with ninety citations in the sample report), and

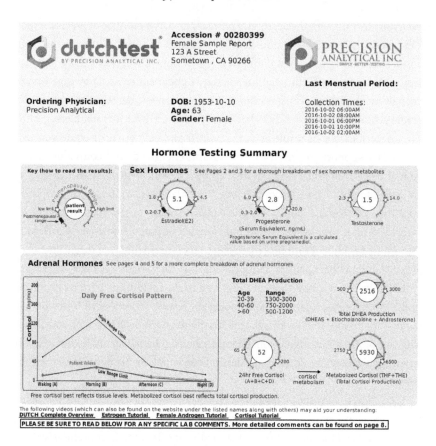

Figure 10. Sample urine test report from DUTCH Dried Urine Test for Comprehensive Hormones. The top panel lists the client's biographical information, the timing of their menstrual cycle (if applicable), and specimen collection times. Below this panel is the "Hormone Testing Summary," with gauge charts showing ideal and measured hormone ranges for sex hormones (*middle panel*) and adrenal hormones (*bottom panel*); the bottom panel also features a graph of the client's daily "free cortisol."

seven pages of notes to the provider on "How to read the DUTCH report." Notably, this final section begins with the disclaimer that "this report is not intended to treat, cure or diagnose any specific diseases," but any customer reading this highly detailed report could be forgiven for believing in its diagnostic power.[44] Indeed, Composed Nutrition's own homepage attests to that power by promising customers that DUTCH testing will "get to the root of any body imbalances" and "create a path to reclaim your health." Using a language of repairing and reclaiming within the logic of restoration, Composed Nutrition and similar sites situate themselves as the gateway to health: without using the companies' at-home tests, people cannot know what is really going on inside their bodies. Further, as long as people do not know how their bodies are doing, they cannot optimize their health. This is why the watchword of at-home wellness testing, according to the similar nutritional testing website The Women's Dietitian, is "Test, don't guess."[45]

There is one more step in Composed Nutrition's hormone testing process, which is the nutritionist's review of the test results with the client. Over one or more sessions, the nutritionist designs meal plans to restore the client's hormonal balance and recommends supplements "if deemed appropriate."[46] Following the consultation, Composed Nutrition's clients are linked directly to an online supplement dispensary that is hosted by the practitioner but powered by a third-party platform, Fullscript. Practitioners who use Fullscript are able to set their own prices and prescribe specific products to individual clients, while Fullscript provides the supplements and fills customer orders. By using Fullscript, Composed Nutrition therefore provides an end-to-end service, moving clients from wellness tracking to data analysis to bespoke nutritional advice and supplements. In turn, Composed Nutrition, like similar online nutrition-diagnostic websites, situates its clients in a closed loop between the pole of restoration, by bringing the body back into "balance," and the pole of enhancement, by making the body ever more "vibrant, energized, and confident."[47]

At-Home Wellness Testing: Viome

Before I turn to wellness hacking, let us look at one more example of wellness tracking. Viome is a web- and app-based testing service that, like Composed Nutrition, offers at-home laboratory testing, but with one crucial difference: it does away with the practitioner. Instead, the service itself stands in as guru-scientist, using stool samples to identify the different microorganisms living in a user's gut and to determine the proportions and balance of each microbe. Based on the testing data, Viome generates a series of reports that users can view in the app, along with customized meal plans and supplement recommendations geared toward optimizing their microbiome. Viome offers several packages, including the entry-level "Gut Intelligence Test," which aims to "balance your gut microbiome with a personalized, 90-day action plan" based on the user's individual test results in categories such as "Digestive Efficiency" and "Metabolic Fitness."[48] Those who choose this package receive specific recommendations for supplements in "precise dosages" ostensibly matched to their unique gut microbiome; initially, Viome would recommend particular manufacturers for certain supplements, but now the company sells them directly. The premiere package on

Viome's website is the "Precision Supplements Complete" subscription, available for US$199 per month, which includes stool testing every six months plus all required supplements based on the client's most recent test results.[49]

The Viome testing process is similar to Composed Nutrition's DUTCH test. Once users receive the test kit, they register its unique ID number with the company and then obtain and prepare the samples. They fill out an electronic questionnaire either on Viome's website or through the app, including hip and waist measurements, and collect their stool sample using the supplied capturing device. Users of certain packages take the additional step of drawing a small blood sample from their fingertip using a supplied lancet and collection tube. Once the biological samples are prepared, customers ship them back to the company along with the appropriate customs paperwork for those who live outside the United States. Three or four weeks later, users can log on to Viome's website or app to view their results and learn about Viome's recommendations for improving their gut health. The way Viome presents its results and recommendations appears to be a significant factor in enhancing the perceived credibility both of the tests themselves and, more generally, of tracking as a means of wellness optimization.

As with the DUTCH test, I did not submit my own sample for testing, but I was able to review sample results reports for Viome's tests, which are posted on Viome's website, as well as an informational video about the app hosted on Viome's YouTube page.[50] I also reviewed video reviews by Viome customers, such as YouTube user Jake Wilkins, a homebuilder in Boise, Idaho, who posted a twenty-six-minute video in spring 2018 about his experience with the basic microbiome test.[51] The dominant message reinforced in all these materials is that Viome delivers precise and personalized results for each Viome user's unique microbial composition. In the version of the app I viewed, for instance, the customer is greeted by name on each of the two main pages, "Recommendations" and "Results"; clicking on either leads users to detailed information that they are reminded is customized just for them. While the app and the downloadable written report are necessarily arranged differently, they are organized by the same categories and provide the same information. I will walk through the "Results" section of the app to show how it reinforces the idea of tracking as personalized, precision wellness.

Selecting "Results" from the Viome app's main page takes the user to a new page with a personalized message beginning "Test Results for," followed by the user's first name in much larger font (fig. 11, left image). Under that heading, the user is presented with their results sorted into three categories: "Needs Fo-

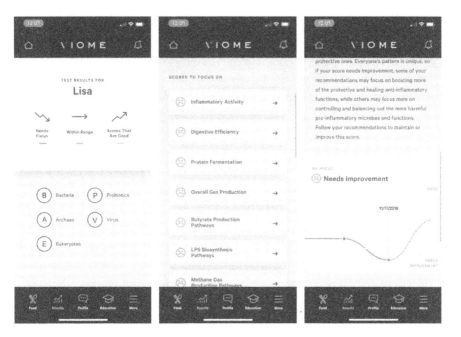

Figure 11. Screenshots of Viome test results. *Left,* "Test Results for Lisa": Listed in the bottom half of the image are the test's areas of assessment: "Bacteria," "Archaea," "Eukaryotes," "Probiotics," and "Virus." The dark panel along the bottom features links to other sections of the app ("Food," "Profile," "Education," and "More"). *Middle,* "Scores to Focus On": The frowning emojis indicate specific areas to address, including "Inflammatory Activity," "Digestive Efficiency," "Protein Fermentation," "Overall Gas Production," "Butyrate Production Pathways," "LPS Biosynthesis Pathways," "Methane Gas Production Pathways," and others not visible on the screen. *Right,* "Viome App Tour Video": This page of the app is accessed by clicking on one of the "Scores to Focus On" (*middle*). The text in the shaded top half of the screen provides a descriptive summary of the specific score that needs to be improved. In the unshaded bottom half is a graph that illustrates where the score for the client's specimen sits in relation to ratings of "Good" at the top of the graph and "Needs Improvement" at the bottom.

cus," which features an arrow shaped like a downward-sloping graph line; "Within Range," with a horizontal arrow pointing forward; and "Scores That Are Good," with an arrow like an upward-sloping graph line. Clicking on one of these links takes users to the corresponding results page, divided into categories, such as "Inflammatory Activity" and "Digestive Efficiency." To the left of each category name is an emoji that corresponds to the category—a frowning face for scores that need improvement, a neutral face for average scores, and a smiling face for good scores (fig. 11, middle image). Clicking on one of these categories in turn takes the user to a general description of the category and places the user's score on a graph showing how it relates to average and good scores (see fig. 11, right image). The descriptions in the text consistently reinforce Viome's delivery of customized results: "Everyone's pattern is unique. . . . Follow your recommendations to maintain or improve this score."[52] The ultimate object for each category seems to be to get your score as high as possible on each specific graph. After all, "good" has no ceiling.

For Jake, the Viome customer who reviewed his experience on YouTube, Viome's customization is its main appeal. Standing in front of a blackboard with an overview of his Viome results, he dismisses the "super dumb blanket diet" that he grew up with, everyone eating the same number of recommended servings from different food groups regardless of their body composition.[53] He believes that for each person there is a unique diet appropriate specifically for them, a diet that can only be discovered by wellness tracking services such as Viome. (Not coincidentally, Viome's own marketing materials consistently reinforce this same claim, explaining in the app's informational video, for example, that "in fact, not all healthy foods are good for every person.")[54] Jake praises Viome for basing its recommendations on a scientific analysis of each person's own gut, an analysis he believes helps him enhance his health by promoting good microbial balance and preventing chronic conditions such as diabetes or Crohn's disease, which he believes are entirely preventable through good gut health. He worries when the app says his microbiome is out of balance but trusts the app's recommendations because they target his own body's needs: "When they give me a recommendation for not only a supplement but a maker and a provider of it, I just trust it. And so, what's cool about that is I don't have to go sift through the millions of supplements that are out there, I can just pick this one because they said it's good for you, because they say it's good and I trust them."[55]

The final point I want to address regarding Viome is who Jake is trusting when he says he trusts "their" recommendations, because the answer links directly back to the life-optimization strategies and to the rhetorics of laboratory testing I discussed earlier in this chapter. In the most general terms, Jake is of course referring to the company that produces and analyzes the tests and offers recommendations. But more precisely, his trust lies in the algorithmic knowledge generated by the tests themselves. As he explains at the top of his review video, Viome's data are highly adaptive and constantly evolving: "As soon as . . . they've taken enough people's tests and as their data pool grows and grows and grows, they're able to change the results that you get. And the reason that is is because the more people that send samples to Viome that they can test, the more accurate the results can be. The bigger the . . . survey pool, the more accurate the results are."[56] A few weeks after he first received his results, for example, he got an email from the company saying that they had received more samples, which changed his results, and so they were able to provide more detailed breakdowns about different aspects of his overall wellness. For Jake, this email signaled Viome's transparency and the reliability of his test results, but his trust is placed primarily in the data themselves, which allow him to optimize his own health and wellness through careful biological tracking.

To return to Martin's concept of "flexible bodies," the direct-to-consumer laboratory wellness tests I have just discussed, and others like them, lock directly into the principle of flexible accumulation, which valorizes "technological innovation, specificity, and rapid, flexible change."[57] Viome's persuasiveness lies partly in its adaptive and constantly evolving database. But the wellness consumer is constantly evolving too—hormones fluctuate, health and habits change, and there is always room to improve on any of the dozens of datapoints we can track about ourselves—and so wellness tracking is an ongoing project. For this reason, retesting is a central plank of many wellness testing services like Viome, which advises users to "see how your scores evolve and update your recommendations by re-testing every 4–6 months."[58] Jake, for one, planned to retest his stool as soon as three months after he received his first test results because he believed his microbiome would change significantly over that time from following Viome's recommendations. The retesting may be expensive, he explains at the end of his video, "but what is it worth to know exactly what fuel your body needs and what is it worth to have a future without chronic diseases? To me, it's priceless. . . . I don't care what it costs. I'm willing to pay it to know exactly what my body needs, to avoid a future of disease and discomfort."[59] Being able to know and track exactly what your body needs is therefore the first step toward wellness optimization. The second step, which I turn to now, is acting on that knowledge with strategically targeted natural health products to "hack" your wellness.

Hacking Wellness

Within the Silicon Valley-influenced culture of life optimization, hacking is fundamentally about systematic and purposeful improvement in virtually any arena of life, whether that includes computers, machines, jobs, household management, relationships, or bodies. Tracking makes that improvement possible by furnishing data that identify and isolate patterns, indicate appropriate interventions to remedy or enhance those patterns, and provide markers of progress. For Tim Ferriss, one of the original popularizers of life hacking, the process of reflecting on and then breaking down the different elements of his own workaholic career selling performance-enhancing supplements allowed him to devise a system for freeing up time and maximizing his effectiveness. In Reagle's telling, Ferriss's bestselling book, *The 4-Hour Work Week*, offers hacks for readers to work less and earn more by eliminating unnecessary busywork, outsourcing as much work as possible, and adopting a systematic approach to streamlining tasks.[60] In Ferriss's case, tracking is intuitive, not scientific; he observes and reflects on his performance rather than monitoring it with digital technologies. The same is true for most wellness seekers too: not everyone who wants to optimize their wellness employs tracking technologies such as lab tests or apps. Most of my interview participants, for instance, reported deciding which supplements to use simply by observing and analyzing how they feel—how their bodies and minds are performing across a range of domains that include physical health, energy, strength, work, personal relationships, and emotional and spiritual well-being. Through a combination of intuition and reflection, they make individualized and strategic choices about when and how to take action to enhance their wellness.

People in both of my main datasets, the Bill C-51 petition comments and the interviews, hack their wellness through targeted supplementation, which I define here as the highly specific use of natural health products to optimize a person's individual faculties. A *hacker* was first defined in 1969 by the Tech Model Railroad Club at the Massachusetts Institute of Technology as someone who, in pursuing efficiency and optimization, "avoids the standard solution."[61] Even though most people who actively seek to optimize their wellness would not describe themselves as hackers, the definition nevertheless fits because targeted supplementation adopts a just-in-time ethos based on a person's perception of what their body needs at a given moment in time, whether that involves fighting an infection or finding extra energy to power through a big task. Bypassing conventional biomedical diagnosis and treatment, wellness seekers draw on hacking culture's maverick mentality to seek solutions that work specifically for them, for their unique bodies, and for their own particular understanding of wellness. I first show how people use supplements to foster conditions of flourishing, and then I turn to how people use supplements to enhance their hormonal and gut health. I close by reflecting briefly on how the collective will toward optimization affects each of us as individuals.

Creating Conditions of Flourishing

As I explained in chapter 4, wellness seekers frequently praise natural health products for optimizing the body by creating conditions under which it can flourish. I illustrated in that chapter that arguments about flourishing often slip from the logic of enhancement to that of restoration as exhausted and over-stretched people seek enough of a boost from products such as Dream EZ and Rescue Remedy to get through the day. Nevertheless, the logic of enhancement remains a powerful driver of wellness discourse. For example, the interview participant Terry, who is in his fifties and works in a medical setting, credits omega-3 and high-dose turmeric supplements for supercharging him both physically and mentally, giving him an edge in his demanding job: "I feel very alert for my age. When I go to work, my brain is just very alert, like even almost more than it was when I was in my thirties and forties. I just feel like I'm ready to get going every day."[62] Although Terry expressed skepticism about the science backing certain natural health supplements, he believes strongly in the supplements he uses daily to enhance his "heart health," "brain health," and "joint health" so his body can function optimally.

Kayla, a 30-year-old tech worker with a doctorate, similarly explained her quest for wellness as driven by a desire for enhancement because "I don't feel that I'm as productive or performing as optimally as I should be." She uses natural health products and tinkers with her diet to align herself more closely with what she described as the "benchmark" of optimal health:

> Eighteen years old, no wrinkles, perfect energy, cannot have hangovers after drinking. You know, sleeps nine hours and feels great and only eats green plants or something like that. . . . Flexible but also with a strong body and everything is, like, firm and perky and no cellulite and that kind of thing. So from this benchmark, then you start feeling like, "Oh, I have a bit of a poochy belly after I eat, maybe my digestion is wrong." Or, "Oh, I have black circles under my eyes. Maybe I'm not sleeping well." Or, "Oh, I don't feel that energetic . . . so maybe I need to do something about that."[63]

By comparing herself with someone more than a decade younger, Kayla invokes the logic of restoration, but her main focus is less on restoring her previous energy, strength, or appearance than on trying to create the best possible conditions for her current body to thrive. She takes high-dose vitamin C to "mediat[e] the collagen production pathway" so her skin stays firm, as well as a range of "weird herbs" such as ashwagandha for "adaptogenic support," which in this case refers to a class of natural health products that purportedly stabilize physiological processes and promote a state of balance within the body.[64]

To track her progress, Kayla uses various digital apps to record details about her mood, weight, body fat, blood pressure, fitness, and other metrics, but she scoffed at the idea of laboratory testing. (She has a friend who does regular blood and saliva tests, but she said there was "no way" she would do them herself.) Kayla was ultimately a little circumspect about whether the products she takes even work because despite her efforts to tracks her wellness, "I can't really quantify how I feel. Like, I don't even know if I get an energy boost from doing the B12 or not, but I just take it because I know it's related to energy."[65] Driven by a sense of obligation that she should try to help her body function as well as it can, Kayla adopts the wellness hacks that seem to work for her, even though she can never be quite sure they really do.

Like the interview participants, many "Stop Bill C-51" petition signatories expressed feelings of obligation to self-optimize, and they similarly believe that natural health products are an important pathway to optimization. The commenters frequently cite their belief that the products not only are free of both toxins and side effects but, equally important, enhance the body's ability to perform by providing holistic, preventive support rather than masking symptoms. Tamara explains that supplements not only treat problems within the body but also create optimal conditions for the body to both heal and thrive, enabling long days at work by providing "the boost I needed to regain my health and vitality."[66] Tamara and other commenters believe that the holistic approach to health afforded by natural health products allows the body to heal itself by providing a balanced nutritional environment. They feel that when the body is in balance it can function efficiently and effectively, without relying on external interventions such as pharmaceuticals to effect a change in the body. The conditions these commenters describe are conditions of optimization that allow supplement consumers to feel good, energetic, strong, and productive.

Those who signed the petition opposing Bill C-51 fear that if their access to natural health products is restricted, they will not be able to support and enhance their wellness. Rhonda, for instance, questions the government's motivation to pursue the legislation: "I have the right to choose if I want to consume proven health diminishers [i.e., pharmaceuticals], why not the choice of health enhancers?" Andrew asks, more pointedly: "Who can legislate away the body's inherent ability to heal itself when given the nutritional support and environment it requires?"[67] Within the petition comments, the concept of optimization is so tightly fused with the concept of risk that any potential limits to supplementation of the physical body are framed as a risk to citizens' fundamental democratic rights to self-realization and autonomy. These commenters are caught in a loop between restoration and enhancement because the risk of illness can never be fully eliminated and the well body can always be improved.

Further, the neoliberal models of self-care and health citizenship discussed in chapter 2 come home to roost in the realm of optimization because we have so internalized health messaging about self-management and cultural messaging about self-enhancement that the failure to sufficiently optimize now constitutes its own form of risk. Not only are wellness seekers exhorted to enhance their wellness at every turn, they are charged with sole responsibility for creating the very conditions of their own flourishing. According to all the primary sources I examined for this book, most people fulfill that responsibility through targeted supplementation.

Targeted Supplementation

In *Hacking Life*, Reagle illustrates that for many health hackers the goal is to become transhuman, to become more than human in capability and function, and thereby "transcend the nominal" of everyday human life.[68] He chronicles how Silicon Valley self-help gurus such as Tim Ferriss and Tony Robbins sell advice and supplements to those who want to optimize their bodies, minds, and productivity. Specializing in nootropics, so-called smart drugs that purportedly enhance cognition, memory, creativity, and motivation, these figures trade in TED Talk–style scientism and capitalize on public cynicism about mainstream medicine to market themselves as maverick entrepreneurs who make special knowledge available to those wise enough to seek it. (A frequent refrain in this discourse is, "Doctors won't tell you this but *I* will.") Reagle explains that life hackers are drawn to supplements alongside self-help quotations and slogans "because they are tools: small, easily consumed boosts to body and brain."[69] For everyday wellness seekers, the goal of self-optimization is usually more mundane than it is for figures such as Ferriss, as individuals such as those I discuss in this book do not seek to become superhuman but simply better, more effective versions of themselves. Despite this difference, wellness seekers are nevertheless drawn to natural health products for the same reasons, because these products are quick, modular hacks for targeted improvement in particular bodily processes or functions.

One way natural health products work as modular hacks, according to everyone I interviewed, is that that they maintain, support, and boost specific organs or systems, helping to optimize their performance. For example, Marilyn, a school support worker in her late fifties, described using a natural kelp supplement for her thyroid gland because she believes it is necessary to take proactive steps "to maintain your hormone level and your thyroid."[70] Previously diagnosed with a thyroid problem that was successfully treated with a pharmaceutical, Marilyn felt that the kelp supplement would keep her thyroid functioning well.

Similarly, Erin, a nutritionist in her mid-twenties, explained that she uses a probiotic supplement because "it helps with enzymes, digestive support. It's levelling out my healthy bacteria in my body so that my immune system stays up."[71] Other participants gave other examples of targeted supplementation, such as "a homeopathic remedy for adrenal gland support," an "herbal tea blend to support a healthy pregnancy," and omega fatty acids "to support your body's release of particular hormones."[72] Further, many participants described supplements as catalysts, kicking the body into a more efficient or effective state. For example, Donna, who is in her late fifties and lives with hypothyroidism, pointed to a product she had heard about that would "boost your thyroid naturally" so it could function more effectively.[73] In all these examples, natural health products lighten some of the body's load, thereby alleviating strain and conserving the body's resources so it can run optimally. For the individuals I interviewed, natural health products are keys that unlock their ability to be as well as they can be.

The principle of balance is at the center of claims that natural health products optimize wellness by maintaining, supporting, and boosting specific organs or systems. Mirroring the marketing for hormone and gut health tests discussed above, interview participants frequently argued that the body needs to be in a state of equilibrium to function effectively and efficiently. Many participants believe, for instance, that when their sex hormones and stress hormones are balanced, their moods will be more stable and positive, and their periods shorter and less painful. For instance, Kayla, the tech worker in her thirties, uses the supplements omega-3 and *Vitex agnus-castus*, also known as chaste tree or chasteberry, along with as a raspberry leaf tea called Balance Tea, to improve the regularity of her menstrual cycle. Jana, a journalist in her early thirties, similarly uses *Vitex*, which she characterized as "the hormone balancing natural supplement," to improve her own menstrual cycle "so that my symptoms wouldn't last longer than they had to. Because I would have, like, really bad cramps for a long time and I had really irregular periods, but then that hormone balancer helped shorten the period and then helped my symptoms last for like only one day." Jana's description here draws primarily on the logic of restoration, of returning the ill body to a prior state of functioning, which in this case refers to the non-menstrual phase of her cycle. Setting aside the question of whether or not a period counts as illness, Jana also invokes the logic of enhancement, framing her decision to use *Vitex* as a way to fine-tune her periods so they "wouldn't last longer than they had to."[74] Like life hackers who fine-tune their productivity and focus, Jana and Kayla use natural health products to target and improve their menstrual cycles.

Balance is also widely believed to be important for optimizing gut health. Echoing the websites for Composed Nutrition and Viome, the interview participants frequently asserted that gut bacteria need to be in balance for the body to be healthy—for the immune system to function properly, for the body to absorb and process nutrients and eliminate waste, and for the person to maintain good energy, mood, and cognition. Recall Erin's explanation above that probiotic supplements help with "levelling out my healthy bacteria in my body" to ensure that the different microorganisms that colonize her body exist in symbiotic proportions.[75] Clara, a retired dance instructor, expressed similar beliefs about the necessity of properly balanced gut microbiota. She was particularly concerned that the heavy metals, preservatives, and antibacterial products we encounter in our everyday lives might throw off her gut's balance of bacteria because her digestive system cannot effectively process those toxins. She explained that the "heavy onslaught of chemicals that are received into the body cumulatively build up [and] definitely affect the gut and the brain, and we know a lot about the gut-brain connection now, and how the microbiome is affected."[76] She believes that natural health products detoxify her body, thereby bringing her gut microbiome back into balance and optimizing its function.

To keep gut bacteria in balance, many participants proactively take probiotic supplements in pill or capsule form and consume foods that contain probiotics, such as yogurt, kombucha (a drink made from fermented, sugared tea), and kimchi (a spicy dish made from fermented cabbage and other vegetables). They cited easy digestion and comfortable elimination as signs of a well-balanced gut, whereas gas, bloating, constipation, and diarrhea are signals that the gut is not working as well as it could be. Many participants were especially concerned about the relationship between the gut and antibiotics and described using probiotics to counteract the harmful effect of the antibiotics on their good gut bacteria. Kayla, for instance, explained that "when you take antibiotics, you should take a probiotic. It's not like the probiotic is helping you clear your infection per se, it's just making sure that you don't ruin your gut biome."[77] Clara described using probiotics to counter antibiotics as an almost moral conflict: when treating an ear infection with penicillin, she said with a smile, "I also took probiotics at the same time to balance the bacteria in the body. The good versus the bad."[78] For some participants, balancing gut bacteria is a lifelong project, not episodic. For example, Tania, who is in her late forties and on sick leave, feels she must offset her history of taking antibiotics by supplementing with probiotics for the rest of her life. Overall, the general consensus among the participants who use probiotic supplements is that the more they consume, the better for their gut and their overall wellness.

All these targeted supplementation strategies connect to the broader culture of life hacking in several ways. Most immediately, participants' use of supplements to optimize their hormones and gut bacteria share with hacking culture an emphasis on surgically precise self-improvement through highly individualized approaches that often fly in the face of convention. (Recall, here, the MIT Tech Model Railroad Club's definition of a hacker as someone who "avoids the standard solution.") Across the interviews, participants said that one-size-fits-all approaches to health and wellness do not easily apply to individuals and that everyone needs to find their own unique path to wellness.

A particularly common story I heard in the interviews was of those who wanted to balance their hormones and gut bacteria having to strike out on their own after unsuccessfully seeking help from their doctors. For instance, Vanita, a consultant in her early thirties, recalled her doctor "chiding and chastising" her for asking about natural options for managing her menstrual cycle, and so she sought her own unique solution: "Ultimately I really just listened to my body and I also talked to some other women . . . and read about . . . their stories" to make the right decision.[79] Glory, a retired schoolteacher in her mid-seventies, recounted a similarly negative experience when she began menopause. After her doctor "fired" her for not agreeing to try hormone replacement therapy, she became determined to find her own way: "I believed so much in my own research rather than just depending on drug companies and . . . in the end it turned out I'm really pleased with the decision I made."[80] For both Glory and Vanita, the path to optimizing their hormones has been one they had to clear on their own, for their own bodies, to suit their own circumstances.

In another key parallel between targeted supplementation and hacking culture, participants emphasized the need to help their bodies work smarter, not harder. They frequently described the human body as an efficient and variable machine that runs more effectively when it is managed in an agile and adaptive way. For example, Kayla explained that managing her hormones and improving her cycle requires her to constantly shift her approach because her body is constantly releasing different ratios of hormones depending on where she is in her monthly cycle. The body figured here is flexible, in Martin's sense of the term, because it is always adapting fluidly to changing circumstances. Any effort to improve its operation must unfold in sync with those evolving circumstances.

Jordana, a graduate student in her late twenties, also approaches her body flexibly, engaging in what she calls "seed cycling," which involves eating different kinds of seeds at different times of her menstrual cycle. This practice helps her optimize her cycle because the different "seeds have different kinds of Omegas in them, and different nutrients as well, that are supposed to support your body's release of particular hormones."[81] Jordana's highly specific approach to optimizing her hormone levels parallels flexible economic models of production and distribution, both of which require careful monitoring and maintenance to ensure maximum productivity. The downside of such a nimble, flexible approach to optimizing wellness, however, is that it can quickly become overwhelming: because there is no ceiling for wellness, there is likewise no ceiling for what we can track and, correspondingly, no ceiling for what we can hack.

Tantalizing Self-Improvement

Let us go back to Suzanne Somers, the actor turned lifestyle guru with whom I began my discussion of wellness as a form of optimization. When she appeared on *Oprah* with her fellow "natural menopause" advocate, the obstetrician-gynecologist Christiane Northrup, Somers assured audience members, most of them women, and viewers at home that they too could take charge of their health and maximize their wellness through regular hormone testing and supplementation. Somers's advice about menopause both on the show and in her many trade books is enticing, but it is founded on three key problems that tie into broader rhetorics of wellness optimization.

The first problem is that Somers describes menopause in terms of illness, as a condition that requires medical intervention. As Margaret Lock and others have shown, this framing of menopause as a pathology is pretty standard in conventional menopause discourse,[82] but it runs counter to Somers's own insistence that menopause done naturally is a wondrous period of self-exploration and improvement—the "Sexy Years," as she described it in her 2003 book of the same name. Even while Somers breathlessly touts menopause as the most empowering phase of a woman's life, she describes it elsewhere as a "crisis" that needs to be addressed with concerted action: "I was not going to let it beat me. I would not go silently into the night . . . so I fought for an answer that would work for me."[83] Here Somers situates menopause in a standard narrative frame of illness as a battle that each woman must fight individually.

In this framing, menopause is not a normal change in the life course but a dysfunction, a condition from which it seems one could even possibly die. Somers recounts, for example, that as a result of menopause, "I was no longer making my full complement of hormones. Because of that, I had no life-restoring nutrients feeding me metabolically. My organs were shutting down from lack of nutrients."[84]

Here Somers shifts resolutely from the logic of enhancement, where menopause is an empowering and sexy experience, to the logic of restoration, where she needs to stabilize her hormones to prevent her organs from "shutting down." The way she cycles fluidly between the two logics of wellness mirrors how the individuals in both of my datasets describe their own efforts to optimize their hormones and gut health. Ultimately, beneath every claim about optimization is a problem that needs to be fixed.

The second key problem with Somers's menopause optimization strategies is that she argues for a strong conceptual separation between conventional pharmaceutical treatments for menopause and the natural regimen she advocates, but that separation frequently collapses in the language she uses to explain natural menopause supplementation. She frequently uses enhancement-oriented terms such as *hormonal change* and *hormonal balance* when praising natural hormones and supplements for alleviating menopausal discomfort and promoting vitality, well-being, and invigorated sexuality, whereas she dismisses conventional hormone therapy as a quick fix that harms women's health more than it helps. Elsewhere, however, these enhancement-oriented terms give way to more conventional pharmaceutical terms that instead emphasize restoration: *hormonal change* becomes *hormonal loss* or *hormonal depletion,* whereas *hormonal balance* becomes *hormonal correction*.[85] Menopause is again framed as a deficiency disease that needs to be fixed, except that natural hormones and supplements now stand as the solution instead of pharmaceuticals. The shifts in Somers's language mirror the datasets in this regard as well: optimizing hormones or gut health is frequently about diagnosing and treating a problem rather than about improving or enhancing wellness. Natural health products become, in effect, pharmaceuticals.

The third key problem with Somers's advice about optimizing menopause is that natural hormone supplementation may not empower women to the extent that she claims. In *Ageless*, she advises aging readers to take action because "you don't want to lose your energy, lose your sexuality, or be put out to pasture by your family much the same way they do old horses. . . . Your best defense to prevent this from happening is to take charge of your health now!"[86] The idea of taking charge of our health is certainly appealing but the strategies Somers advocates hardly seem empowering. Recall, for example, that after explaining on *Oprah* her routine of taking more than sixty supplements a day, in addition to using various hormonal creams and routinely testing her hormones through blood and urine tests, Somers added: "You don't have to take all this. Although the deeper you get into [this regimen], the more you're apt to want to keep adding to it."[87] For Somers, optimizing her wellness consumes a considerable amount of her time and attention, and for the average person it would be a prohibitively expensive prospect too. The people I interviewed similarly struggled with the temptation to "keep adding to" their wellness routines, knowing that there was always something else they could or should do to optimize themselves. Ultimately, self-optimization is a project without an end.

These examples from Somers help illustrate my larger argument in this chapter, which is that we are exhorted to optimize our wellness in the same way that we are exhorted to optimize our finances, productivity, relationships, and housekeeping; to perfect our hormone levels and our gut health as we do our pancakes. Wellness optimization is tantalizing because it is always just out of reach. And if we only become our true authentic selves through self-exploration and self-improvement, then we, ourselves, are also perpetually out of reach, and so we are left to keep on striving. I often think about this never-ending project of becoming the best *me* I can be when I fold laundry late at night and try to psych myself up to fold my clothes in small self-standing rectangles as recommended by decluttering guru Marie Kondo. I almost never do fold them that way, but I do always feel guilty about it. And that guilt can tell us something about how optimization works as a vector of wellness discourse. As Lupton, Reagle, and Cederström and Spicer all illustrate, the cycle of self-improvement is fueled by the very anxiety, self-doubt, disappointment, feelings of loss of control, and confusion that we seek to quench through self-improvement.[88] And so the cycle goes.

We are left with an overwhelming feeling that improvement is right around the corner if only we can find our way to it. Like Delaney in *Wellmania*, some of us may burn ourselves out with the effort, which only encourages us to redouble our efforts. Or like Jasmine, a policy professional in her thirties whom I interviewed, we may feel trapped in a permanent state of confusion, overwhelmed by all the choices around us, such as whether gluten is okay to eat or whether to try this supplement or that.[89] Or, like Suri, a graduate student in her mid-twenties, we might ask ourselves, "How did people be happy and support brain health and support gut health before the advent of these products?"[90]

The route to self-optimization through natural health and wellness is fraught because it changes us in important ways. Wellness tracking gives the illusion of control, but as Reagle illustrates, measurement distorts, and not everything that matters can be measured.[91] Tracking also changes how we think about ourselves. If I order a stool test through Viome, the results will tell me more about me, and whether or not the results have any scientific relevance, they *become* me, in the same way that brain scans and medical diagnoses change how people see and understand themselves.[92] Wellness hacking creates a sense of obligation that never ends because we can always be more effective, more efficient, and more productive. That obligation is also concerningly individualized because it reframes collective social problems as individual shortcomings to be remedied through self-education and self-improvement. For people with the time, financial resources, and inclination required, optimizing wellness with natural health products may be a reasonable prospect, but the obligation to self-improve leaves anyone without similar privileges in a lurch, converting their failure to optimize into a personal failing. Wellness as a form of optimization may not, in the end, be our route to the good life but simply a role we feel compelled to perform in the looping cycle of becoming who we are.

CHAPTER SIX

Wellness as Performance

Over the course of this book, I have mapped five of the key vectors of wellness as a self-generating rhetorical system—wellness as incipient illness, self-management, harm reduction, survival strategy, and optimization. These five vectors give rise to and shape the sixth and final vector, wellness as performance. By describing wellness as "performance," I mean that wellness is enacted and embodied, unfolding at particular times and places to particular effects. Performances of wellness, both for the self and for others, are animated by something of a script that is constituted by the previous five vectors. These vectors together establish a framework for languaging wellness that corresponds to rhetorician Kenneth Burke's concept of piety, summarized here by Marika Seigel: "Pieties are orientations that determine [in a given context] what people can or cannot say and do."[1] Performances of wellness are scripted by pieties that tell us what we should and should not do for our wellness, how we should think and feel, whether and how we measure up in our personal, emotional, and professional lives, and how we can improve our wellness across domains.

Pieties of wellness are rooted in what Cederström and Spicer characterize as the "moral demand" of wellness, the deeply felt but invisible tug many of us feel to be "good" by working toward wellness, whether or not we choose to or even can respond to that tug. The invisible tug of wellness is what tells me I should be exercising when I am scrolling on Twitter. It is what makes me feel guilty when I struggle to focus at work, regardless of what else is going on in my life. It is what makes me feel virtuous when I resist making midnight nachos—and what gives me a thrill of sneaky pleasure when I give in. Most of us experience feelings of right and wrong when we make decisions about our health and wellness, feelings that tell us what is moral to do or to resist in the name of being good. But where do these feelings come from? How do they work? And how do they affect how we view one another and ourselves? In this final chapter, I explain how the moral demand of wellness works, how it circulates, and how it informs who and how we are.

Let me start with an example of the invisible scripts of wellness we perform in our everyday lives. Before I had my daughter in 2006, I had never given vaccines a second thought. I did not know much, or care, about the supposed link between vaccines and autism, despite extensive media coverage in the years immediately prior about disgraced doctor Andrew Wakefield's fraudulent 1998 study in the *Lancet* medical journal, which falsely linked autism with the measles, mumps, and rubella (MMR) vaccine. Although the study was retracted in 2004, by the time I was pregnant in 2006 stories were circulating widely in parent circles and celebrity media about apparently neurotypical children who had "regressed" after receiving vaccines, forever changing their lives and their parents' lives. I did not pay much attention to these stories, although they were hard to avoid. When it came time for my first well-baby visit at six weeks postpartum, my family doctor weighed my baby and took other vitals and then explained the vaccine schedule to me. I remember clearly what happened next: to my own surprise, I asked her whether vaccines were safe.

I remember not being all that concerned about vaccine safety in the moment. I trusted my doctor. Nevertheless, negative vaccine coverage was very much in the air, and as an anxious new mother, I thought I *should* be concerned about vaccines, especially if so many other dedicated parents and public figures were concerned. Western culture is steeped in pieties about what constitutes good motherhood: that good mothers are concerned about their children's health; that they ask the right questions; that they are not afraid to question authority. In that doctor's appointment, I acted in accordance with these pieties because it seemed like the right thing to do, even though I felt like an actor committed to neither her script nor her role. My doctor responded to my question with composure and compassion, and reassured, I vaccinated my daughter on schedule and never gave it another thought.

This story illustrates how we perform wellness according to invisible scripts that are themselves animated by pieties circulating in public culture. During my pregnancy and immediately postpartum, I picked up on the pieties of good motherhood that surrounded me in my everyday life—in the headlines of grocery store magazines, in conversations I overheard at baby groups and coffee shops, in online discussions I drifted across in my late-night baby-googling, in chyrons running across the screens of twenty-four-hour news channels in the waiting rooms and transit stations I passed through. I encountered these materials in my daily life, and although they barely registered, they nevertheless taught me much about my role as a new mother. As I have argued elsewhere, following Judy Segal, we are collectively affected by the stories about health and wellness that circulate in public even if we do not read or tell those stories ourselves.[2] Those stories nevertheless register in our daily lives, even at a distance, because they manifest around us in our discursive environment. The ambient rhetorics of wellness shape us in ways that can be difficult and sometimes impossible to see.

Of course, vaccine safety is only a piece of this story about my well-baby visit because concerns about vaccines are also nested, partly, within the larger milieu of white, progressive, west coast motherhood in which I was learning to parent. This was a world of politically minded liberals who valued babywearing, on-demand and extended nursing, and co-sleeping. A world of organic produce, co-op markets, natural cleaning products, and juice cleanses, as well as pricey SUV-like strollers, über-safe car seats, and breezy, free-range toddlers. This broader parenting milieu was both governed by and productive of associated pieties about proper and authentic childrearing, and these pieties shaped what I did, said, and felt as a new parent. I learned and internalized the piety that good, authentic mothers breastfeed exclusively and that nursing difficulties, while normal, must be overcome. I learned the piety that good, authentic mothers keep their babies well by using organic, if not homemade, food and body care products, as well as cloth diapers (ideally) or unbleached, compostable diapers (minimally). All these pieties about the "well mother" informed my own emerging identity as a parent, prompting me to ask my doctor if vaccines were safe simply because the question was part of the script I had internalized from the parenting world around me.[3]

To return to the broader themes of this book, wellness is not any one thing, it is not found in a specific place, nor is it achieved in a single way. As both an idea and a moral demand, wellness is everywhere around us: it is ambient, to use rhetorician Thomas Rickert's term. The pieties of wellness—the scripts according to which we perform wellness—are therefore not produced in isolation by particular products or pressures from particular sources. This is why debunking wellness products and services only takes us so far toward understanding and mitigating the cultural hegemony of wellness because pieties associated with wellness exceed the conscious efforts of those trying to sell wellness to us. Pieties of wellness circulate freely in newspapers and magazines, on radio and television, and across the web. They circulate among friends, family, salespeople, and strangers in shops, cafés, and baby groups; they circulate in the products we see in advertisements and on store shelves; and they circulate in the ways we live and the ways we see others live. These pieties draw on the argumentative resources of both logics of wellness, the logics of restoration and enhancement, sometimes by alternating between them and sometimes by drawing on them simultaneously. These pieties affect how we envision the good life, and they tell us that to be good and to be well, we must be and think and do in certain ways, and not others.

In this chapter, I illustrate how wellness constitutes both public and private performance and how these performances are scripted by knowledge of what it is right, or pious, to do for our health. I begin by defining the three terms that guide what follows: *piety*, *ritual*, and *performance*. I link these terms to the cultural gap that wellness fills in secular twenty-first-century life as it transforms nature into a para-religious force and agent of self-transformation. I then examine in more detail how we perform wellness in part through the choices we make, which become synecdochic of who we are: the health products we do or do not consume become markers of identity, both as personal branding (e.g., "I am a virtuous, healthy person") and as enactment of health citizenship (e.g., "I accept responsibility for my own health"). I explain how we perform wellness through embodied experience—how we live in and interpret our bodies—and by internalizing and transforming the "sick role" into the "well role."[4] Over this chapter, I show how piety informs performances of wellness by telling us who and how we ought to be.

Natural Health as Ritual Performance

In wellness culture, one of the most persistent narratives is that of the daily wellness routine. In this narrative, wellness seekers summarize the steps they take each day to restore and enhance their wellness, describing in often reverent terms the supplements and other products they use. Recall, for example, Suzanne Somers's daily routine from *Oprah*, discussed in chapter 5. Somers performed for cameras the carefully orchestrated sequence she undertakes each morning and night to optimize her hormones, every step designed to stave off the effects of aging and enhance her mood, energy, and sexuality.[5] Despite her assurance that viewers did not need to take dozens of supplements to support their wellness, the clip's message was nevertheless clear: if *Oprah* viewers wanted to be as vibrant and youthful as Somers, the way to get there was to follow her intensive hormone-optimization routine.

Narratives of daily wellness routines have become so prevalent in contemporary culture that the genre of the narrative has itself become routine. These narratives are found in magazine accounts of celebrities' favorite anti-aging, mood-enhancing, and stress-busting rituals. They are found in the Instagram posts of women snowboarders I follow, who share (often sponsored) stories about the supplements, fortified foods, and related products they use to improve their sleep, energy, and performance. These narratives are found in friends' shared tips about new kombucha drinks for settling their digestion or CBD gummies to quiet their minds. In each of these cases, the narrative of the daily wellness routine does several important things at once: first, it tells a story about what wellness is and means; second, it tells a story about the storyteller's path to wellness, in turn providing a path for others to follow; and, third, it tells a story about the storyteller themself, about the kind of person they are (one who is good and also well). Even people who do not explicitly identify with wellness culture both participate in and perpetuate that culture when they read or listen to those kinds of stories or relay stories of their own.

As people respond to and share tips for restoring or enhancing health, they simultaneously reinforce values about wellness that circulate in everyday public life. In this first half of the chapter, I characterize these values as *pieties* that work as scripts that determine where, when, and how we perform wellness. When I say that we *perform* wellness, I am not contrasting performance to authentic experience or suggesting that performance is in any way illusory or phony. Instead, I am working from the tenet of performance studies scholarship that performance constitutes an embodied form of doing, a dynamic mode of action in the world. Accordingly, I argue that we perform wellness for ourselves and for others through our daily wellness routine (even if that routine only involves brushing our teeth) and that we also perform wellness through our narration of those routines, whether online or in the media, within our social groups, or only for ourselves.

Our performances of wellness are animated by pieties that circulate in public culture. Such performances take on an element of ritual that charges the language of wellness with a potential for transformation because these performances tell us that if we follow a particular set of steps or actions, we can become better versions of ourselves. As I outline in this section, wellness therefore sells, in part, by selling us pieties to perform in rituals of self-transformation that are aided by natural health products. Of course, if wellness has no ceiling, we may never arrive at a state of transformed *being*, remaining instead perpetually in a state of transformational *becoming*, no matter how elaborate our daily wellness routines. Nevertheless, to understand why wellness sells, we need first to understand how wellness becomes so charged with meaning that using a certain supplement or remedy can feel akin to a religious or spiritual experience.

Pieties of Wellness

When Kenneth Burke developed the rhetorical concept of piety, he was not thinking about religious salvation or adherence to church doctrine or anything we might associate with being "good." Instead, as rhetoric scholar Jordynn Jack recounts, Burke came to the idea of piety by thinking about illicit drugs. At the time, he had been working at the US-based Bureau of Social Hygiene, a philanthropic organization founded to study criminality and policy reform in the realms of sex work, drug use, corruption, and more. As Jack explains, Burke's work at the bureau was a key influence motivating his 1932 treatise *Permanence and Change*, in which he examines the invisible scripts, or pieties, that motivate and animate human action. In Jack's account, Burke drew on his observations regarding deviant behavior to explain how the terms we use to organize and understand the world are interpretive, ideological, and powerfully persuasive and thereby resistant to change. Burke was thinking in particular about how difficult it is for people to change their patterns of association and behavior because human beings infer what is appropriate to do or say from the situations or circumstances they are in.[6] To use Burke's example, the crude behaviors of men involved in criminal gangs, such as swearing, spitting, and harassing women, go with the territory, so we might usefully consider those behaviors as part of an allegiance to a collective moral logic internal to the situation rather than an individual moral failing. In other words, such men behave in accordance with "a deeply felt and piously obeyed sense of the appropriate" within a situation wherein "vulgarity is pious."[7]

In broader rhetorical terms, piety involves a situationally attuned "sense of what properly goes with what," in Burke's oft-cited definition, rather than fidelity to a generalized moral or religious code.[8] Piety is a useful heuristic for understanding wellness as performance because it explains how and why wellness seekers are motivated to take action to restore and enhance their wellness. Viewed through the prism of piety, natural health products fit among a suite of approaches to wellness that generally "go with" one another, such as preferring natural consumer goods, selective diets, certain parenting styles, and so on. Furthermore, as a sense of what goes with what, piety links wellness culture to identity because piety organizes our idiosyncratic traits and haphazard experiences into patterns that make sense to us. This is why piety so powerfully scripts the ways we move in the world and the people we are. As rhetorician Anne George explains, "Piety names the force that drives people to create coherence in their lives, to form a unified identity as supermom or computer nerd or obsessive cat lover."[9] Pieties of wellness create an important sense of identity and purpose for individuals who use natural health products to support and enhance their wellness. Indeed, these pieties were what helped my interview participants recognize themselves in the recruitment materials I circulated asking, "Are you interested in wellness?"

Pieties are produced and affirmed rhetorically, both through discourse and through materialities of the lived environment. Seigel illustrates beautifully how we can "read" piety even in a mundane cultural text such as a user manual for a blender, which she argues shows not only what a person can do with a blender but also *what is pious* to do with it.[10] For example, the manual's instructions and illustrations indicate the piety that women "go with" cooking, as well as other related pieties: that the pious user of the blender is a housewife and parent, that she prepares primarily processed foods, that she is neat and clean, and that she frequently hosts guests in her home. Similarly, Seigel finds that pregnancy manuals evince a range of related pieties that come to script how people experience pregnancy, how they care for their infants, and how they understand their own place in medical and gendered hierarchies.[11] Seigel shows how these pieties also shape pregnant people's identities as individuals and parents. Similarly, we can read wellness discourse to understand how it comes to define what the pious wellness seeker must be and do.

So what are the pieties of wellness? Advertisements are a good place to look because, as my analysis in previous chapters has shown, advertisements are powerful sites of ideological influence in the realm of wellness. We can reframe that influence here through the concept of piety because ads speak largely in terms of values that tell us how to live the good life.[12] For example, the commercials for Rescue Remedy discussed in chapter 4 convey pieties about gender, motherhood, hard work, and stress, most notably the pieties that "women should be calm even under pressure" and "wellness is manageable with natural, plant-based remedies." Similarly, the YouTube commercial for the sleep aid Natrol, also discussed in that chapter, trades on pieties about sleep, performance, and health, particularly the piety that people who are healthy and successful sleep easily without interruption each night. If pieties act as scripts that tell you what goes with what, then the Natrol commercial tells viewers that using that supplement is of a piece with health and success. For someone who wants to be healthy and successful, the pious thing to do is to take the product daily.

The Instagram accounts of supplement companies are another rich site for examining pieties of wellness. These accounts are advertising engines at their core, but embedded within the other personal and commercial posts that appear in any user's feed, they read less as ads than they do as "content," simply part of the steady supply of eye candy for Instagram scrollers. The conflation of corporate promotion with lifestyle media is entirely by design, of course. The images posted to these accounts tap into and replicate prevalent trends on social media—the right lighting, angles, graphics, setting, body types, poses, beauty and styling, and in the accompanying captions, phrasing, and emojis. Posts from these accounts call their viewers into community by marrying the products promoted with viewers' lifestyles, as if to say, "Those who use our products look and live like us."

The California-based company Vegamour, for example, promotes its supplements and serums on Instagram to its 275,000 followers and through paid advertisements in users' feeds under the tagline "A 360 approach to hair wellness."[13] The tagline's reference to "hair wellness" is itself both curious and telling: it anthropomorphizes hair by suggesting that it can be "well," shifting the burden of care so that prospective Vegamour customers become doubly responsible for wellness—both their own and that of their hair. Vegamour's marketing and packaging supports this anthropomorphic reading of hair wellness. For example, when consumers open Vegamour's product boxes, they are greeted with a message on the inside lid that says "your hair thanks you," gratitude presumably for their purchase of the product.[14] By anthropomorphizing the wellness seeker's hair, Vegamour evinces two key pieties associated with its products: that hair needs to be well and that individual consumers are responsible for ensuring that it is.

Other posts on Vegamour's Instagram page pick up on these pieties of wellness and add others to them. One post, for instance (fig. 12), promotes Vegamour's GRO Biotin Gummies. The image features a labeled product bottle on its side with heart-shaped gummies with the company "V" logo stamped in the center spilling out on a warmly lit surface, all in soft pinks and pastels. Black text indicates the various vitamins and minerals they contain. The caption accompanying the image begins with the assertion that "Just like healthy, glowy skin starts from the inside out, so does hair wellness." Here, glowy skin and shiny hair become external signals of internal health: if you are beautiful, you must be well. (The corollary, of course, is that wellness in turn requires beauty.) The caption further explains that the product will "help support your body's production of keratin and collagen," proteins that Vegamour says on its website will strengthen and thicken hair.[15] This image, together with Vegamour's other posts on Instagram— which primarily feature women with a range of body sizes and ethnic backgrounds, but all with conventionally feminine hairstyles—indicates that the pious user of the company's products is a woman who has thick, lustrous hair; that that she uses natural products rather than chemicals; and that she takes active steps to resist ag-

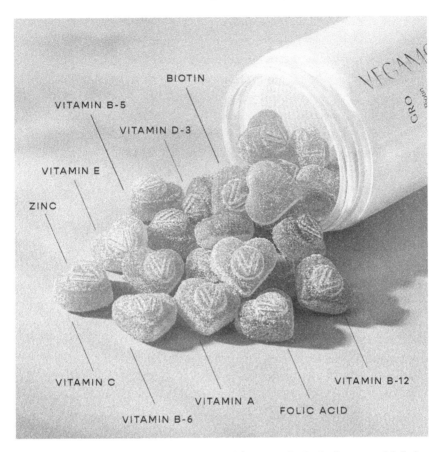

BIOTIN

VITAMIN B-5

VITAMIN D-3

VITAMIN E

ZINC

VITAMIN C

VITAMIN A

VITAMIN B-6

VITAMIN B-12

FOLIC ACID

Figure 12. Detail of Vegamour Instagram post. The gummies in the image are labeled with the product's contents, including zinc and biotin, folic acid, and other vitamins. VEGAMOUR (@vegamour). "Just like healthy, glowy skin starts from the inside out, so does hair wellness. So what makes our GRO Biotin Gummies so great? Our. . . ." Instagram photo, May 7, 2021. https://www.instagram.com/p/COlWHqZsoAW/.

ing. In the Vegamour universe, there seems to be a right way to age, which includes maintaining hair thickness, whereas thinning hair or choosing not to use the products implies surrender.

When those who use Vegamour products post their own Instagram images tagged "#vegamour," they both embody and reproduce the wellness pieties advanced by Vegamour's promotional materials. Searching that hashtag produces a stream of user-generated content that is almost indistinguishable from that of Vegamour's own feed, with beautifully lit and framed photographs of users' hair and captions praising Vegamour for supporting users' journeys toward longer, stronger, fuller hair. Some users post before-and-after comparisons, highlighting how much younger they look and feel after using Vegamour's products and how happy they are to use products free of harmful chemicals. These user-generated posts illustrate how the pieties of wellness associated with Vegamour effectively script what its users say, echoing Seigel's observation that pieties determine "what people can or cannot say and do."[16] Furthermore, these pieties are tightly bound to personal identity: Vegamour customers credit the products for transforming their lives, not just their hair. For example, a user with nearly twenty thousand followers credited Vegamour in a tagged post with helping her find herself as she grew out her natural grey hair after years of coloring it: "It's about WAY more than the growth of your hair. It's the growth of WHO YOU ARE. The internal transformation that happens over time is full of great surprise and wonder. The realization of accepting yourself exactly the way you are."[17]

The yoking of piety with identity is important for understanding wellness culture because it illustrates that wellness is never just about the supplements you take or the diets you follow: wellness is entirely bound up with who you are as a person. To explain the link between piety and identity before moving to supplement rituals, I want to pause here to introduce three interrelated types of piety that apply to wellness, which I return to later in the chapter. First, pieties of wellness are constitutive in that they call us forth as particular types of people. This is because, as Kenneth Chase argues, "symbolic realities have within them valences and attraction directing the [pious] agent toward certain duties and away from others."[18] In other words, we *become* wellness seekers in part by acting in accordance with pieties of wellness culture. Second, pieties of wellness invite and even require adherence to deeply held beliefs about wellness as a form of responsible health citizenship, a concept discussed in chapter 2 that links here to the concept of civic piety. The good, or pious, wellness citizen is one who accepts responsibility for their own wellness and that of their family (and in this case also that of their hair). Finally, the pieties of wellness espoused by Vegamour tie into what Emma Bloomfield terms neoliberal piety, an overarching schema that in wellness discourse classifies protecting and promoting wellness as a matter of individual, market-oriented policies and practices rather than a matter of collective social action. Vegamour's pieties of wellness frame the thinning of women's hair with age as an individual failing that is best addressed by using Vegamour products rather than by countering the ageist and sexist beliefs that frame thin hair as a problem in the first place. These three varieties of piety—constitutive, civic, and neoliberal—all inflect the pieties of wellness that circulate in the world of natural health.

As I have illustrated thus far, wellness culture is shaped by distinct pieties that govern how people think about their health and their bodies, as well as how they think about themselves. These pieties script performances of wellness, both for the self and for others. However, the relationship between script and performance is never linear, moving from script to performance. Every time a script is performed, it changes, and those changes in turn change subsequent performances, ad infinitum. As in theater, cultural performances both produce and reproduce the scripts that animate them. Enactments of wellness constitute performance of a very specific sort, more akin to a rite of passage or religious ceremony than to a stage play. The pieties just discussed aim to move those who heed them toward a state of physical, psychological, and even spiritual transformation because wellness is, at its core, a form of ritual.

Performing Supplement Rituals

To illustrate the links between piety and ritual performance in the language of wellness, I want to return to the interviews I conducted with Canadians who use natural health products to enhance their wellness. In those interviews, I heard a range of narratives of daily wellness routines, both at the start of the interview, when I asked each participant to talk about the supplements they use regularly (daily or weekly) for at least part of the year, and when they discussed other aspects of their beliefs about and use of natural health products. Many of those narratives were brief and straightforward lists, such as these:

Serrapeptase, conenzyme Q10, nitric oxide, natto, apple cider vinegar, kombucha, teas, HD, targeted vitamins.[19]

Vegan multivitamins, milk thistle, concentrated turmeric, magnesium, probiotics, cranberry extract, herbal teas, essential oils.[20]

Vitamin B, vitamin A, vitamin D, vitamin K, nutritional yeast, riboflavin, saw palmetto, lavender, rosemary, thyme, cedar wood oil, peppermint.[21]

Vitex, Balance Tea, Bach Flower Remedy Rescue Drops, dandelion root tea, Saje products, tea tree oil, vitamin B, vitamin D.[22]

Several participants brought to their interviews handwritten records of the products they use regularly to make sure they remembered to list all of them. Numerous participants became self-conscious about the number of products they consume, and some even expressed surprise on hearing themselves say the full list out loud. For instance, Gene, the construction worker in his fifties, responded with a good-natured laugh when asked about his regular supplements and said, "I have a list—I came prepared. So I will get my glasses on and then I will let you know. It's kind of long, I was surprised. But here we go."[23] Gene's routine included daily vitamins, probiotics, fish oil, and other supplements, as well as specialized products he uses when he needs specific types of support, such as when he has trouble sleeping or feels a cold coming on. Multiple participants expressed concern about whether an element of their routine, such as taking multivitamins or drinking soups made from Chinese medicinal herbs, would "count" for my study, but whatever their routine, all forty participants had a clear sense of their routine *as* a routine, as a repeated pattern of behaviors undertaken for a specific end.

While some participants simply listed off their supplements as above, numerous people instead offered full-bodied narratives rendered in careful detail, not only enumerating the supplements they use but also describing how and why they use them. For instance, Ariel, an acupuncturist in her early thirties, explained that she could not offer a simple summary of the supplements she uses: "I do a rotation actually. So I don't take the same thing, usually, for more than two months. I don't want my body to get used to it." She explained that because her wellness requires precise, ongoing maintenance, she must tailor her supplement strategy to her present needs. At the time of the interview, for example, she was using the botanical product ashwagandha, which purportedly helps bodies respond to periods of stress, "just in case there's, like, some burnout there."[24] For Ariel, the daily wellness routine is more than a list of products to take; because her routine is carefully optimized to meet her evolving needs, it is deeply invested with meaning about how she cares for her body and for herself. Ariel believes that by rotating products based on what she feels she needs at a given time, she can have control over her wellness.

All forty interview participants framed their efforts to achieve wellness in accordance with pieties such as those I have already discussed, including the pieties that wellness is best managed daily with natural, plant-based remedies and that women should be calm even under pressure. Animated by these pieties, the daily supplement routine functions for these individuals as a ritual that, performed step by step, serves as a gateway to wellness. This ritual holds deep cultural and personal significance because it promises to effect change within the wellness seeker's world. For this reason, it is useful to view wellness and supplementation in terms of ritual theory that emerges out of the field of performance studies.[25] Scholars in this field examine the continuities between formal rituals, such as coming-of-age rites, marriages, and religious ceremonies, and informal rituals, such as giving high-fives, rising for the national anthem, and smashing a bottle on the hull of a new boat. Both formal and informal rituals constitute a form of cultural performance in that they involve the enactment of social roles in dynamic action that unfolds according to scripts and sequences of behavior that are to some extent predetermined and repeated across performances. These formal and informal rituals can be sacred or secular, performed alone or in groups, but they are all oriented to achieving some state of permanent or temporary transformation. Examples of such transformation range from changes in legal status (in the case of marriage) or social status (in the case of coming-of-age rites) to expressing positive affect and affirming relationships (in the case of high-fives).

Viewing ritual as performance situates ritual within the broader tradition of how people *do* things in the social world. For Turner, arguably the key figure in early studies of ritual as performance, ritual is an *"enactment"* along the same line as performance, wherein "to perform is thus to bring something about, to consummate something, or to *'carry out'* a play, order or project. But in the 'carrying out,' I hold, something new may be generated. The performance transforms itself."[26] In other words, ritual is a form of cultural performance that is aimed at effecting some sort of transition or change, some kind of "doing" in the world. Just as saying a certain set of words or phrases in a specific order can perform the speech act of pronouncing a marriage, performing a certain set of ritual actions (words but also gestures, sounds, and manipulation of objects or space) can perform the action of becoming an adult, showing respect, or mourning.

The parallels between ritual performance and speech acts is no mistake: early ritual scholars recognized that rituals perform action just as words do. By aligning ritual with speech acts (which, incidentally, J. L. Austin dubbed "performative utterances" or *"performatives"*), we can situate ritual within the realm of human action more generally.[27] When we view wellness routines as ritual, we are therefore able to ask, What do these routines *do*? How do they effect transformation? What is the nature of that transformation? Is transformation permanent or fleeting? What cultural values do these routines generate, maintain, or disrupt? What meanings do they produce?

To begin to answer these questions, let us look at how June, a call center worker in her late fifties, responded to my request at the start of her interview for a list of products she takes regularly to enhance her wellness. Instead of running through her supplements like items on a grocery list, as so many other participants did, she walked methodically through her daily routine, which I quote here in full:

> I start every morning taking three capsules of NAC [N-acetyl cysteine], and that does something for the mind, I forget. It was recommended by my naturopath. And I take two capsules of theanine, which is supposed to be a relaxant. And then I wait a half an hour, and then I start eating and then, with my first meal of the day, I take an advanced B complex, and then I take that again at lunch. Um, I take the advanced [vitamin] B's to help me relax. I take two calcium and a magnesium, which is pretty obvious, probably—you know, osteoporosis prevention. I do that again at lunchtime.
>
> And . . . what else do I take? I take 3000 vitamin C. This is, believe it or not, for my mental health but it also helps to ward off disease. What else do I take? I take cinnamon. I actually started the cinnamon at the same time as I started Jenny Craig last year and cinnamon is known to have an effect on blood sugar. So, sometimes I think, I don't know if it was Jenny Craig, maybe it was the cinnamon but, anyhow, I'm not going to stop taking the cinnamon [*laughs*].
>
> I take chromium, which is supposed to have an effect on the blood sugar as well, as far as my understanding is. And I take that at breakfast and I take that during the lunchtime. . . . I take a multi-SAP [sodium ascorbyl phosphate], which is a multivitamin. I take that during the morning as well in the afternoon, and I take two teaspoons of fish oil, super EFA [essential fatty acids]. Yeah, so that's what I take daily.[28]

There are several key, overlapping elements in June's narrative of her daily wellness routine that crystallize the ritual performance of wellness through the use of natural health products. Let us look at five of these elements briefly in turn.

First, June's wellness routine is carefully rationalized and sequenced: she has a goal (wellness), she knows the particular challenges she faces in her pursuit of this goal (stress, decreasing bone mass, weakened immunity, high blood sugar), and she follows a clearly determined sequence to meet that goal (consuming certain supplements at certain times in a certain order). These characteristics of June's routine fit within anthropologist Roy Rappaport's landmark definition of ritual as "the performance of more or less invariant sequences of formal acts and utterances not entirely encoded by the performers."[29] June's natural health routine is not as structured and invariant as a formal ritual such as a liturgy (Rappaport's example), but its ordered sequence, timing, and goals resonate with formal rites in religious and spiritual practice.

Second, paralleling communion and other ritual practices of ingestion, June follows a pattern of concrete physical acts that include taking substances into her body, all in the service of an outcome that may not register in immediate physical experience. As with taking the Eucharist, June can see, touch, and potentially smell and taste the natural health products she consumes, but as with Communion, the outcome of her ritual is neither sharply defined nor concrete. She does not know *for sure* that the NAC positively affects her mind or that cinnamon does indeed lower her blood sugar. Rituals associated with supplementation are thus future-oriented and optimistic: the wellness seeker performs a sequence of embodied actions in the service of a goal that may not register in physical experience. The daily enactments of this ritual—opening a container, parceling out a dose, preparing and swallowing it, timing the next dose, as well as the associated rituals of researching, choosing, and obtaining products—therefore become not only a part of what June does but, equally importantly, part of who she is.

Third, June's routine is repeatable. It consists of a set of behaviors that she performs in roughly the same sequence each day and that closely resemble the behaviors of other wellness seekers although June may be unaware of those resemblances. To put this in terms of performance theory, June's daily wellness routine consists of what Richard Schechner calls "restored behavior" or "twice-behaved behavior." For Schechner, all performances have already been performed in some way before; everything we do or say, even when we think we are being spontaneous and original, has, in effect, been done and said before. He described restored behavior as "living behavior treated as a film director treats a strip of film," which can be cut, rearranged, and spliced together. He argues that strips of behavior are separate from their political, intellectual, and technological origins because restored behavior is "out there," separate from the performer; it is "'me behaving as if I were someone else,' or 'as I am told to do,' or 'as I have learned.'"[30]

For June and others who engage in supplement rituals, the performance is made up of strips of behavior that come largely from medicine. These behaviors often resemble rituals associated with clinical consultations with health professionals, including the "plot" of the office visit, which moves from identification of symptoms to diagnosis to treatment; the setting, which moves from reception to waiting area to consultation room; the script, which includes conversations between patients and practitioners, the use of honorific titles, the unfolding of diagnostic processes and tests (palpating the body, drawing blood), and the prescription of treatments; the wardrobe, including lab coats and paper gowns; and props, such as stethoscopes, tongue depressors, and various gadgets. Even more significant, supplement routines involve rituals associated specifically with pharmaceuticals, including the "prescription" (whether by self or practitioner), obtaining the product from a pharmacy or specialty supplement store (which often resemble pharmacies), ingesting the product as instructed, and so on. Furthermore, in most cases, supplements, like pharmaceuticals, come in bottles of pills (e.g., capsules, tablets, softgels) that are also swallowed with water according to a specified schedule and dose.

The acts just described—visiting a clinic, receiving a prescription or recommendation, obtaining a treatment, swallowing a dose—constitute strips of behavior that together in some combination make up most of the rituals associated with supplementation. Indeed, these rituals so closely resemble those standard in medicine that although the wellness seekers studied in this book vehemently maintain that natural health products are fundamentally distinct from pharmaceuticals, the language they use to describe them routinely renders them indistinguishable. Further, the blurry boundary between natural health rituals and those in mainstream medicine contributes significantly to the strength and importance of supplement routines because those routines are animated by pieties associated with *both* medicine and wellness. That is, wellness seekers not only pick up and respond to the pieties of wellness that circulate in public culture such as those I discussed above (e.g., "Wellness is manageable with natural, plant-based remedies"); they are also affected by those that circulate, somewhat differently, in biomedicine (e.g., "The body is always at the edge of illness or failure and in need of external intervention to maintain function"; see chapter 1).

Fourth, June's wellness routine is motivated by a strong element of faith—faith in her naturopath's advice, in her own instincts, and in the supplements' effectiveness. The performance of any ritual, whether sacred or secular, is powered by belief that the ritual will be effective even when we cannot have concrete proof that it has achieved its intended effect. June is not always certain about the purpose of each of the products she uses or its effectiveness, but she takes them all the same because she believes they will have a positive impact on her wellness. Each morning, for instance, she takes capsules of N-acetyl cysteine (NAC) because she thinks the product "does something for the mind, I forget. It was recommended by my naturopath." June admits that she is unsure what NAC does, but she still takes it regularly because she trusts her naturopath and, in turn, the product itself. Similarly, she takes supplementary cinnamon because she believes it might help lower her blood sugar, a belief that is based on her own previous experience of successful weight loss by combining the Jenny Craig diet with cinnamon supplements. Balancing inference with hope, she reflected: "I don't know if it was Jenny Craig, maybe it was the cinnamon but, anyhow, I'm not going to stop taking the cinnamon." Chromium is another product in June's daily wellness routine that she is unsure about but uses anyway: "I take chromium, which is supposed to have an effect on the blood sugar as well, as far as my understanding is."[31] Her use of *supposed* here indicates her uncertainty about chromium's effects. She thinks it will improve her blood sugar, but she does not know for sure. All she can do is follow the routine and hope it has an effect.

Fifth, June's daily supplement routine is an embodied act that she performs to initiate her transformation into a state of wellness. At least part of this potential for transformation, if not all of it, stems from the fact that the enactment alone of any ritual can affect the person enacting or experiencing it.[32] The power of ritual *as* ritual is evident not only in religious or mystical rites but also in more earthbound situations such as health and healthcare. Biomedical healing rites have been shown to improve patient outcomes even in cases of nonspecific symptoms and symptoms without immediately recognizable biological causes (e.g., pain, fatigue). Although these improvements are often dismissed as placebo effects (improvement based on expectation and belief) or as interactive effects (improvement based on interpersonal care),[33] they can also be attributed in part to the ritual "strips of behavior" associated with biomedicine discussed above, from doctor's visits to exams, diagnostics, treatments, and technologies. These rituals precipitate a performative "magic" that translates quite directly to wellness and natural health: the enactment of a supplement ritual may itself initiate a shift in a person's perceived well-being.[34] In June's case, sorting through her supplements, timing them with meals, touching and swallowing the tablets and capsules, and waiting for the next dose are all physical enactments of a ritual that, through its daily repetition, sharpens her conviction regarding the ritual and its effects.

Because June's supplement routine is loaded with symbolic potential for helping her achieve an enhanced state of wellness, it can usefully be considered as what Turner and later ritual scholars term a *liminal* act, a rite intended to facilitate a person's passage from one state of being to another. Liminal acts are "threshold" acts (*limen* means "threshold") in that they occur on the threshold between states. Liminal rites such as coming-of-age ceremonies, marriages, and graduation ceremonies formally transform their participants through culturally standardized rituals with clearly demarcated states of "before" and "after," as well as a period during the rite itself in which participants are suspended between states. (Mid-rite, one is no longer a child but not yet an adult, no longer single but not yet married, no longer a student but not yet graduated.) It is tempting to focus on the before and after of liminal rites, but ritual scholars remind us that the in-between period is particularly rich with signification. For wellness, the in-between state is key to understanding its cultural power and prevalence because those who seek wellness arguably remain perpetually suspended in a liminal state: since wellness has no ceiling, they never fully transform. For instance, although June earnestly follows her supplement routine each day, she never *becomes* well. For this reason we might more properly consider supplement routines as *liminoid* rituals, to use Turner's term, rather than liminal, as the transformations they initiate are only ever temporary.[35]

Whether we call the daily rituals associated with wellness liminal or liminoid, they are an important part of understanding how we perform wellness culturally. These rituals are embodied, they are repeated and repeatable, they organize our experiences of our bodies and our health, and they facilitate our efforts toward finding wellness. These rituals are performed individually and collectively at kitchen tables, in bedrooms and bathrooms, at clinics and drugstores, online, in books and magazines, and elsewhere, animated by shared scripts that emerge out of collective material-discursive practices. As these piety scripts are performed and reperformed, they circulate widely in culture and inform individual behavior by telling us what the pious wellness seeker ought to do. Further, these pieties and their public and private enactments also precipitate the feelings of obligation that manifest in and drive wellness culture as a self-generating discourse.

Performing at the Altar of Wellness

If natural health routines constitute a ritual performance scripted by cultural pieties, then the altar of wellness is the conceptual space within which these performances unfold. For Burke, altars are a key metaphor for understanding rhetorical piety. In religious rites, the altar serves as a physical surface upon which devotional practices are prepared and performed, whereas in rhetorical performances of piety the altar is a metaphorical locus of devotion, an organizing point toward which the pious person directs their attention. In Seigel's analysis of pregnancy, for instance, the pious pregnant person organizes their actions around the altar of pregnancy and what they believe it is pious to do and not do as a pregnant person.[36] In the world of natural health, those who manage their health and well-being with supplements gather at the altar of wellness alongside those who adopt other approaches, such as mind-body practices, nutritional programs, apps, coaches, gurus, optimization systems, and more. Seeking to restore and enhance their wellness, these individuals act in accordance with the pieties of wellness they have picked up from the world around them, adhering to their sense of what is appropriate to say and do so they can approach the altar of wellness with "clean hands," as Burke puts it.[37] By following the pieties that script their ritual enactments, wellness seekers aim to join themselves with their object of devotion, to *be* well. Wellness therefore functions for its devotees as a form of faith, of "spiritual sustenance," as Brigid Delaney explains in *Wellmania*.[38] Natural health supplements serve as both rites of purification and expressions of devotion at the altar of wellness. The altar is the focal point of the wellness seek-er's attention as well as the abstracted space where piety manifests as action.

In this second half of the chapter, I draw together the threads I laid out in the first half to show how piety and ritual actualize in performances of wellness and how those performances script our lives and shape our obligations. I have orga-nized this section under three main heads that together explain what we worship when we worship at the altar of wellness: nature, medicine, and the self. In each of these subsections, I examine wellness as it is performed both publicly and pri-vately, drawing on a range of sources that include the interviews and Bill C-51 petition comments discussed throughout this book as well as Instagram posts from corporate and individual accounts. Instagram posts are steeped in ritual; they involve reaching for a device (most often a phone), logging in, establishing setting and lighting, choosing angles and poses, selecting photos, posting and editing them, writing captions and hashtags, and so on. Using Instagram likewise involves rituals—opening the app; scrolling on images, accounts, and ads; liking and commenting on posts; and sending and receiving messages. Ad-ditionally, Instagram posts are produced and consumed in tension with the pre-vailing pieties of wellness that both shape and are shaped by their content. Ins-tagram is therefore a critical site for understanding how pieties of wellness script its performance; as Delaney observes, if natural health provides "spiritual suste-nance," Instagrammers serve as "patron saints who demonstrate how it is done."[39]

Because my analysis below gathers and extends observations I have made both earlier in this chapter and in previous chapters, my discussion moves briskly at times to avoid repetition. However, the first subsection, on nature worship, takes a little more time to set up because the primary texts I examine are new and take my discussion in some new directions. The varying lengths of the three subsec-tions that follow thus do not reflect their relative complexity or significance, but simply the degree to which I have discussed their contents and effects in other parts of this book.

Worshipping Nature

Approaching the altar of wellness with "clean hands" means living in accordance with the pieties of wellness that surround us. Two of the most dominant associ-ated pieties are that wellness is natural and that natural is authentic. In con-temporary Western life, nature has become such an object of worship that the adjective *natural* has become a "theological term," according to religion scholar Alan Levinovitz, because nature has transformed into a para-religious force that signals holiness, purity, and virtue, as well as health, truth, and authenticity.[40] Recall, for instance, that the "Stop Bill C-51" petition signatories passionately argued that natural health products were safe and pure because they came straight from nature, a pristine, God-like originary force. As a marketplace descriptor, Levinovitz argues, *natural* now works as "an earnest metaphor for goodness," harkening back to an Eden-like state of purity that suggests how we ought to look, eat, and behave, and so it serves as a consumer "shorthand" for a food or product's origin and production.[41] As a shorthand descriptor, *natural* therefore operates in product marketing as an enthymeme, an implicit argument that relies on an audience to complete its logical chain of reasoning.[42] Products labeled "natural" generally do not specify what that means, leaving consumers to infer that the product is pure, healthy, and authentic. By extension, conventional products not classified as "natural" become in comparison unholy—evil—and to be avoided. As consumers, we are regularly exhorted to believe that buying natural health products means we are being true to nature, true to our wellness, and true to ourselves. Through nature, we can be born anew, unpolluted and pure.

The public performance of wellness is shot through with implicit arguments regarding the superiority of natural health products, most notably that they are cleaner, safer, and more effective than their conventional alternatives. For example, Delaney dedicates a full third of *Wellmania* to understanding the power of "clean" products and services, particularly supplement-supported cleanses. On the eleventh day of her 101-day cleanse described in chapter 5, Delaney enthuses about her "lovely, clean, clear, superfast brain," which feels as if it "has been thoroughly rinsed, tuned and given extra component parts."[43] Here, *clean* has overlapping meanings—that her brain is free of toxins, banished from her body during the cleanse, and that her mind is unencumbered by metaphorical dirt and debris from overuse (toxic thoughts, feelings) and so is, in effect, brand-new. After undergoing the physical and spiritual trial of a grueling, low-calorie, supplement-supported regimen, Delaney feels purified and reborn even while she remains critical of cleanses and the wellness culture they support. In wellness culture, Delaney argues, the clean brain is the natural brain.

On Instagram, posts about wellness trade on natural products' associations with purity and redemption, promoting what Levinovitz terms *consecrated consumption*, or the ritual of shopping for retail products anointed with spiritual properties of nature.[44] Consider, for example, the Instagram presence of the lifestyle and wellness company goop (stylized without capital letters) from the

American actress turned guru Gwyneth Paltrow. As an e-commerce website and an in-house brand selling health, beauty, and home goods, goop forges associations with a clean lifestyle wherever possible, from its "clean" design palate on its website, products, and social media channels (muted colors; simple, clear lines; generous white space; minimalist typography) to its product descriptions and promotions, which emphasize clean products and clean living. Scholar of religion and ritual Dana W. Logan explains that in valorizing "clean" products, goop promotes a form of asceticism for the privileged as consumers turn to its products to help them cleanse themselves spiritually, socially, emotionally, and physically.[45] For Logan, it was no surprise that goop's most searched term in 2016, the year prior to the publication of Logan's article, was *detox*. goop trades on a promise to help its customers purify and redeem themselves through the goodness of nature.

Paltrow's own public Instagram account complements goop's account by reinforcing and personalizing the company's claims to clean, natural living. She frequently features snapshots from her own daily life—Gwyneth floating on an air mattress on a lake, Gwyneth making a goofy face on a talk show, Gwyneth with her kids—among posts featuring her company's products. In one post from August 2020, Paltrow uploaded an image of a tightly framed shot of her white medicine cabinet lined with clear glass shelves, which held a range of tinctures in droppers and spray bottles, some tubes of creams, what appears to be blue mouthwash, and an electric toothbrush alongside a regular plastic toothbrush in a white ceramic cup. The cabinet is unremarkable aside from the fact that the many items contained within it are goop products. Beside the image is a caption that reads, "I think pretty much everything in my medicine cabinet is non-toxic and clean by our standards at @goop. We work hard to make and curate products that really work and are better for you. #goopglow," followed by an orange heart emoji.[46] This Instagram post conveys a pair of interrelated pieties, that the products we use should be pure ("nontoxic and clean") and that we should use products that really do work, while at the same time Paltrow's ordinary-looking medicine cabinet demonstrates that those pieties are within reach for ordinary people. Paltrow may be glamorous, but like the rest of us, she uses a disposable plastic toothbrush.

Clean and its sibling term *detox*, the process of "making clean," recur throughout the world of Instagram wellness, both on official accounts of supplement companies and on accounts of celebrities, influencers, and private consumers.[47] For example, goop frequently uses the hashtag "goodcleangoop" to promote products such as its collagen supplement called GOOPGENES Marine Collagen Superpowder, a drink mix promoted on goop's sales website as a way to counter the unnatural effects of exposure to pollution and UV rays, as well as age.[48] (Notably, in wellness culture age itself is as good as unnatural.) The former *Glee* star Lea Michele similarly promotes detoxification products and services on her personal Instagram account, including charcoal products from goop along with supplement-supported cleanses, infrared saunas, and cryotherapy chambers. Michele promotes these activities as ways to purify herself from exposure to unnatural substances and activities such as air travel, work stress, and prescription pharmaceuticals. In one post from 2018, for instance, Michele posted an image of mason jars filled with liquid with a caption reading, "Starting a 4 day cleanse from @owlvenice today! After taking medicine and not feeling well it's so important to detox your system! Let's do this!"[49] For Michele, the cleanse becomes the centerpiece of a purification ritual that will restore her to her natural state, free of illness or medication.

The worship of nature is much more overt on the Instagram account for INBLOOM, American actress Kate Hudson's line of drinkable "nutritional powders." INBLOOM's biography on the main account page reads, "Live in Full Bloom with @katehudson / Inside out wellness and nutritional powders from nature. / Non-GMO [green-leaf emoji] Plant-based [Earth emoji] Earth-friendly."[50] This biography statement situates nature as an object of worship at the altar of wellness by emphasizing the products' purity (no genetically modified organisms, no animal products), their "naturalness" (they are "from nature," made from plants, and "Earth-friendly"), and their sustaining qualities ("nutritional," "Inside out wellness"). INBLOOM's Instagram feed continues these themes in images featuring the company's products both on their own and with Hudson holding them in various settings at home (by the pool, in the bath, in bed, playing with her children). These images are accompanied by captions that insistently refer to nature, plants, "green" power, natural beauty, and "Mother Nature." For example, a post about INBLOOM's Brain Flow cognition blend is captioned, "Our formulas are inspired by the powerful properties of the earth's most incredible plants," followed by a green plant emoji.[51] INBLOOM's products are powerful because they are made of plants that come directly from nature. Further, because these products are "Earth-friendly," made without toxins or genetically modified organisms, when we use INBLOOM, we in turn take care of Mother Nature.

Even the method of delivery of INBLOOM's products—powder—becomes part of the company's argument that its supplements are powerful because they are natural. For example, the caption of a short video posted on the company's Instagram page showing how to mix the products with liquid explains, "Because INBLOOM powders are made from whole foods, plants, and herbs, they perform their best when whisked, shaken, or blended into liquid."[52] The main argument in the caption is that powders, rather than capsules or pills, are the most natural form for your body to absorb because, again according to the caption, "they have higher bioavailability in this form. That basically means they enter your digestive system almost immediately." Overall, INBLOOM's Instagram posts tell viewers that the pious wellness seeker uses natural products to reach their wellness goals and should seek INBLOOM because, as another caption explains, "our products are an example of what you can make when you work with nature, the right way. . . . Enjoy nature's bounty as it was intended."[53] Put more simply, worshipping nature is the most natural thing you can, and should, do.

The governing pieties that have emerged so far in my discussion of wellness as nature worship are that wellness is natural and that natural is authentic because it is close to nature.[54] The first of these pieties corresponds with my discussion in other chapters, most notably in chapter 3, of arguments that emerge in the comments on the petition against Bill C-51. These arguments include the positions that because natural health products are natural, they are safe and effective; that because pharmaceuticals are unnatural, they are unsafe and/or ineffective; and that because people are responsible for their own health and wellness, they must make the right choice by choosing natural products. The second piety, that natural products are authentic and original, suggests to consumers that if you use natural health products, you are yourself more authentic than if you used unnatural products such as pharmaceuticals.

This piety, that we become natural and authentic when we use natural, authentic products, is a type of constitutive piety because it calls us forth, or *constitutes* us, as certain types of people.[55] This piety resonates throughout the other research sites I examine in this book, including the interviews I conducted with Canadian wellness seekers. For instance, Tania, who is in her late forties and on medical leave from her job, explained that "I don't want to be that youngish person with all these prescription bottles, you know? I'd rather do it naturally if I could."[56] Here Tania associates the health products she uses with the type of person she is. For her, choosing natural products becomes a form of community identification and participation, and so to be authentically her age and to be authentically well, Tania wants her health interventions to align with her sense of self. Of course, the forms of authenticity sold by supplement producers such as goop and INBLOOM do not come cheaply, so as Levinovitz argues, "Being real becomes a luxury," one that not everyone can access.[57]

The final piety I want to discuss in association with nature worship in the performance of wellness is that natural health products are vessels of divine community. We see this piety at work in Instagram posts that emphasize wellness as a form of collective worship, where those who use natural health products engage in shared practices of ritual ingestion that are mobilized by faith in nature. One image from INBLOOM, for example, features Kate Hudson swimming in a deep turquoise pool that is superimposed by the text of positive product reviews from customers. Next to the image is a caption that says, "We're all on our own wellness journeys but together, we're a community Being INBLOOM."[58] We also see the piety that supplements constitute divine community reflected in goop captions that address consumers as part of a nature-worshiping community, signaled by the use of inclusive first-person pronouns such as *we, us,* and *our.* And we see this piety at work in hashtags promoted by Lea Michele such as "#wellness-wednesday" and goop's "#goodcleangoop," which gather posts from different corporate, public, and private users to assemble a wellness congregation of sorts. These individual performances of wellness on Instagram cohere into collectives that in turn script for others how to be well.

The piety that natural health products are vessels of divine community is also performed through a recurring type of image that appears frequently in the Instagram feeds of wellness influencers and celebrities in poses reminiscent of Holy Communion in Christian religious traditions. In these religious traditions, Communion is a form of consecrated consumption in its most literal sense, as worshippers consume wafers and wine (or juice) that have been consecrated as the body and blood of Christ. In the realm of Instagram wellness, users post images in which they hold a natural health product before their open mouths, receiving the product on their tongue almost as if it were a Communion wafer. Sisters and American reality TV stars Khloé and Kim Kardashian (fig. 13), for instance, posted photos of themselves holding gummies from the supplement company Sugarbear Hair in front of their parted lips. These gummies are marketed as "hair vitamins" shaped as gummy bears and sold under the tagline "Get healthy hair, eat the blue bear."[59] Sugarbear Hair does not associate its products with nature as explicitly as INBLOOM and goop do, but the company nevertheless signals its products' purity through proxy indicators, such as identifying them as vegan and cruelty free and using emojis of green leaves.

In these images, which are tagged on Instagram as advertisements in paid partnership with Sugarbear Hair, both women pose with the product in a highly stylized format, each with full makeup, sleek, straight hair, and minimal clothing (Khloé wears a turquoise bodysuit; Kim is in a tan bandeau and tan sweatpants). Khloé holds a bottle of Sugarbear Hair vitamins with a turquoise label toward the viewer, whereas Kim has a similar bottle beside her on the back of the

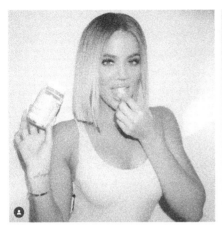 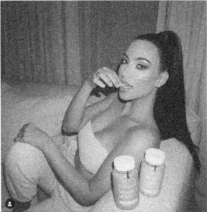

Figure 13. Screenshots of Khloé Kardashian (*left*) and Kim Kardashian (*right*) promoting Sugarbear Hair gummies on Instagram. (@khloekardashian) Instagram photo, August 15, 2017, from Longhetti, "That's Some Pocket Money!"; (@kimkardashian) Instagram photo, December 13, 2018.

couch, next to a bottle of multivitamins by the same company. Complicating the images' associations with Communion, the lighting, wardrobe, styling, and pose of each image is also reminiscent of soft porn advertising at the back of free weekly newspapers. The sisters each hold their lips open as they place the gummies in their mouths while looking directly at the camera, signaling the presence in these posts of other cultural scripts regarding conventional femininity, hetero-sexual desire, and consumer culture.[60] Nevertheless, the Communion-style posing in these images (and in the many others like them on Instagram) reinforces visually the place and significance of natural health products in many wellness seekers' lives. As with June's wellness routine, supplementation is here depicted visually as a ritual practice of ingestion mobilized by faith in nature, illustrating the para-religious weight of natural health rituals for those who engage in them.

Another way that social media posts about supplement rituals foster divine communities of nature worship is by prompting subsequent users to internalize and reproduce their orienting pieties. We can see how this process of uptake occurs in a 2017 article by Virginia Van De Wall posted to the website of *Life & Style* magazine, "We Tried Those Kardashian-Approved SugarBearHair Vitamins and Here's What Happened."[61] The article's main premise is that Sugarbear Hair gummies are newsworthy simply because the Kardashian sisters posted about them on their Instagram pages. This fact alone illustrates the significance of public performances of wellness. More revealing is Van de Wall's invitation to readers to "check out our reviews and cute photos (because it's pretty much mandatory that you have a photo shoot with them, duh)." Her parenthetical aside that "it's pretty much mandatory" to take pictures of yourself with the supplements explicitly acknowledges how social media posts script future communications about wellness. Individuals who see posts from the Kardashian sisters, or from INBLOOM or goop, may internalize and subsequently perform the pieties conveyed in those posts. Even more to the point, Van de Wall's own article follows her edict to do a photo shoot by including images of the author and four of her magazine colleagues each posing with the gummies à la the Kardashians. The quality of the photos is not comparable to that of the Kardashians' Instagram posts—the lighting, camera angles, make-up, and wardrobe are all amateurish by comparison—but each image reproduces the same type of shot and pose. These images illustrate visually how social media performances of wellness produce a kind of script (here, "wellness as a form of Communion") that others can then follow.[62]

By tracking the uptake of cultural scripts of wellness, we gain insight into how performances of natural health function ritually as "lived codes that reinforce the temporal, social, and moral frameworks that define our identities."[63] We learn how to live the good life from idealized scripts of nature worship that tell us how to become purer and more authentic versions of ourselves. These scripts operate largely within the logic of enhancement, as evidenced by upbeat Instagram posts touting natural health products as tools for optimizing health, beauty, energy, sex, and more. Importantly, however, the selves we become through natural health rituals are never fully optimal because our performances of wellness always rest, at least partly, on the sense that we are not as good as we once were—that we are not as energetic or well rested, as sharp or resilient, or as buoyant and youthful. Although Sugarbear Hair gummies promise to make our hair thick, strong, and silky, they only do so by implying that our hair is currently not those things (it is instead, perhaps, thin, weak, and scraggly). Similarly, INBLOOM's "cognition blend" of nutritional powders, Brain Flow, promises to enhance our thinking, but only by implying that our brains are not, currently, "flowing."[64] Vacillating between the logics of enhancement and restoration, and between health and illness, performances of wellness always involve to some extent the worship of medicine.

Worshipping Medicine

The performance of wellness is necessarily animated partly by pieties that are imprinted by medicine itself. These pieties operate in the logic of restoration,

figuring wellness as an incipient illness that must be managed through medicalizing practices of surveillance and intervention. Even idealized images on
Instagram that emphasize the logic of enhancement still imply a deficiency at
their core (thin hair, sluggish brains) that must be addressed for access to the
good life. The tension between the logics of enhancement and restoration is even
more apparent off Instagram, in the less-varnished realm of everyday life, where
performances of wellness are not idealized but steeped in the messiness of
human experience. This is the realm where we get sick, we age, we become
overwhelmed, and we lose sleep, strength, and function. Medicine is therefore
at the center of why wellness sells: when we perform at the altar of wellness,
part of what we do is worship medicine. In what follows, I return to arguments
I have made in different terms in previous chapters, which I refract here
through the lens of wellness as the performance of four interrelated pieties.

The first piety that guides the performance of wellness as medicine worship
is that natural health is medicine. This piety emerges out of the rituals of diagnosis and treatment that shape discourse surrounding the use of natural health
products. This discourse medicalizes wellness as a condition that requires monitoring, intervention, and care. When June takes two capsules of the supplement
theanine each morning, for example, she is guided by the belief that stress is a
pathology that can be treated by an external intervention. Similarly, as I explained
earlier in this chapter, June's daily supplement routine is made up of "strips of
behavior" from medicine that include assessment, diagnosis, intervention, and
so on. Her supplements in turn function as hyperreal simulacra (or, more-than-
real simulations) of pharmaceuticals that become charged with the same social,
cognitive, and emotional significance as prescription medications.[65] Although
supplements do not contain the same ingredients as pharmaceuticals and many
lack scientific evidence to support their use, they too are synthesized in labs, come
in bottles of tablets, capsules, or powders, and are ingested orally to produce desired effects in the body. Indeed, as I have illustrated over the previous chapters,
natural health products frequently serve as pharmaceutical proxies, substitutes
that many wellness seekers believe are safer and more effective. (Recall, for instance, the interview participant who described using boric acid for vaginal yeast
infections instead of commercially available treatments, or another who used
white willow bark capsules instead of ibuprofen.) In the ritual performance of
wellness, natural health products function as the central liturgical object
around which individuals enact the piety that natural health is medicine.

The second piety of medicine worship in performances of wellness is that
medicine is absolution. This piety is evoked in the Kardashian sisters' promotion

of Sugarbear Hair as a form of spiritual Communion, as well as in goop's and INBLOOM's assertions that busy and overwhelmed consumers become sharper and more energetic after using their products. This piety also underlies the supplement-supported cleanses examined in chapter 3, in which individuals redeem their bodily sins through ritual purification, and is evoked in the remedies for sleep and stress examined in chapter 4. Those who seek help with sleep or concentration may simultaneously be seeking relief from guilt for being less energetic or less focused than they would like to be. The piety that medicine is absolution comes straight from rhetorics that accord to doctors and pharmaceuticals the reverence, authority, and respect once accorded to religious and spiritual figures.[66] As science and secularism expanded in Western culture over the twentieth century, medicine assumed some of the ministerial functions of the church because, as Levinovitz argues, "sick humans are not just broken machines."[67] Our experience of illness is not just physical but emotional and existential as well: when we are sick, it is not merely our bodies that are sick, it is *us*, and so we require care that can absolve us of our discomfort. That care might come in the form of a conversation with a health practitioner, but in contemporary culture it more often comes from a pill. Regardless of whether that pill contains pharmaceutical ingredients or ground-up plants, when we enter the ritual of treatment, we are guided by the piety that it will give us *relief.*

Stepping away from rituals of diagnosis and treatment, the third piety of medicine worship in performances of wellness is the civic piety that the good health citizen takes responsibility for their own health (and wellness). When June performs her daily health routine, for example, she enacts the role of the good health citizen by doing her part to maintain her bone strength, cognitive function, immunity, and blood sugar. She accepts responsibility for addressing her body's deficiencies in accordance with predominant neoliberal discourses that frame ill health as a personal, rather than public or systemic, failure. Similarly, when Delaney recounts in *Wellmania* the extreme cleanse she undertook with the guidance of her traditional Chinese medical practitioner, Dr. Liu, she explains that she became fixated on his recognition of her "good" behavior: "I know he is monitoring my daily weigh-ins and I obscurely want to please him. I'm not doing it for me; I'm doing it for Dr Liu."[68] When she overeats even months after her fast, she wonders to herself, "What would Dr Liu think?" What Delaney craves is an acknowledgment of her responsible wellness citizenship. We also see this piety that good health citizens take responsibility for their health in the "Stop Bill C-51" petition, as commenters assert that choosing which health interventions to use is a democratically protected right that allows them to fulfill their obligations of health citizenship.

The final piety of medicine worship at the altar of wellness is that we are not who we are, but who we could be with appropriate intervention. This piety runs in parallel with medicalization because the expansion of medical categories increasingly reframes ordinary parts of everyday life as medical problems that require treatment. Sugarbear Hair is again a good example: the authentic self is not the you who is reading these words right now but the one who takes appropriate steps to ensure their hair is as strong and thick and silky as it can possibly be. This is the you who is always out of reach in pharmaceutical culture as well as wellness culture, the one whose moods are more even, the one without acne, the one with full erectile function, the one with an unflinching attention span.

Writer and disability activist Eli Clare frames this piety of the idealized future self in his gorgeous book *Brilliant Imperfection: Grappling with Cure* as the fantasy of the other-bodied future. In this fantasy, we become so obsessed with becoming who we think we should be through "always-just-around-the-corner cures"[69] that we fail to serve those who need help in the present. For Clare this looks like focusing on cures for disability rather than investing in inclusionary measures such as accessibility, social supports, or poverty reduction. For individuals such as June this means spending hundreds of dollars on supplements when systemic-institutional supports may be more effective for maintaining her bone density, weight, and blood sugar through, say, appropriate urban design and infrastructure for active living and healthy eating. As Clare points out, when a treatment for a given health condition is available, it creates pressure that, in echoes of bioethicist Carl Elliott, exhorts us to become better than well. All we can do is accept or resist that pressure. The piety that we become ourselves through the interventions we choose leads me to the final form of worship I want to examine in the ritual performance of wellness, the worship of the self.

Worshipping the Self

When we view natural health products as liturgical objects for ritual performance at the altar of wellness, we tap into rhetorics of conversion and transcendence that center on the restoration and enhancement of the self.[70] Take the daily health routine, which is an embodied liminal act that involves performing a series of steps in accordance with cultural scripts of wellness to initiate a transformation in a person's state of being. When June takes her daily dose of theanine, she does so to transform from a state of stress to one relieved of stress. Similarly, when

INBLOOM customers use the Brain Flow cognition blend, they seek passage into an improved state of thinking, memory, and attention. In these examples, the logic of restoration becomes, in effect, a rhetorical process of conversion: we are low, depraved, and need salvation, and so we perform wellness rituals to initiate self-transformation. Correspondingly, wellness routines are also rituals of transcendence operating in the logic of enhancement because they aim to move us beyond the limitations of our present, a process that never ends because we can always be more pure, more devoted, and more self-actualized than we currently are. Operating within rhetorics of conversion and transcendence, wellness in contemporary culture is therefore ultimately about the individual who seeks it. Wellness promises each of us repair, autonomy, purification, respite, and optimal functioning, and it also provides us a script for becoming better versions of ourselves.

At the altar of wellness, the orienting piety for worship of the self is that the good self is authentic, virtuous, and well. Wellness serves as a form of personal branding in terms of both our public presentation and our own self-understanding. This piety tells us that by looking good and feeling good, we *are* good, and it gives people a way of affirming to themselves and others that "I am a virtuous, healthy person." Further, because wellness discourse figures natural health products as more authentic than pharmaceuticals, using those products makes us, by extension, more authentic people. Recall, for example, Tania's statement that "I don't want to be that youngish person with all these prescription bottles, you know? I'd rather do it naturally if I could."[71] Natural products make Tania feel truer to herself, more virtuous and authentically her age, whereas prescribed medicines make her feel prematurely old. Being good, authentic, and well is animated by an invisible script that determines who we should be and how we perform wellness.

A related piety of self-worship in natural health rituals is that you become yourself through wellness. This piety scripts wellness not as a destination but as a mode of becoming, a portal for transforming into who we (really) are. This is one of the biggest appeals of wellness because, as Delaney observes, "in the wellness industry we can self-actualise: follow our bliss and find individual contentment, be the best version of ourselves we can be."[72] Natural health rituals facilitate personal transformation on the order of religious or spiritual awakening, making possible our passage into revelatory new, more complete modes of being. Tania becomes herself when she uses natural mood stabilizers rather than Ativan, for example, and turmeric rather than ibuprofen, because these products better align her with her own self-understanding as a "youngish," well person rather than one with lots of prescription bottles. I feel something similar myself when I take the supplements recommended by my neurologist to ward off migraine attacks, relieved that at least they are not pharmaceuticals and I am not by association sick.

The pious self in wellness is one that accords with Burke's own characterization of piety as "the yearning to conform with the 'sources of one's being.'"[73] By seeking wellness, we in effect find our true selves. This is why even wellness skeptics such as Delaney can become captivated by "yoga sermons" and the other quasi-spiritual trappings of the highly lucrative commercial wellness market. She explains that even the most superficial, Instagram-ready forms of faux spiritualism can "lose their potential to annoy and instead can hit you in tender, devastating places. You drink them up. You didn't realise you were so thirsty."[74] I experienced that same sense of thirst when I first started writing this book, as I shared in chapter 4, when my own deep cynicism about wellness culture was outmatched by my deeper state of exhaustion. Significantly, the wellness seeker's thirst is never quenched. Becoming yourself is an ongoing process of restoration and enhancement, guilt and redemption; it is a lifelong project.

This last point brings us to the final piety of wellness I want to discuss regarding the worship of the self, that being yourself takes ongoing commitment and work. Wellness seekers are caught in an endless cycle of guilt and redemption that is at the heart of wellness as an autopoietic, or self-generating, system. Writing on neoliberal pieties of American climate discourse, Emma Bloomfield observes, citing Burke, that because "piety can be understood as a 'system-builder' that organizes reality and guides appropriate behavior, [in] keeping pious, people maintain the order, meaning that the order soon becomes a 'self-perpetuating structure, creating the measures by which it shall be measured.'"[75] Even when people work consciously to be pious, they inevitably trip up, but the beauty of piety is that "the construction of a piety carries with it the ability to authorize forgiveness."[76] If we correct our behavior to align with the pieties that govern our circumstances, we can become pious once again. Therefore, although we can never fully arrive at being "well" as it is defined in contemporary Western culture, if we want to be a pious wellness *self*, we must continue to try.

The pressure to continually work on ourselves comes from all around us in the rhetorical ecosystem of wellness; it is simply in the air, ambient. The pressure comes from particular products and people; from magazines, television, radio, and the internet; from friends, family, salespeople, strangers on the street. It comes from how others live, and in turn from ourselves in our feeling that to be good we must also live that way. We also learn the scripts of wellness from those who surround us, as June explained: "I remember I was living at a yoga center in '97 and this was a really good experience. I quit smoking cigarettes at that time and it was a very, very strictly healthy environment. . . . I was eating their diet. . . . There was one woman who was making her own yogurt and there were a lot of people with a lot of sensitivities, and I just really got into thinking along those lines even though I don't have particular sensitivities, thank goodness. I just really, you know, it was the milieu."[77] While June described feeling pressure to continually work on herself from her surrounding "milieu," others experience pressure from more specific sources, such as family and friends, health practitioners, marketing, popular media, film and television, and even their own perfectionist tendencies or health anxiety.

Collectively, we experience pressure from all sides to be as natural, authentic, beautiful, healthy, responsible, virtuous, and committed to our wellness as we can be. This pressure underlies the "moral demand" of wellness that Cederström and Spicer identify, the demand that to be good people we must constantly strive to improve ourselves. We may choose not to respond to that pressure, or we may be indifferent to it, or we may strain under it yet lack the time or resources to act, but the pressure to transform ourselves through wellness surrounds us all the same.

The irony of wellness as a form of self-worship, of course, is that true self-transformation requires not an obsession with the self but a destruction or forgetting of the self, so to remake it anew. As the cliché goes, you need to lose yourself to find yourself. In relentlessly centering the self, performances of wellness are therefore effectively short-circuited by the "infectious narcissism" of wellness culture, which fuels, rather than quells, our thirst for self-transformation.[78] Delaney describes just this experience of wellness-driven self-absorption during her extreme fast with Dr. Liu when she laments that she does not have the promised visions or feeling of being at one with the universe. Instead, she says, "I'm self-absorbed, and hyper-focused on my body and its processes. Such narcissism is surely the enemy of any sort of spiritual experience."[79] If wellness is a rhetorical performance of self-transformation, the cruel irony is that we never truly emerge on the other side of it, transformed. As we perform natural health rituals by acting out the pieties that tell us who and how to be, we can never quite become the one thing we seek above all: *well*.

Conclusion

I noticed my first gray hairs in November 2020, about eight months into the coronavirus pandemic, a small patch of silver blooming dead center above my forehead. I joked that the grays were caused by the pandemic, but in truth, I was neither surprised nor alarmed by their appearance, given my age. I paid them no further mind until the following summer, when I sat down one morning to write this conclusion and came across a newspaper article about the effects of pandemic stress on our bodies. The author, Wendy Leung, begins her article thus: "Your joints feel creakier. Your hair looks markedly greyer. The bags under your eyes seem to have become permanent fixtures. You're not just imagining it: The stress of the pandemic may have aged you prematurely."[1] Leung explains that the chronic stress of a prolonged crisis destroys the body's ability to repair itself, particularly by damaging mitochondria in our cells, protective caps on the ends of our chromosomes, and other cellular structures and processes. This damage apparently speeds up our cells' natural aging cycles, resulting in a phenomenon called cell death. This problem is compounded, according to Leung, by what one researcher she interviewed describes as a "threat spiral," when cell-damaging inflammation caused by stress causes our brains to become ever more vigilant and reactive to stress. This vigilance further exacerbates cellular damage and leads, among other things, to one's hair losing pigment and becoming gray. It turns out that my joke about pandemic grays may not have been far off the mark.

There is more to Leung's story about the pandemic's effect on stress and aging, however. Leung warns that our own behavior can also precipitate premature aging because when are stressed we tend to sleep and exercise less, as well as drink more alcohol and eat less well. This is problematic because the stress hormone cortisol affects how we metabolize food (including the bread that Americans and Canadians collectively devoured to the point of flour shortages early in the pandemic),[2] putting us at risk of gaining dangerous visceral fat around our organs. Further, notes Leung, reduced sleep and exercise can also increase our cortisol levels, magnifying the impact of stress on accelerated aging. But there is some good news too, Leung reports: "You can slow and perhaps, to some extent, turn back the clock, researchers say. Healthy habits, like eating and sleeping well, and especially physical activity, help mitigate the aging effects of stress." Leung explains, for example, that graying hair can sometimes be reversed if a person can avoid stress or mitigate its effects with cortisol-reducing activities such as exercise, sleep, and going on vacation. Leung therefore advises readers, "If you haven't been doing these things already, now is the time."[3]

The thing is, I had already been doing those things during the pandemic. While I was experiencing more stress than usual, I had taken pretty good care of myself. I slept a lot and exercised vigorously; I took up old-timey hobbies and read for pleasure; I tried to maintain perspective. I worked hard to manage my stress during the pandemic, and yet my hair still started to turn gray. Likely, it was just age. But perhaps I could have done more to reduce stress? Maybe if I had worked a bit harder to restore and enhance my wellness, I could have protected the cells in my hair follicles? Leung's article made me wonder if I had let myself down by assuming I was doing okay rather than investigating whether I was not. For a moment, only briefly, I felt both responsible for my new gray hairs and disappointed in myself. Wellness culture strikes again.

To conclude *Why Wellness Sells*, I circle back to how I began, with the global coronavirus pandemic first declared in March 2020, because Leung's story of pandemic stress and premature aging captures the essence of my overall argument. The momentary mix of doubt, responsibility, anxiety, and disappointment I experienced after reading the article could have been about anything that happened during the pandemic—graying hair, weight gained, productivity lost. Leung's article does not blame the reader for the pandemic, but it does, to some extent, hold the reader responsible for responding appropriately to the pandemic. The article suggests that I could, and should, have done more to restore and enhance my body after such sustained exposure to stress and that there is more I could still do. However, just as the pandemic was beyond my control, the most effective ways of reducing stress, such as reducing my workload or keeping my child's school open, were likewise beyond my control. Articles like Leung's—and they are legion—give us individual solutions to massive, systemic problems. These are problems better addressed through collective action, such as expanded public health infrastructure for disease surveillance and prevention, adequate healthcare funding and equipment, efficient and equitable vaccine production and distribution, and robust public assistance programs. Instead, we got calls for individual action, self-surveillance, and self-care. In the midst of crisis, we were encouraged to concentrate on what we could control, to look after ourselves, to take time out. We were encouraged, above all, to seek wellness.

As I have argued in the foregoing chapters, wellness sells because it has a horoscopic quality that invites individuals to find within it opportunities for self-determination and access to the good life, in whatever form those opportunities manifest for any individual person. The path to wellness may involve restoring your body to a perceived prior state of ideal health and functioning or enhancing it to become even better than it already is—faster, stronger, more productive, more resilient. Far more likely, the path to wellness involves seamless movement between these two logics, the logics of restoration and enhancement, one always slipping from grasp as the other comes into view. Returning to Leung's article, for example, if I had done more to reduce my cortisol levels during the pandemic, the article implies, I might have been able to restore the mitochondria in my hair follicles enough to regain my hair color. And yet, no matter what steps I took to restore my pre-pandemic self, there was still more I could do because I could always enhance my body's ability to ward off stress-related problems altogether. I could, for example, take supplements or follow a specific diet to optimize my body's resistance to stress-related inflammation. Regardless of what or how much I do, in this framing of pandemic wellness I am never doing enough. This is how arguments about wellness self-generate and grow, because they are driven by the tension between the logics of restoration and enhancement, forming a closed rhetorical system where wellness has no end point, no ceiling. Wellness is ever out of reach.

My main argument in *Why Wellness Sells* has therefore been that wellness is a self-generating rhetoric, that it is *autopoietic*. This argument emerges out of and builds on Lisa Keränen's initial introduction of autopoiesis to rhetorical studies, a concept she draws from social systems theory to explain how rhetorics of bioterror spiral and grow as perceptions of risk and subsequent risk surveillance grow. Rhetorics of wellness similarly self-generate as discourse about what it means to be well cycles through the opposing logics of restoration and enhancement. Like rhetorics of bioterror, rhetorics of wellness operate at the level of systems rather than at the level of individual rhetors, weaving through and across different the viral vectors of wellness examined in the previous chapters.

Chapter 1, for instance, illustrates how wellness discourse reframes wellness as a state of incipient illness that requires ongoing surveillance and intervention.

This reframing of wellness as illness-to-be is fueled by the logic of restoration, leaving individuals who use natural health products scrambling toward an ever-receding horizon of wellness. In this vector of wellness, even enhancement becomes a form of (pre-)illness that requires treatment. Chapter 2 examines wellness as a form of self-management that draws on both logics of wellness to call upon individuals to take responsibility for their own health and wellness as a condition of good citizenship. Supplements become in this vector a moral duty and a consumer right that shifts attention from systemic factors that affect wellness toward individual behaviors that appear to offer consumers autonomy precisely as they limit it. Both chapters highlight how wellness culture disavows the terms of pharmaceutical culture while operating within those very same terms.

Chapters 3 and 4 focus on how wellness discourse, through natural health, works as a means of offsetting the devastation of everyday contemporary life. Wellness becomes in chapter 3 a form of harm reduction, a way for individuals to avoid toxic contamination from pharmaceuticals and rid themselves of toxins accumulated from their lived environments. This vector is powered by both logics of wellness simultaneously as individuals use supplement-supported cleanses to restore their bodies to a prior state of purity and to enhance their defenses against future contamination. In chapter 4 we see how wellness becomes a way of carving out space for rest and recovery in overburdened lives, a means of surviving exhaustion. As much as rhetorics surrounding resilience operate in terms of enhancement, the primary logic that drives this vector of wellness discourse is that of restoring the self and the body in order to keep going.

The final two chapters bring us full circle in considering wellness as an autopoietic rhetoric. Chapter 5 examines wellness as a form of optimization, fueled by the logic of enhancement. In this vector, those who seek wellness do so through both tracking and hacking: they track their wellness using apps, diaries, wearables, and laboratory tests of biological specimens, and then they hack their wellness using specialized supplements and strategies to optimize their bodily systems and process. The principles of optimization that underly this vector of wellness move us from the logic of enhancement back into the logic of restoration, as the failure to optimize constitutes a risk state that must itself be managed, or restored, through subsequent intervention. Chapter 6 examines wellness as a form of performance that is animated by scripts of wellness, or pieties, that emerge out of the previous five vectors of wellness. Natural health supplements function in this vector as ritual objects that facilitate self-transformation, defining who and what sort of people we are—and can be.

For readers in rhetorical studies, *Why Wellness Sells* expands our understanding of how arguments can self-generate in public discourse. Working from an integrative perspective that draws on a range of rhetorical approaches as well as scholarship from related fields, I extend Keränen's initial study of autopoiesis in risk preparedness discourse to show, in closer detail, how systems-level arguments operate and grow. Rhetorics of wellness are diffuse, saturating the fabric of contemporary public life. Approaching these rhetorics through the lens of autopoiesis draws together a range of key foci in the field of rhetoric and the subfield of rhetoric of health and medicine, including institutional, regulatory, and commercial rhetorics about health; rhetorics of medical and alternative health practice; rhetorics of the body and lived experience; and discursive distinctions between individual and public health, cure and care, and illness and health.

My theoretical approach aligns with and complements scholarship on ambient, networked, and percolation rhetorics in that it allows me to show how wellness discourse appears to oppose pharmaceutical rhetorics of illness surveillance and intervention but in fact operates within those same terms.[4] In more explicitly rhetorical terms, we may think of wellness as a counter-rhetoric to mainstream pharmaceutical medicine, but as Jenny Edbauer argues, although "counter-rhetorics directly respond to and resist the original exigence, they also expand the lived experience of the original rhetorics by adding to them—even while changing and expanding their shape."[5] Because rhetorics and counter-rhetorics often have the same mutually reinforcing effects, the drive in wellness culture to avoid and oppose pharmaceutical culture instead largely reinforces it. The language of wellness frames natural health within idioms of illness and optimization that therefore situate wellness as always just beyond our grasp.

For readers in health humanities and related fields such as science and technology studies, social studies of medicine, and beyond, *Why Wellness Sells* explains what public interest in wellness can tell us about ourselves—about our culture, our health, our bodies, and our ways of being in the world. Instead of focusing on what wellness is or why it is problematic, I employ humanities-based methods and scholarship to open to inquiry intractable problems in health and medicine, such as the uneasy relationships between wellness, self-surveillance, and self-care that are enacted through institutional, regulatory, and public rhetorics of health.

As a work of biocriticism that engages with how, in Keränen's words, "discursive formations and material practices comprise 'life,'"[6] this book provides textured qualitative explanations of why people choose wellness products, what they use them for, and why they find them valuable, an approach that would not be possible through quantitative analysis or skeptical debunking. One of the things we learn, for instance, is that interest in wellness often serves as a proxy for broader concerns about health and healthcare, concerns that have not been well addressed by policymakers, practitioners, or public commentators. Widespread interest in wellness and natural health comes from somewhere, and not just from corporations and practitioners with wickedly successful marketing departments or consumers who do not know any better. As I have shown, those who seek wellness products and services are rational people with real needs and good reasons for seeking the products and services they use. Starting from that position allows us to better address their needs both within and beyond the bounds of formal healthcare.

Let us return to the two positions I outlined in my introduction regarding my own view of wellness and natural health: that most wellness products, such as natural health supplements, probably either do not work or do relatively little; and that people who use those products are neither gullible nor scientifically illiterate but are instead seeking support, motivation, empowerment, and care they are not finding elsewhere. While I have not sought to investigate or defend the first position, that supplements likely do not do (most of) what they purport to do, I hope I have demonstrated the second, that people have good reasons for seeking wellness. So where do we go from here? I would venture to say that if wellness is a self-generating discourse that operates on a closed rhetorical loop, the only way out is to change the conditions under which that rhetorical loop operates. I wish I could be more optimistic, but what it comes down to is that wellness, as it manifests in twenty-first-century consumer culture, is not itself a problem but a symptom of a larger problem, or set of problems.

Examining wellness as it manifests within and across the six vectors of wellness examined here—incipient illness, self-management, harm reduction, survival strategy, optimization, and performance—shows us that we can only absorb the shock and the stress of everyday life for so long before we seek ways of reducing that shock and stress, even if just a little. It may be tempting to critique public desire for local, organic, fair-trade, and non-toxic products, but leering portrayals of consumer ignorance fail to recognize that people are engaging in activism through the only socially sanctioned means available to them in contemporary life: through consumer choice. Under global capitalism, people can speak far more powerfully with their wallets than with words for their vision of another way of life, for a more authentic, more fulfilling, more nourishing way of being. Given that there is little opportunity for meaningful, lasting change in the contemporary market of privatization, sponsored content, and brand influencers, wellness seekers leverage their own livelihoods in an effort to remake their lives.

As anthropologist Anna Tsing and philosopher Alexis Shotwell illustrate so elegantly in their respective works, human beings are scrambling to find new ways of living in the face of cultural, economic, and environmental devastation. Writing about mushrooms that flourished in Fukushima, Japan, after the 2011 nuclear meltdown there, Tsing remarks that "blasted landscapes are what we have, and we need to explore their life-promoting patches."[7] Wellness can be seen, in this view, as a life-promoting patch in the landscape of late capitalism, although of course what we need more than detoxes and sleep aids is humane communities and workplaces where we can foster wellness by redesigning healthcare and public health, transit infrastructure, social supports, and mental health services and address systemic discrimination based on race, origin, gender, sexual orientation, and ability. We can draw a parallel here with breast- and chestfeeding support campaigns that cheerfully exhort that "breast is best" and provoke fear of formula in new parents while not investing in infrastructure to reduce the trade-offs that nursing requires, such as reduced mobility, workplace obstacles, and new parents' mental and financial health.[8] Corporate mindfulness programs similarly shift responsibility for collective problems to individuals by encouraging people to meditate rather than lobby for higher pay or reduced working hours.[9] Packaged as "self-care," wellness is a powerful cultural signifier of what we want, and what is missing, in everyday life.

The problem of wellness is ultimately not an individual problem, however, and so it cannot be solved by individual actions. Shotwell, Tsing, and environmental and forest biologist Robin Kimmerer have each written about individual versus collective flourishing in the face of widespread devastation, and they have shown in different ways how collaborative action is the only means of producing sustainable and equitable health and happiness for all people. In her essay "The Council of Pecans," for example, Kimmerer uses the phenomenon of mast fruiting—when trees simultaneously produce fruit en masse—to illustrate her book's core argument that "we make a grave error if we try to separate individual well-being from the health of the whole."[10] Explaining how trees communicate with one another through fungal networks and know as collectives when to produce and drop fruit, Kimmerer explains that their cycles of production initiate a circle of benefit—squirrels amass nuts, foxes feed on the squirrels, more trees grow, and the cycle continues. She writes, "If one tree fruits, they all fruit—there are no soloists. Not one tree in a grove, but the whole grove; not one grove in the forest, but every grove; all across the county and all across the state. The trees act not as individuals, but somehow as a collective. Exactly how they do this, we don't yet know. But what we see is the power of unity. What happens to one happens to us all. We can starve together or feast together. All flourishing is mutual."[11] Wellness as it is realized in the texts I have analyzed in this book is largely a solo act, a pharmaceutical solution enacted through capitalist means that comes at a cost to the collective: some feast, while others starve. To expand the "life-promoting patches" that Tsing describes, we need to move beyond wellness.

As I think about everything wellness does for and to us, both positively and negatively, I return to Eli Clare, whose *Brilliant Imperfection: Grappling with Cure* is discussed in chapters 1 and 6. Writing on our collective cultural obsession with "always-just-around-the-corner cures," Clare asks, not just of disabled people but of all people, "What do we need to make peace with our visceral selves today, to let go of the fantasies, even if we hope beyond hope that our flesh and bones, organs and neurons might be different someday down the line? I ask because I don't know the answers."[12] I do not know the answers either, but following rhetoric scholar Blake Scott, I do think we can find ways to intervene in harmful discourse by providing viable possibilities for resistance and change.[13] Of course, as I argue in chapter 4, sometimes all we can do is draw attention to things that need attention, but that in itself is a form of action, a means of *doing* in the world. Rhetoric makes it possible to see things that can otherwise be harder to see. When we can see them, the odds are better that we can change them.

Wellness rhetoric governs, in part, what individuals believe, say, and do. It is a rhetoric that transforms wellness into a commodity that appears to offer what we seek, at least within the suspended present of consumption. However, the commodification of wellness does little to move the needle for our sustained, collective welfare because relying on the market is insufficient for effecting change. As geographer Julie Guthman writes of alternative-food culture that valorizes local and organic products, "commodified alternatives to regulatory failure tend to accentuate class inequality rather than ameliorate it."[14] Similarly, religion scholar Alan Levinovitz observes that the purity offered by natural health and self-care products "becomes a luxury" accessible only to a few.[15] If we view wellness culture as simply a problem of fraudulent marketing and naive consumption, we miss the point. Products do not invent markets out of thin air. They tap into existing needs and desires, even if their solutions are only available to a few. Understanding what those needs and desires *are* is our first step toward addressing them with lasting, equitable, systemic solutions.

While others can address the transformations of policy, social practice, power, funding, education, healthcare training and practice, and more that are necessary to dampen the overpowering effects of wellness culture, my point of intervention as a rhetoric scholar is at the level of discourse. What I can offer to the larger conversation about the potential harms of wellness is a way of reframing the conversation itself. By examining wellness rhetoric as autopoietic, I shift the focus from individual discursive players, such as supplement producers, marketers, health practitioners, citizen-consumers, policymakers, and more, toward the flows of wellness rhetoric between and among them. By examining what drives that rhetoric—the tension between the logics of restoration and enhancement— we gain a better sense of how to disrupt that tension, to break the cycle across the different vectors through which wellness rhetoric accrues strength and spreads.

Disrupting the power of wellness culture means disrupting the discursive scripts, or pieties, of wellness that animate it. It means breaking that discourse into its component parts by engaging in what rhetorician Kenneth Burke describes as "verbal 'atom cracking,'" a process that in breaking it up defamiliarizes and denatures the whole.[16] Viewing wellness through six different vectors at essentially the same time does exactly this. It gives us the benefit of what Burke calls perspective by incongruity, a way of putting opposite things together to see each more clearly in relief.[17] When we see that wellness can be so many different things simultaneously, we can see that it is not the monolith it seems to be. Cracking the "atom" of wellness as an autopoietic discourse makes it both trickier and easier to intervene in wellness culture's harmful effects—trickier because we learn that there are many places to start rather than just one, yet easier because cracking the atom of wellness discourse gives us the knowledge and the tools to begin.

Introduction

1. Stokols, "Establishing and Maintaining Healthy Environments"; Watt, Verma, and Flynn, "Wellness Programs"; Nichter and Thompson, "For My Wellness"; Kannan et al., "Medical Utilization among Wellness Consumers"; Cederström and Spicer, *Wellness Syndrome*.

2. For examples of this kind of definition, see Kraft and Goodell, "Identifying the Health Conscious Consumer," 18; Schuster et al., "Wellness Lifestyles I"; and Zimmer, "Wellness."

3. Kannan et al., "Medical Utilization among Wellness Consumers"; Schuster et al., "Wellness Lifestyles I"; Derkatch, "'Wellness' as Incipient Illness"; Dickinson and MacKay, "Health Habits and Other Characteristics"; Nichter and Thompson, "For My Wellness."

4. Armstrong, "Rise of Surveillance Medicine," 401. See also Cederström and Spicer, *Wellness Syndrome*; Conrad, "Wellness as Virtue"; Elliott, *Better than Well*; Metzl and Kirkland, *Against Health*; Bunton and Petersen, *Foucault, Health and Medicine*; and Spoel, Harris, and Henwood, "Moralization of Healthy Living."

5. See, e.g., Caulfield, *Cure for Everything*; Caulfield, *Is Gwyneth Paltrow Wrong about Everything?*; Cederström and Spicer, *Wellness Syndrome*; Delaney, *Wellmania*; Ehrenreich, *Natural Causes*; and Hodge, *User's Guide to Cheating Death*.

6. Gwyneth Paltrow is an Academy Award–winning actress who launched her wellness empire *goop* in 2008; Dr. Mehmet Oz is a cardiothoracic surgeon turned television personality and 2022 Republican Senate nominee for Pennsylvania who among other things has hosted his own talk show and published his own magazine, both about health and wellness.

7. Segal, "Rhetoric of Health and Medicine."

8. Elliott, *Better than Well*.

9. Keränen, "How Does a Pathogen Become a Terrorist?"

10. Luhmann, "Autopoiesis of Social Systems"; Luhmann, "Concept of Society"; Blaschke, "It's All in the Network"; Keränen, "How Does a Pathogen Become a Terrorist?"

11. Keränen, "How Does a Pathogen Become a Terrorist?," 83.

12. I am mindful of Donna Haraway's caution in *Staying with the Trouble* that in practice nothing actually can be autopoietic, in the sense of autonomously making or organizing itself. Haraway prefers the broader concept of *sympoiesis*, which she describes as a form of "making-with" nested in "complex, dynamic, responsive, situated, historical systems" (58).

Haraway makes a compelling case for adopting sympoiesis as a theoretical lens through which to see how different parts of complex systems interact, but I prefer the greater conceptual clarity afforded by autopoiesis as a form of self-generation. Understanding wellness rhetoric as autopoietic narrows our focus from all the players and factors that drive wellness discourse to the rhetorical power of the discourse itself. See also Zoltan Majdik's 2019 study of systems-based climate communications, "A Computational Approach to Assessing Rhetorical Effectiveness."

13. The terms *sickness*, *syndrome*, and *epidemic* are from Hanson, "Goop and the Anxiety of Wellness"; Cederström and Spicer, *Wellness Syndrome*; and Larocca, "How 'Wellness' Became an Epidemic," respectively.

14. My guiding metaphor of vectors draws on philosopher of science Ian Hacking's use of the concept to explain how "transient" mental illnesses spread only at certain times and places; his use of the metaphor in turn comes from epidemiology and viral biology to explain the spread of disease across populations. I am grateful to Alan Richardson and Judy Segal for reminding me of this connection. Hacking, *Mad Travelers*.

15. "From Body Mechanics to Mindfulness."

16. Bloodworth, *Hired*; Kaori Gurley, "Amazon Denies Workers Pee in Bottles"; Klippenstein, "Documents Show Amazon Is Aware Drivers Pee in Bottles "; Long, "Amazon, Contractors Settle Wage-Theft Lawsuit."

17. Gault, "Amazon Introduces Tiny 'ZenBooths'"; see also J. Kelly, "Social Media Savaged"; "Amazon Offers 'Wellness Chamber' for Stressed Staff."

18. See Dietary Supplement Health and Education Act of 1994.

19. At the time of this writing, Canadian legislation surrounding the regulation of natural health products is undergoing significant changes, but the previous legislation, from 2012, features the two separate streams for approval of natural health products mentioned here. The avenue for approval of products for "traditional use" in practices such as ethnomedicines of the First Nations, Ayurveda, and traditional Chinese medicine requires evidence of historical use but not formal scientific evidence of safety or efficacy, whereas the avenue for "modern health" claims does require differing degrees of scientific support depending on the risk classification of the product. Health Canada, "2.6 Efficacy Evidence Recommendations"; Health Canada, "2.7 Safety Evidence for Traditional Medicines."

20. Nichter and Thompson, "For My Wellness," 183.

21. Derkatch, *Bounding Biomedicine*; Derkatch, "'Wellness' as Incipient Illness"; Nichter and Thompson, "For My Wellness."

22. In this book, I use the terms *natural health product* and *dietary supplement* interchangeably, even though they are somewhat distinct. The Canadian regulatory term *natural health product* includes a broader range of interventions than its US counterpart, *dietary supplement* because it includes not only materials ingested orally, per FDA regulations, but also products delivered topically, such as nasal sprays, creams, and ointments. Health Canada, "About Natural Health Products"; US Food and Drug Administration, "Questions and Answers on Dietary Supplements."

23. Somers, "Newsweek Attack."

24. Somers, *Sexy Years*, 28.

25. Somers, *Ageless*, 16.

26. Kirmayer, "Mind and Body as Metaphors," 57.

27. This definition is adapted from Derkatch, *Bounding Biomedicine*, 13.

28. Scott, *Risky Rhetoric*.

29. In my undergraduate course on rhetorical criticism, I often include two epigraphs on the syllabus that usefully characterize my integrative approach to rhetorical criticism in this book. The first is from playwright Bertolt Brecht, who wrote in 1920, "A man with one theory is lost. He needs several of them, four, lots! He should stuff them in his pockets like newspapers, hot from the press." Quoted in Parker, *Bertolt Brecht*, 155. The second epigraph, from Kenneth Burke, gets even closer to my own approach in rhetoric: "The main ideal of criticism, as I conceive it, is to use all that is there to use." K. Burke, *Philosophy of Literary Form*, 23.

30. Keränen, "Addressing the Epidemic of Epidemics," 225.

31. Keränen, "Addressing the Epidemic of Epidemics," 238.

32. Berlant, "Risky Bigness"; Berlant, *Cruel Optimism*.

33. Rickert, *Ambient Rhetoric*, 16.

34. Rickert, *Ambient Rhetoric*, xiii.

35. For an example of rhetoric as a distributed assemblage, see Nicotra, "Assemblage Rhetorics." For models of rhetorical circulation as networked, ecological, and percolative, see Edbauer, "Unframing Models of Public Distribution"; and Jensen, "Ecological Turn in Rhetoric of Health Scholarship."

36. Ehrenfeld, "Ecological Investments and the Circulation of Rhetoric," 43 (emphasis added).

37. Edbauer, "Unframing Models of Public Distribution," 14.

38. Edbauer, "Unframing Models of Public Distribution," 14 (emphasis in original).

39. Rickert, *Ambient Rhetoric,* 91. For the example of increasing or reducing hair growth, see Clare, *Brilliant Imperfection*, 95–97.

40. I am grateful to one of this book's anonymous peer reviewers for improving my conceptual framing and phrasing here.

41. Dumit, *Drugs for Life*.

Chapter 1 · *Wellness as Incipient Illness*

1. Smith, *Wellness Prescription*, 79.

2. Smith, *Wellness Prescription*, 79.

3. *The Wellness Prescription* was self-published in a run of a thousand copies. Tim Fransky, phone conversation with author, July 16, 2021. Despite its modest print run, it is in the holdings of numerous major university libraries across Canada and the United States, as well as those of the Library and Archives Canada and the US National Institutes of Health's National Library of Medicine.

4. Armstrong, "Rise of Surveillance Medicine," 401; see also Clarke et al., "Biomedicalization," 172.

5. Dumit, *Drugs for Life*, 55.

6. Data on regional differences in both the United States and Canada show that public interest in and use of natural health products such as supplements is 10–20 percent higher in western regions than in eastern ones. Statistics Canada, "Health Fact Sheets"; Rozga et al., "Dietary Supplement Users." For this reason, I conducted an equal number of interviews in Western Canada and Eastern Canada to capture a potentially broader range of perspectives on wellness and natural health. Because of the study size, however, I did not analyze regional variations among the responses.

7. Dickinson and MacKay, "Health Habits and Other Characteristics"; Guo et al., "Use of Vitamin and Mineral Supplements"; Statistics Canada, "Health Fact Sheets."

8. This study received institutional research ethics approval. Participants were recruited in each city through online advertisements on Facebook, Twitter, and my website and through physical posters placed on bulletin boards in public spaces, including community centers, coffee shops, and natural food stores. This study was approved by the Toronto Metropolitan University (formerly Ryerson University) Research Ethics Board. Prospective participants were screened for inclusion via email according to the following criteria: (a) 18 years or older; (b) actively interested in wellness; (c) use natural health products (e.g., herbal medicine, vitamins other than regular multivitamins, homeopathic remedies) regularly (i.e., daily or weekly, for at least part of the year); (d) would be physically present for the interview; (e) at arm's length from the researcher (e.g., not first-degree friends, colleagues, or family members). The first twenty prospective participants in each city who met the inclusion criteria were scheduled for interviews; all forty interviews were conducted by paid graduate-level research assistants in a private office on a university campus. Participants received a twenty-five-dollar VISA cash card as an incentive for their participation.

9. The transcripts include features of spoken language such as repetition, false starts, pauses, and filler words (e.g., *um*, *like*), but I did not factor these elements into my analysis unless they seemed significant. All quotations have been lightly edited to exclude these elements except where noted. Participants are identified in the text by number and interview location (*E* for East, *W* for West).

10. When I began this project, I analyzed the transcripts first by participant and question and then by themes that I identified primarily inductively, using an iterative process that involved identifying overarching themes in the transcripts until no new themes emerged and then reanalyzing all the transcripts in terms of those broad themes. My approach was not solely inductive, however, as I also brought theoretical frameworks to bear on my inquiry throughout the process of writing this book. To orient and ground my analysis in this first chapter, for example, I considered whether and how participants' responses accorded with my earlier observation, regarding a different set of primary texts, that wellness is often figured discursively as a state of incipient illness that requires careful observation and intervention. Derkatch, "'Wellness' as Incipient Illness"; Derkatch, *Bounding Biomedicine*. Additionally, as I came to see that Keränen's concept of rhetorical autopoiesis offers a robust theoretical framework for explaining how wellness discourse is propelled by the intertwined logics of restoration and enhancement, I reanalyzed the materials specifically through that theoretical lens. See Keränen, "How Does a Pathogen Become a Terrorist?" My early thinking for the remainder of the book was similarly shaped largely by the themes I identified in the interview dataset, although as later chapters illustrate, I found comparable patterns throughout the primary sources I discuss.

11. Clare, *Brilliant Imperfection*, 179.

12. Cliffe (@Nicole_Cliffe), "Person who came up with 'wellness.'"

13. Berlant, *Cruel Optimism*.

14. For more on conceptions of wellness and natural health products, see Derkatch, *Bounding Biomedicine*; Derkatch, "'Wellness' as Incipient Illness"; and Nichter and Thompson, "For My Wellness."

15. Interview with research participant W-01, 2015.

16. Interview with research participant W-16, 2018.

17. Interview with research participant E-13, 2018.

18. Interview with research participant W-15, 2018.

19. Interview with research participant W-18, 2018.

20. Interview with research participant E-02, 2015.

21. Interviews with research participants E-03, E-05, E-06, E-07, and W-02, all 2015.

22. Interview with research participant W-18, 2018.

23. Interview with research participant E-04, 2015.

24. Interview with research participant E-04, 2015.

25. Interview with research participant W-06, 2015.

26. Interview with research participant W-13, 2018.

27. Interview with research participant W-12, 2018.

28. Interviews with research participants E-14, 2018; W-03, 2015; W-06, 2015; W-15, 2018; E-05, 2015; E-13, 2018; E-04, 2015; E-01, 2015; E-09, 2015; E-16, 2018; W-06, 2015; W-10, 2015; W-16, 2018; E-19, 2018; and W-03, 2018.

29. Interviews with research participants E-07 and W-08, both 2015.

30. Interview with research participant W-15, 2018.

31. Interview with research participant W-05, 2015.

32. Interview with research participant E-08, 2015.

33. Interview with research participant W-09, 2015.

34. Interview with research participant E-12, 2018.

35. Interview with research participant E-11, 2018.

36. Interview with research participant E-03, 2015.

37. Interview with research participant W-10, 2015 (emphasis added).

38. Interview with research participant E-16, 2018.

39. Interview with research participant E-08, 2015 (emphasis added).

40. Interview with research participant W-03, 2015 (emphasis added).

41. Interview with research participant W-05, 2015.

42. Interview with research participant W-04, 2015.

43. Conrad, *Medicalization of Society*. See also Armstrong, "Rise of Surveillance Medicine"; Rose, *Politics of Life Itself*; and Dumit, *Drugs for Life*.

44. Interview with research participant W-10, 2015.

45. Interview with research participant W-07, 2015.

46. Interview with research participant E-09, 2015.

47. Interview with research participant E-02, 2015.

48. Interview with research participant E-03, 2015.

49. Interview with research participant W-08, 2015. Here, Jordana echoes disability studies scholar Lennard Davis's conceptualization of the unattainable "ideal" body of the divine as a contrast to the "normal" or average body, on the one hand, and to disabled or ill bodies, on the other. Davis, *Enforcing Normalcy*.

50. Interview with research participant W-01, 2015.

51. Armstrong, "Rise of Surveillance Medicine"; Rose, *Politics of Life Itself*; Scott, *Risky Rhetoric*; Scott, "Kairos as Indeterminate Risk Management"; Dumit, *Drugs for Life*.

52. Interview with research participant E-03, 2015.

53. Bunton and Petersen, *Foucault, Health and Medicine*; Cederström and Spicer, *Wellness Syndrome*; Spoel, Harris, and Henwood, "Moralization of Healthy Living."

54. Interview with research participant E-02, 2015.

55. Interview with research participant W-06, 2015.

56. Interview with research participant W-06, 2015.

57. Interview with research participant W-01, 2015.

58. Interview with research participant E-07, 2015.

59. Interview with research participant E-02, 2015.

60. Interview with research participant W-06, 2015.

61. Interview with research participant W-10, 2015.

62. Conrad, *Medicalization of Society*; Dumit, *Drugs for Life*; Rose, *Politics of Life Itself*.

63. Armstrong, "Rise of Surveillance Medicine"; Belling, *Condition of Doubt*; Cheek and Porter, "Reviewing Foucault"; Dumit, *Drugs for Life*; Lowenberg and Davis, "Beyond Medicalisation-Demedicalisation"; Lupton, "M-Health and Health Promotion"; Moynihan and Cassels, *Selling Sickness*; Rose, *Politics of Life Itself*.

64. Interview with research participant E-06, 2015.

65. Interview with research participant E-10, 2015.

66. Perelman and Olbrechts-Tyteca, *New Rhetoric*, 117.

67. Perelman, *Realm of Rhetoric*, 36.

68. Elliott, *Better than Well*.

69. Interview with research participant W-10, 2015 (emphasis added).

70. Cederström and Spicer, *Wellness Syndrome*; Conrad, *Medicalization of Society*; Elliott, *Better than Well*; Hyde, *Perfection*; Bunton and Petersen, *Foucault, Health and Medicine*; Spoel, Harris, and Henwood, "Moralization of Healthy Living."

71. Kosova and Wingert. "Live Your Best Life Ever!"

72. Interview with research participant E-01, 2015.

73. Interview with research participant E-05, 2015.

74. Interview with research participant E-01, 2015.

75. Interview with research participant W-08, 2015.

76. Interview with research participant E-03, 2015.

77. Interview with research participant E-09, 2015.

78. Derkatch, "'Wellness' as Incipient Illness," 3.

79. Interviews with research participants E-01, E-07, E-02, E-01, E-03, E-06, and W-08, respectively, all 2015.

80. Interview with research participant E-03, 2015.

81. Interview with research participant E-03, 2015.

82. Interview with research participant E-01, 2015.

83. Interview with research participant E-07, 2015.

84. Armstrong, "Rise of Surveillance Medicine," 401. See also Brownlee, *Overtreated*; Hadler, *Worried Sick*; Moynihan and Cassels, *Selling Sickness*; and Welch. Schwartz, and Woloshin, *Overdiagnosed*.

85. Conrad, *Medicalization of Society*, 141.

86. Interview with research participant E-03, 2015.

87. Dumit, *Drugs for Life*, 67.

88. Interview with research participant E-03, 2015.

89. Dumit, *Drugs for Life*, 65.

90. Dumit, *Drugs for Life*, 113.

91. Dumit, *Drugs for Life*, 7.

92. Clare, *Brilliant Imperfection*, 179.

93. Clare, *Brilliant Imperfection*, 57.

Chapter 2 · Wellness as Self-Management

1. An Act to Amend the Food and Drugs Act.

2. Picard, "Legislation Worthy of Our Support."

3. Klingbeil, "Stop Bill C-51."

4. A. Burke, "ACT NOW!"

5. "Stop C-51 Forever," The Official Stop C-51 Website. The website has been discontinued but is accessible via the Internet Archive. It is worth noting that the Stop C-51 website was later exposed as sponsored by the supplement producer Truehope, a company with longstanding legal trouble with Health Canada, as has been reported in Blackwell, "Firms Back Campaign against Health Bill."

6. Tiedemann, "Bill C-51," discusses the potential impact of the public opposition on the bill itself.

7. See Petersen et al., "Healthy Living and Citizenship"; Bunton and Petersen, *Foucault, Health and Medicine*; Clarke et al., *Biomedicalization*; Conrad, *Medicalization*; Conrad, "Wellness as Virtue"; and Rose, *Politics of Life Itself.*

8. For more on the discursive foundations of self-governance and the politics of health within biomedicine, see Spoel, Harris, and Henwood, "Moralization of Health Living"; Petersen et al., "Healthy Living and Citizenship"; and Rose, *Politics of Life Itself.*

9. My initial analysis of the petition comments followed an iterative process that involved first identifying overarching topics in the comments until no new topics emerged and then reanalyzing all the comments in accordance with the five topics identified: health, nature, choice, greed, and government. I then examined each individual topic to identify its specific arguments and subarguments. For example, under *health*, commenters advanced five key arguments in protest of the proposed legislation, including that (1) health is a holistic concept; (2) natural health products (NHPs) are as effective as pharmaceuticals and preventive in effect; (3) NHPs are safe, while pharmaceuticals are dangerous; (4) NHPs reduce the burden of formal medical care; and (5) the government should not limit NHP access out of concern for health because it also permits many unhealthy things such as smoking. This initial analysis of topics and arguments in the "Stop Bill C-51" petition now forms the basis of a separate study underway at the time of this writing.

10. See Derkatch, *Bounding Biomedicine*, 141.

11. For outlines of these general shifts, see M. Brown, "Don't Be the 'Fifth Guy'"; Bunton and Petersen, *Foucault, Health and Medicine*; Cederström and Spicer, *Wellness Syndrome*; Conrad, "Wellness as Virtue"; Derkatch and Spoel, "Public Health Promotion of 'Local Food'"; Elliott, *Better than Well*; Hyde, *Perfection*; Spoel and Derkatch, "Resilience and Self-Reliance"; and Spoel, Harris, and Henwood, "Moralization of Healthy Living."

12. Spoel, Harris, and Henwood, "Moralization of Healthy Living," 620.

13. See Stambler, "Eating Data," for discussion of rhetorics of employee wellness programs and a summary of current evidence of their return on investment.

14. British Columbia Ministry of Health, *BC Health Guide.*

15. Klingbeil, "Stop Bill C-51." Quotations from the petition are largely reproduced here as they appear in the original, including errors in spelling and punctuation and extra or missing spaces; in a few cases I have made silent changes in spacing to improve readability.

I have preserved these idiosyncrasies to reflect the comments' generic and situational origins in the petition as an online text.

16. Klingbeil, "Stop Bill C-51."

17. Motta, Callaghan, and Sylvester, "Knowing Less but Presuming More."

18. Cederström and Spicer, *Wellness Syndrome*, 3.

19. Shotwell, *Against Purity*, 24; Crawford, "Healthism and the Medicalization of Everyday Life."

20. Shotwell, *Against Purity*, 29.

21. Biss, *On Immunity*, 40; see also Levinovitz, *Natural*. I discuss the restorative power of nature at greater length in chapter 6.

22. Klingbeil, "Stop Bill C-51."

23. Klingbeil, "Stop Bill C-51."

24. Klingbeil, "Stop Bill C-51."

25. Klingbeil, "Stop Bill C-51."

26. Klingbeil, "Stop Bill C-51."

27. Klingbeil, "Stop Bill C-51."

28. Klingbeil, "Stop Bill C-51."

29. Spoel and Derkatch, "Resilience and Self-Reliance"; Spoel, Harris, and Henwood, "Rhetorics of Health Citizenship."

30. Klingbeil, "Stop Bill C-51."

31. Klingbeil, "Stop Bill C-51."

32. Klingbeil, "Stop Bill C-51"

33. Klingbeil, "Stop Bill C-51" (ellipsis in original).

34. Klingbeil, "Stop Bill C-51."

35. Klingbeil, "Stop Bill C-51."

36. Porter, *Quacks*, 45, 46, 50.

37. Porter's *Quacks* was first published as *Health for Sale: Quackery in England, 1660–1850.*

38. Hargreaves-Heap et al., *Theory of Choice*, 88. While Hargreaves-Heap and colleagues theorize choice in economic terms, Elwyn and Edwards extend that model of choice to medicine to problematize consumerist approaches to health and health care. Elwyn and Edwards, "Evidence-Based Patient Choice?"

39. Klingbeil, "Stop Bill C-51."

40. Klingbeil, "Stop Bill C-51."

41. Klingbeil, "Stop Bill C-51."

42. Cooper, *Rhetoric of Aristotle.*

43. Klingbeil, "Stop Bill C-51" (emphases added).

44. Klingbeil, "Stop Bill C-51."

45. Klingbeil, "Stop Bill C-51."

46. If we phrased this argument as a rhetorical syllogism, or an argument reasoned from premises to a conclusion, here is how it would go:

Premise 1: People would not use something for hundreds/thousands of years if it did not work.

Premise 2: X product has been used for hundreds/thousands of years.

Conclusion: X product works.

There are at least two logical problems with this argument. First, it is not true that people would necessarily stop using something if it did not work. They might, for example, *believe* that it works even in the absence of proof, and that might be reason enough to continue its use. Or they might continue to use it simply because there are no other available options and they feel it is better to do *something* rather than nothing. Second, many products that are purported to be ancient in origin have not, in fact, been in use for long at all.

47. Most notoriously, a 2015 episode of the Canadian Broadcasting Corporation television newsmagazine show *Marketplace* investigated Health Canada's approval process for natural health products. The show's investigative journalists successfully applied for a natural product number to sell a bogus homeopathic remedy that contained nothing but tap water, submitting only several photocopied pages of a homeopathic handbook as evidence of its effectiveness. CBC, "Licence to Deceive."

48. Klingbeil, "Stop Bill C-51."

49. Klingbeil, "Stop Bill C-51."

50. Klingbeil, "Stop Bill C-51."

51. Klingbeil, "Stop Bill C-51."

52. Klingbeil, "Stop Bill C-51."

53. Klingbeil, "Stop Bill C-51."

54. Klingbeil, "Stop Bill C-51."

55. Klingbeil, "Stop Bill C-51."

56. Klingbeil, "Stop Bill C-51."

57. Klingbeil, "Stop Bill C-51."

58. Klingbeil, "Stop Bill C-51."

59. For incisive overviews of problems in pharmaceutical research, approval, and marketing, see Angell, *Truth about the Drug Companies*; Dumit, *Drugs for Life*; and Elliott, *White Coat, Black Hat*.

60. Hurley, *Natural Causes*.

61. Klingbeil, "Stop Bill C-51."

62. Klingbeil, "Stop Bill C-51."

63. Klingbeil, "Stop Bill C-51."

Chapter 3 · *Wellness as Harm Reduction*

1. Nichter and Thompson, "For My Wellness."

2. Renew Life Canada, "Renew Life® First Cleanse."

3. Renew Life Canada, "Renew Life® CleanseSMART®."

4. Campbell, *Dr. Oz Show*, episode 80, "Toxic Home."

5. Pezzullo, *Toxic Tourism*, 59 (emphasis in original).

6. Pezzullo, *Toxic Tourism*.

7. Dumit, *Drugs for Life*.

8. Smith and Lourie, *Slow Death by Rubber Duck*; Lourie and Smith, *Toxin Toxout*.

9. Jensen, "Theorizing Chemical Rhetoric," 433, 432.

10. Conrad, *Medicalization of Society*, 151 (emphasis in original).

11. Dumit, *Drugs for Life*, 55, 1.

12. Dumit, *Drugs for Life*, 1, 2.

13. Scott, *Risky Rhetoric*, 131.

14. Keränen, "How Does a Pathogen Become a Terrorist?"
15. Dumit, *Drugs for Life*, 60.
16. Belling, *Condition of Doubt*, 62.
17. Lourie and Smith, *Toxin Toxout*, 3.
18. Lourie and Smith, *Toxin Toxout*, 107.
19. For further discussion of colloquial and chemical definitions of toxicity, see Biss, "Illusion of 'Natural'"; and Jensen, "Theorizing Chemical Rhetoric."
20. Lourie and Smith, *Toxin Toxout*, 87.
21. MacKendrick, *Better Safe than Sorry*.
22. Lourie and Smith, *Toxin Toxout*, 89, 90.
23. Lourie and Smith, *Toxin Toxout*, 97.
24. Smith and Lourie, *Slow Death by Rubber Duck*, 4.
25. Lourie and Smith, *Toxin Toxout*, 2–3.
26. Lourie and Smith, *Toxin Toxout*, 39.
27. Lourie and Smith, *Toxin Toxout*, 105.
28. Lourie and Smith, *Toxin Toxout*, 58, 119.
29. Nichter and Thompson, "For My Wellness."
30. Interview with research participant E-07, 2015.
31. Interview with research participant E-18, 2018.
32. Klingbeil, "Stop Bill C-51."
33. Klingbeil, "Stop Bill C-51." The original text has *comprised*, although it is clear from the surrounding context that *compromise* was the intended word. I emended the quotation for clarity.
34. Jensen, "Theorizing Chemical Rhetoric."
35. Interview with research participant E-16, 2018.
36. Interview with research participant E-18, 2018.
37. Klingbeil, "Stop Bill C-51."
38. Klingbeil, "Stop Bill C-51."
39. Interview with research participant E-15, 2018.
40. Newmaster and colleagues found in a study of forty-four natural health products from twelve different companies that one-third of their tested products "contained contaminants and or fillers not listed on the label." Newmaster et al., "DNA Barcoding Detects Contamination and Substitution," 1.
41. EZ Lifestyle, "Over EZ."
42. Klingbeil, "Stop Bill C-51."
43. Klingbeil, "Stop Bill C-51."
44. See Kolata, "Hormone Studies."
45. Angell, *Truth about the Drug Companies*; Conrad, *Medicalization of Society*; Dumit, *Drugs for Life*; Elliott, *White Coat, Black Hat*; Lexchin, *Doctors in Denial*; Moynihan and Cassels, *Selling Sickness*.
46. Angell, *Truth about the Drug Companies*, offers a summary of the Vioxx scandal.
47. Klingbeil, "Stop Bill C-51."
48. See Hurley, *Natural Causes*.
49. Interview with research participant W-15, 2018.
50. Klingbeil, "Stop Bill C-51."
51. Interview with research participant W-18, 2018.

52. Klingbeil, "Stop Bill C-51."

53. Interview with research participant E-15, 2018.

54. Interviews with research participants W-13, 2018, and E-02, 2015.

55. Interview with research participant W-18, 2018.

56. Interview with research participant E-05, 2015.

57. Klingbeil, "Stop Bill C-51."

58. Interview with research participant W-18, 2018.

59. Interview with research participant E-14, 2018.

60. Interview with research participant E-05, 2015.

61. Interview with research participant E-01, 2015.

62. Interview with research participant E-11, 2018.

63. Interviews with research participant E-01and E-04, both 2015.

64. Interview with research participant E-04, 2015.

65. Interview with research participant E-01, 2015.

66. Interview with research participant E-15, 2018.

67. Klingbeil, "Stop Bill C-51."

68. Klingbeil, "Stop Bill C-51."

69. Interview with research participant E-17, 2018.

70. Dumit, *Drugs for Life*, 16.

71. Interview with research participant E-17, 2018.

72. Interview with research participant W-18, 2018.

73. MacKendrick, *Better Safe than Sorry*, 4.

74. MacKendrick, *Better Safe than Sorry*, 3.

75. MacKendrick, *Better Safe than Sorry*, 7.

76. MacKendrick, *Better Safe than Sorry*, 97.

77. Moynihan and Cassels, *Selling Sickness*, xvii.

78. MacKendrick, *Better Safe than Sorry*, 34, 35.

79. Levenstein, *Fear of Food*; Whorton, *Inner Hygiene*; Whorton, "Civilisation and the Colon."

80. MacKendrick, *Better Safe than Sorry*; Oreskes and Conway, *Merchants of Doubt*.

81. MacKendrick, *Better Safe than Sorry*, 37.

82. Biss, "Illusion of 'Natural'"; Crowe, "Toxically Clean"; Guthman, *Weighing In*; Levenstein, *Fear of Food*; MacKendrick, *Better Safe than Sorry*; Reich, *Calling the Shots*; Shotwell, *Against Purity*.

83. MacKendrick, *Better Safe than Sorry*, 8.

84. Biss, "Illusion of 'Natural,'" 3.

85. MacKendrick, *Better Safe than Sorry*; Shotwell, *Against Purity*.

86. MacKendrick, *Better Safe than Sorry*, 4.

87. Renew Life Canada, "Renew Life® First Cleanse."

88. Lourie and Smith, *Toxin Toxout*, 120, 233.

89. Lourie and Smith, *Toxin Toxout*, 113, 122.

90. See, e.g., Pezzullo, *Toxic Tourism*.

91. Nichter and Thompson, "For My Wellness."

92. MacKendrick, *Better Safe than Sorry*, 107.

93. Interview with research participant W-13, 2018.

94. Lourie and Smith, *Toxin Toxout*, 216.

95. Even the researcher and media skeptic Timothy Caulfield experienced euphoric effects after completing a cleanse from Gwyneth Paltrow's wellness lifestyle company goop. Kirkey, "Delusion of Detoxing."

96. Renew Life Canada, "Renew Life® Rapid Cleanse."

97. Renew Life Canada, "Renew Life® CleanseSMART®."

98. Guthman, *Weighing In*; MacKendrick, *Better Safe than Sorry*; Shotwell, *Against Purity*.

99. MacKendrick, *Better Safe than Sorry*, 4.

100. Levenstein, *Fear of Food*, 123.

101. Belasco, *Appetite for Change*; Guthman, *Weighing In*; Hurley, *Natural Causes*; Levenstein, *Fear of Food*; Levinovitz, *Natural*; MacKendrick, *Better Safe than Sorry*; Shotwell, *Against Purity*.

102. MacKendrick, *Better Safe than Sorry*, 12.

103. Klingbeil, "Stop Bill C-51."

104. Shotwell, *Against Purity*, 7.

105. Shotwell, *Against Purity*, 79.

Chapter 4 · *Wellness as Survival Strategy*

1. Berlant, "Risky Bigness," 27.

2. World Health Organization, "Burn-out an 'Occupational Phenomenon.'"

3. Ahmed, "Time of Complaint."

4. Berlant, *Cruel Optimism*.

5. Some examples of recent scholarship in this area are McGreavy, "Resilience as Discourse"; Spoel and Derkatch, "Resilience and Self-Reliance"; and Stormer and McGreavy, "Thinking Ecologically about Rhetoric's Ontology."

6. Berlant, "Risky Bigness," 30.

7. Glasbergen, "Due to unusually high call volume."

8. Meme Generator, "Conspiracy Keanu."

9. Agamben, *State of Exception*. A key example in Agamben's analysis is the US Patriot Act, adopted in 2001 following the 9/11 attacks in New York and Washington, an ostensibly temporary emergency measure that "authorized the 'indefinite detention' and trial by 'military commissions' (not to be confused with the military tribunals provided for by the law of war) of noncitizens suspected of involvement in terrorist activities" (3). For useful examples of the state of exception as it is applied to bodies and health specifically, see Davis and Murphy, "Intersex Bodies as States of Exception"; Latimer, "Bio-Reproductive Futurism"; and Reeve, "Biopolitics and Bare Life."

10. Martin, "End of the Body?," 133.

11. Berlant, "Risky Bigness," 26.

12. Sontag, *Illness as Metaphor*.

13. Bayes, "IV Drips Are the Latest Overpriced Bullshit Wellness Fad."

14. Delaney, *Wellmania*, 14.

15. For more on nineteenth-century rhetorics of hypochondria and neurasthenia, see Segal, *Health and the Rhetoric of Medicine*. For a broader discussion of neurasthenia and its links to contemporary understandings of health and happiness, see J. Beck, "'Americanitis.'"

16. McGreavy, "Resilience as Discourse," 105–6.

17. Interview with research participant E-07, 2015.

18. Interview with research participant W-13, 2018.

19. Interview with research participant W-18, 2018.

20. Interview with research participant W-15, 2018.

21. Interview with research participant E-19, 2018.

22. Interview with research participant E-18, 2018.

23. Interview with research participant E-20, 2018.

24. Interview with research participant W-10, 2015.

25. Interview with research participant E-16, 2018.

26. Interview with research participant E-12, 2018.

27. Interview with research participant E-12, 2018.

28. Interview with research participant E-07, 2015.

29. Interview with research participant W-11, 2018.

30. Rescue Remedy, *Rescue Remedy Mother and Interview*, 0:12–0:16.

31. Interview with research participant E-15, 2018. See also Rescue Remedy, "RES-CUE Remedy® Dropper."

32. Bach Remedies, "About The Bach® Essences." The seven "emotional groups" identified by Bach are "Fear," "Uncertainty," "Insufficient interest in present circumstances," "Loneliness," "Oversensitivity to influences and ideas," "Despondency and despair," and "Overcare for the welfare of others."

33. Thaler et al., "Bach Flower Remedies."

34. Rescue Remedy, "Discover The RESCUE® Range" (emphasis added).

35. Bach Remedies, "Bach & RESCUE Remedy®."

36. For discussion of pharmaceutical marketing strategies, see Conrad, *Medicalization of Society*; Dumit, *Drugs for Life*; and Moynihan and Cassels, *Selling Sickness*.

37. Bach Remedies, "Bach & RESCUE Remedy®."

38. For the YouTube channel, see Rescue Remedy, "Rescue Remedy." For individual commercials, see Rescue Remedy, *Rescue Remedy Mother and Exam, Rescue Remedy Mother and Interview; Rescue Remedy TVC Mother, Bride and Exam,* and *Rescue Remedy TVC Mother, Bride and Interviewee.*

39. Rescue Remedy, *Rescue Remedy Mother and Interview*.

40. Spoel and Derkatch, "Resilience and Self-Reliance."

41. Dumit discusses these pharmaceutical promotional practices at length in *Drugs for Life.*

42. Berlant, "Risky Bigness."

43. Rescue Remedy, "RESCUE® On the Go"; "RESCUE Remedy®—Our Every Day Essentials."

44. I want to thank my colleague Beck Wise for offering context about Australian secondary education for interpreting this element of the commercials.

45. Interview with research participant E-07, 2015.

46. Interview with research participant E-19, 2018.

47. Interview with research participant E-19, 2018.

48. EZ Lifestyle, "About Us."

49. EZ Lifestyle, "Over EZ."

50. EZ Lifestyle, "Fuel EZ Natural Energy Supplements"; EZ Lifestyle, "Dream EZ Sleeping Pills."

51. EZ Lifestyle, "About Us."
52. Natrol, "Melatonin For Sleep."
53. Natrol, *What is Healthy Sleep?*
54. Foucault, *History of Sexuality,* 141.
55. Importantly, the evidence does not clearly show that workplace wellness programs necessarily produce these positive effects. For a detailed discussion of economic versus wellness and medical framings of employee wellness programs, see Stambler, "Eating Data." See also Cederström and Spicer, *Wellness Syndrome,* 35–37.
56. Toronto Metropolitan University, "Recharge."
57. Cederström and Spicer, *Wellness Syndrome,* 34, summarizing Johnathan Crary's argument in *24/7.*
58. Berlant, "Risky Bigness," 27, 30.
59. Interview with research participant E-12, 2018.
60. Berlant, "Risky Bigness," 26.
61. REVIV, "IV Therapies."
62. REVIV, "Royal Flush Deluxe IV."
63. REVIV, "Ultraviv Recovery IV Therapy."
64. REVIV.
65. EZ Lifestyle, "Over EZ."
66. Melman, *Grey's Anatomy.*
67. Gibney, *Billions.*
68. Interview with research participant E-12, 2018.
69. Interview with research participant E-12, 2018.
70. Segal, "What, in Addition to Drugs."
71. Ahmed, "Feeling Depleted?"; Ahmed, "Time of Complaint."
72. Frost, *Biocultural Creatures,* 4, 23.
73. Klein, "What Is Health and How Do You Get It?," 15.
74. The Nap Ministry, "About." I am grateful to one of this book's anonymous peer reviewers for pointing me to this website.
75. The Nap Ministry (@thenapministry), "Public Service Announcement for the weekend"; The Nap Ministry (@TheNapMinistry), "It is our right to rest. #thenapministry."
76. Wells and Hamblin, "Listen: You Are Worthy of Sleep."
77. Ahmed, "Selfcare as Warfare."
78. DeRango-Adem, "Self-Care Is a Radical Act."
79. Love, "Dark Truths behind Our Obsession with Self-Care."
80. Cederström and Spicer, *Wellness Syndrome,* 8.
81. For a sample of critiques of resilience rhetoric, see Walker and Cagle, "Resilience Rhetorics."

Chapter 5 · Wellness as Optimization

1. Elliott, *Better than Well.*
2. Northrup, *Wisdom of Menopause*; Somers, *Ageless*; Somers, *I'm Too Young for This!*; Somers, *Suzanne Somers' Fast and Easy.*
3. Somers, *Sexy Years,* 33.
4. Mayo Clinic, "Bioidentical Hormones."
5. Naftulin, "Oprah's Best and Worst Health Advice."

6. "Great Debate."

7. Somers, *Ageless*, 16.

8. K. Burke, *Language as Symbolic Action*, 44.

9. Nisly et al., "Dietary Supplement Polypharmacy."

10. Baluja and Hammer, "How to Build a Healthier, Smarter Student"; L. Beck, "Video: How to Pick a Healthy Snack"; Riedl, "Video: Chef Basics"; *Globe and Mail*, "Video: BBQ Basics."

11. For excellent summaries of that criticism, see Cederström and Spicer, *Wellness Syndrome*; Lupton, *Quantified Self*; and Reagle, *Hacking Life*.

12. Foucault, *History of Sexuality*, 141.

13. Martin, "End of the Body?," 122.

14. Martin, "End of the Body?," 121.

15. Delaney, *Wellmania*, 76, 77, 76.

16. Cederström and Spicer, *Wellness Syndrome*; Lupton, *Quantified Self*.

17. Lupton, *Quantified Self*, 50.

18. Reagle, *Hacking Life*, 3.

19. Reagle, *Hacking Life*, 13–14.

20. Derkatch, *Bounding Biomedicine*; Nichter and Thompson, "For My Wellness."

21. "Secrets to Healthier Aging."

22. Viome, "Gut Microbiome Testing."

23. Segal, *Health and the Rhetoric of Medicine*, 86.

24. An excerpt from Composed Nutrition's disclaimer reads:

Nutritional, fitness, and wellness information provided on the site is designed for educational purposes only. This information is not a substitute for, nor does it replace professional medical advice, diagnosis or treatment. If you have any concerns or questions about your health, you should always consult with a physician or other healthcare professional. Do not disregard, avoid, or delay obtaining medical or health-related advice from your healthcare professional because of something you may have read on this site.

Any claims made with respect to dietary supplements, including those made with respect to supplements available in the Composed Nutrition Shop, have not been evaluated by the Food and Drug Administration, and is not necessarily based on scientific evidence from any source. Dietary supplements are not intended to treat, diagnose, cure or prevent medical conditions or disease. You should consult with a healthcare provider before beginning any dietary supplement program.

Viome's disclaimer in 2021 reads:

Any statements or claims that appear on the supplements or probiotics+prebiotics packaging, subscription service descriptions, Viome website, or in documentation relevant to supplements, probiotics+prebiotics, or other services have not been evaluated by the Food and Drug Administration. The supplements, probiotics+prebiotics, or the kits are not intended to diagnose, treat, cure, or prevent any disease.

Composed Nutrition, "Disclaimer"; Viome, "Terms & Conditions" (in full caps in the original).

25. Metabolic Renewal, "Overview."

26. G. Wolf, "Know Thyself"; see also Quantified Self, "Homepage."

27. G. Wolf, "Know Thyself."

28. K. Kelly, "What Is the Quantified Self?"

29. Lupton, *Quantified Self*, 78; Reagle, *Hacking Life*.

30. Lupton, *Quantified Self*, 95.

31. Lupton, *Quantified Self*, 68.

32. Dumit, *Picturing Personhood*; Gardner, "Let's Send That to the Lab"; Segal, *Health and the Rhetoric of Medicine*.

33. Jutel, *Diagnosis*, 136. See also Jutel, *Putting a Name to It*; and Segal, *Health and the Rhetoric of Medicine*.

34. Canadian Association of Naturopathic Doctors, "Common Questions: Naturopathic Visits"; Irving et al., "International Variations in Primary Care Physician Consultation Time."

35. Canadian Association of Naturopathic Doctors, "Common Questions: Naturopathic Visits."

36. Rocky Mountain Analytical, "RMA FST™-IgG Food Sensitivity Test."

37. Martin, "End of the Body?," 122. Another example of food sensitivity testing in naturopathic care is electrodermal screening (EDS), or VEGA testing, which is commonly used to diagnose food sensitivities and allergies as well as vitamin and mineral levels, toxins, infections, and other conditions by tracking the movement of electricity through the human body. According to a blog post from a naturopathic clinic in Campbell River, British Columbia, food sensitivities are frequently "hidden" from those who suffer them, leading to sustained ill health. According to the blog post, EDS allows practitioners to recommend an elimination diet and clinical follow-up with regular retesting because "food sensitivities are always changing." Perceptive Health, "Hidden Food Sensitivities."

38. Canadian Association of Naturopathic Doctors, "What Exactly Is Alternative Medicine?"

39. 23andMe, "Health + Ancestry Service."

40. Reagle, *Hacking Life*, 83.

41. Lindsay O'Reilly Nutrition; Ruth, "Welcome!"

42. Composed Nutrition, "Composed Nutrition."

43. Precision Analytical, "DUTCH: Dried Urine Test for Comprehensive Hormones."

44. Precision Analytical, "DUTCH: Dried Urine Test for Comprehensive Hormones."

45. Ruth, "Welcome!"

46. Composed Nutrition, "Composed Nutrition."

47. See Ruth, "Welcome!"; and Lindsay O'Reilly Nutrition.

48. Viome, "Gut Intelligence Test™."

49. Viome, "Customized, Precision Supplements."

50. *Viome App Tour Video*. I was not able to create a Viome account without subscribing to the service, so I was not able to directly access the Viome app.

51. *My VIOME Results*.

52. *Viome App Tour Video*, 1:59.

53. *My VIOME Results*, 20:02.

54. *Viome App Tour Video*, 0:49.

55. *My VIOME Results*, 11:48–12:14.

56. *My VIOME Results*, 1:10–1:43.

57. Martin, "End of the Body?," 122.

58. Viome, "Viome's Health Intelligence™ Service."

59. *My VIOME Results*, 22:27–25:45.

60. See Reagle, *Hacking Life*.

61. Reagle, *Hacking Life*, 15.

62. Interview with research participant W-14, 2018.

63. Interview with research participant E-11, 2018.

64. Interview with research participant E-11, 2018; Healthline, "12 Proven Health Benefits of Ashwagandha"; Cleveland Clinic, Health Essentials, "What Is Ashwagandha?"

65. Interview with research participant E-11, 2018.

66. Klingbeil, "Stop Bill C-51."

67. Klingbeil, "Stop Bill C-51."

68. Reagle, *Hacking Life*, 87.

69. Reagle, *Hacking Life*, 98.

70. Interview with research participant E-03, 2015.

71. Interview with research participant W-10, 2015.

72. Interview with research participants E-12, 2018, and W-03 and W-08, 2015, respectively.

73. Interview with research participant W-01, 2018.

74. Interview with research participant E-17, 2018.

75. Interview with research participant W-10, 2015.

76. Interview with research participant E-15, 2018.

77. Interview with research participant E-11, 2018.

78. Interview with research participant E-15, 2018.

79. Interview with research participant W-19, 2018.

80. Interview with research participant W-12, 2018.

81. Interview with research participant W-08, 2015.

82. See Lock, "Anomalous Ageing."

83. Somers, *Sexy Years*, 4.

84. Somers, *Sexy Years*, 29.

85. There are many examples of this use of language in Somers, *Sexy Years*, esp. on pp. 41 and 121.

86. Somers, *Sexy Years*, 14.

87. Naftulin, "Oprah's Best and Worst Health Advice."

88. Lupton, *Quantified Self*; Reagle, *Hacking Life*; Cederström and Spicer, *Wellness Syndrome*.

89. Interview with research participant E-12, 2018.

90. Interview with research participant E-02, 2015.

91. See Reagle, *Hacking Life*.

92. Dumit, *Picturing Personhood*; Jutel, *Diagnosis*.

Chapter 6 · *Wellness as Performance*

1. Seigel, *Rhetoric of Pregnancy*, 25. See also K. Burke, *Permanence and Change*; and Jack, "'Piety of Degradation.'"

2. Derkatch, *Bounding Biomedicine*; Segal, *Health and the Rhetoric of Medicine*.

3. Contemporary constructions of the "well mother" share strong parallels with those of "organic" mothering. See Cairns, Johnston, and MacKendrick, "Feeding the 'Organic Child.'"

4. Parsons, *Social System*.

5. "Great Debate."

6. Jack, "'Piety of Degradation.'"

7. K. Burke, *Permanence and Change*, 77.

8. K. Burke, *Permanence and Change*, 74.

9. George, *Kenneth Burke's "Permanence and Change,"* 34.

10. Seigel, *Rhetoric of Pregnancy*, 26.

11. Seigel, *Rhetoric of Pregnancy*, 69.

12. Segal, "What, in Addition to Drugs."

13. VEGAMOUR (@vegamour), "VEGAMOUR."

14. VEGAMOUR (@vegamour), "Your hair thanks you." The built-in ephemerality of Instagram stories such as these posts by Vegamour poses an issue for citational practice: stories are typically accessible for twenty-four hours only. Exceptions to this rule are Story Highlights, which allow users to make selected stories permanently visible on their page. Where possible, I cite an Instagram user's highlight reel if it contains the story in question; in all other cases, the story is cited, but because it has expired, the URL merely leads to the user's account. For discussion of the methodological difficulties and opportunities immanent in Instagram stories, see Bainotti, Caliandro, and Gandinni, "From Archive Cultures to Ephemeral Content, and Back."

15. VEGAMOUR, "Science of VEGAMOUR."

16. Seigel, *Rhetoric of Pregnancy*, 25.

17. @shegotawildhair, "[Gray-hair emojis] It's about WAY more than the growth of your hair."

18. Chase, "Constructing Ethics through Rhetoric," 241.

19. Interview with research participant W-18, 2018.

20. Interview with research participant W-19, 2018.

21. Interview with research participant E-14, 2018.

22. Interview with research participant E-15, 2018.

23. Interview with research participant E-07, 2015.

24. Interview with research participant E-01, 2015.

25. For surveys of scholarship on ritual as performance, see G. Brown, "Theorizing Ritual as Performance"; Rappaport, *Ritual and Religion*; Schechner, *Performance Studies*; Stephenson, *Ritual*; and Turner, *From Ritual to Theatre*.

26. Turner, *From Ritual to Theatre*, 79 (emphasis in original).

27. Austin, *How to Do Things with Words*.

28. Interview with research participant E-05, 2015.

29. Rappaport, *Ritual and Religion*, 24.

30. Schechner, *Performance Studies*, 10.

31. Interview with research participant E-05, 2015.

32. Rappaport, *Ritual and Religion*; Schechner, *Performance Studies*; Stephenson, *Ritual*.

33. Derkatch, *Bounding Biomedicine*.

34. Here is Stephenson on the "performative magic" of medicine:

The effort to explain and understand the efficacy of the placebo effect, Western bio-medicine's own form of magic, generally points to the symbolic qualities common to both "modern" medical treatment and "traditional" healing rites. Falling ill and being healed involve interactions between patient, healer, family, community, and, in some cases, spirits, demons, or the sacred. These interactions are both instrumental (cleaning a wound, for example)—the physiological and pharmacological know-how present in traditional healing rites has long been underestimated—but also decisively symbolic and performative, providing a culturally sanctioned vocabulary, explanation, or narrative in making sense and effectively dealing with illness.

Stephenson, *Ritual*, 67–68.

35. Schechner explains that for Turner, liminal rites are obligatory within a culture, often determined by the calendar, and part of collective social process, whereas limonoid rites are voluntary, ongoing, often informal, more individual and can occur at the margins of society. Schechner calls these temporary changes "transportations" rather than transformations. Schechner, *Performance Studies*, 148.

36. Seigel, *Rhetoric of Pregnancy*, 25.

37. Here is Burke on approaching altars with "clean hands": "If there is an altar, it is pious of a man to perform some ritual act whereby he may approach this altar with clean hands. A kind of symbolic cleanliness goes with altars, a technique of symbolic cleansing goes with cleanliness, a preparation or initiation goes with the technique of cleansing, the need of cleansing was based upon some feeling of taboo—and so on, until pious linkages may have brought all the significant details of the day into coordination, relating them integrally with one another by a complex interpretative network." K. Burke, *Permanence and Change*, 74–75.

38. Delaney, *Wellmania*, 175.

39. Delaney, *Wellmania*, 175–76.

40. Levinovitz, *Natural*, 134.

41. Levinovitz, *Natural*, 37.

42. Here is an example of an enthymeme: A long-lost friend of mine once began an email by saying "I'm emailing an English professor so I have to be careful what I say. ;)." She was making an argument that called on me as her audience to complete its chain of reasoning by "hearing" its unstated first premise, that all English professors care about grammar. This implied first premise leads to the second, explicitly stated premise, "You are an English professor," and then to the corresponding conclusion that, therefore, "You care about my grammar."

43. Delaney, *Wellmania*, 76–77.

44. Levinovitz, *Natural*, 35.

45. Logan, "Lean Closet."

46. Paltrow (@gwynethpaltrow), "I think pretty much everything."

47. Wellman, "What It Means to Be a Bodybuilder." An "influencer" is someone who positions themselves as a public persona and who shares branded content with their followers. They may be compensated for their posts financially or in kind, or not at all.

48. @goop, "GOOPGENES: What's inside?"; Goop, "Goop Beauty GOOPGENES."

49. Leah Michele (@leamichele), "WELLNESS."

50. INBLOOM Nutrition (@tobeinbloom), "INBLOOM Nutrition."

51. INBLOOM Nutrition (@tobeinbloom), "Elevate the every day."

52. INBLOOM Nutrition (@tobeinbloom), "It really is this easy [smiley face emoji with tongue out]."

53. INBLOOM Nutrition (@tobeinbloom), "Our products are an example."

54. Levinovitz, *Natural*, 38.

55. Chase, "Constructing Ethics through Rhetoric." Chase's discussion of constitutive piety builds on the concept of constitutive rhetoric, which is a rhetoric that constructs identities for the very subjects it addresses. In responding to a given rhetorical text, subjects accept and assume the identities it constructs, effectively becoming the people called forth by the text itself. See Charland, "Constitutive Rhetoric."

56. Interview with research participant W-11, 2018.

57. Levinovitz, *Natural*, 133.

58. INBLOOM Nutrition (@tobeinbloom), "We're all on our own wellness journeys."

59. Sugarbear Hair (@sugarbear), "Get healthy hair, eat the blue bear." The image in figure 13, from August 15, 2017, has been deleted from Khloé Kardashian's Instagram account since it was screen-captured, but it is archived in numerous media articles. See, e.g., Longhetti, "That's Some Pocket Money!"

60. For example, the images of supplement users placing the product in their mouths is reminiscent of the "tasting shot" in cooking shows, which Andrew Chan links to the "money shot" in pornography, showing the grand climax of a sexual performance, a shot that often centers on seminal ejaculation. Chan, "'La Grande Bouffe.'"

61. Van De Wall, "We Tried Those Kardashian-Approved SugarBearHair Vitamins and Here's What Happened."

62. Even the presence of "finsta" accounts (fake Instagram accounts that some users maintain for smaller audiences of followers where they post more candid, and less flattering, images of their lives than on their "rinsta," or "real Instagram," accounts) confirms the prevalence and cultural influence of these scripts of wellness, as users consciously push back on conventional performances of wellness as enhancement. For more on "finsta" accounts, see Molina, "Does Your Kid Have a 'finsta' Account?" Another good example of simultaneous resistance to and reinforcement of online influencer and wellness culture is the comedian Celeste Barber's "challenge accepted" series, in which she spoofs images posted by models and celebrities to highlight the idealism and inaccessibility of images posted on social media. In exaggerated poses that highlight her "real" body (she is a woman in her forties with children), Barber mimics the styling, posing, and composition of selected images, trading couture outfits for improvised "budget" alternatives. Barber (@celestebarber), "Celeste Barber (@celestebarber)."

63. Levinovitz, *Natural*, 82.

64. INBLOOM Nutrition (@tobeinbloom), "Elevate the every day."

65. Baudrillard, *Simulacra and Simulation.*

66. Barnard, "Physician as Priest, Revisited."

67. Levinovitz, *Natural*, 123.

68. Delaney, *Wellmania*, 86.

69. Clare, *Brilliant Imperfection*, 87.

70. For a survey of scholarship on conversion rhetorics, see Lynch, "'Prepare to Believe'"; for more on piety and transcendence, see Bloomfield, "Rhetoric of Energy Darwinism."

71. Interview with research participant W-11, 2018.
72. Delaney, *Wellmania*, 177.
73. K. Burke, *Permanence and Change*, 69.
74. Delaney, *Wellmania*, 184.
75. Bloomfield, "Rhetoric of Energy Darwinism"; K. Burke, *Permanence and Change*, 75, 262.
76. Bloomfield, "Rhetoric of Energy Darwinism," 325.
77. Interview with research participant E-05, 2015.
78. Cederström and Spicer, *Wellness Syndrome*, 133.
79. Delaney, *Wellmania*, 83.

Conclusion

1. Leung, "Stiff Joints, Grey Hair."
2. VanDerWerff, "How to Bake Bread"; Mull, "Americans Have Baked All the Flour Away."
3. Leung, "Stiff Joints, Grey Hair."
4. See Rickert, *Ambient Rhetoric*; Edbauer, "Unframing Models of Public Distribution"; and Jensen, "Ecological Turn in Rhetoric of Health Scholarship," respectively.
5. Edbauer, "Unframing Models of Public Distribution," 19.
6. Keränen, "Addressing the Epidemic of Epidemics," 238.
7. Tsing, "Blasted Landscapes," 108; see also Tsing, *Mushroom at the End of the World*.
8. J. Wolf, "Against Breastfeeding (Sometimes)," 83.
9. Cederström and Spicer, *Wellness Syndrome*, 25.
10. Kimmerer, *Braiding Sweetgrass*, 16.
11. Kimmerer, *Braiding Sweetgrass*, 15.
12. Clare, *Brilliant Imperfection*, 87.
13. See Scott, *Risky Rhetoric*, 21.
14. Guthman, *Weighing In*, 152.
15. Levinovitz, *Natural*, 133.
16. K. Burke, *Attitudes toward History*, 308.
17. K. Burke, *Attitudes toward History*; K. Burke, *Permanence and Change*.

Agamben, Giorgio. *State of Exception*. Translated by Kevin Attell. Chicago: University of Chicago Press, 2005.

Ahmed, Sara. "Feeling Depleted?" *Feministkilljoys* (blog), November 17, 2013. https://feministkilljoys.com/2013/11/17/feeling-depleted/.

———. "Selfcare as Warfare." *Feministkilljoys* (blog), August 25, 2014. https://feministkilljoys.com/2014/08/25/selfcare-as-warfare/.

———. "The Time of Complaint." *Feministkilljoys* (blog), May 30, 2018. https://feministkilljoys.com/2018/05/30/the-time-of-complaint/.

"Amazon Offers 'Wellness Chamber' for Stressed Staff." *BBC News*, May 28, 2021, Technology. https://www.bbc.com/news/technology-57287151.

An Act to Amend the Food and Drugs Act and to Make Consequential Amendments to Other Acts. Bill C-51. https://parl.ca/DocumentViewer/en/39-2/bill/C-51/first-reading.

Angell, Marcia. *The Truth about the Drug Companies: How They Deceive Us and What to Do about It*. New York: Random House, 2005.

Armstrong, David. "The Rise of Surveillance Medicine." *Sociology of Health & Illness* 17, no. 3 (1995): 393–404. https://doi.org/10.1111/1467-9566.ep10933329.

Austin, John Langshaw. *How to Do Things with Words*. 2nd ed. Cambridge, MA: Harvard University Press, 1975.

Bach Remedies. "About The Bach® Essences." Accessed March 3, 2022. https://www.bachremedies.com/en-ca/about/.

———. "Bach & RESCUE Remedy®." Accessed March 3, 2022. https://www.bachremedies.com/en-gb/about/bach-and-rescue-remedy/.

Bainotti, Lucia, Alessandro Caliandro, and Alessandro Gandini. "From Archive Cultures to Ephemeral Content, and Back: Studying Instagram Stories with Digital Methods." *New Media & Society*, September 20, 2020. https://doi.org/10.1177/1461444820960071.

Baluja, Tamara, and Kate Hammer. "How to Build a Healthier, Smarter Student." *Globe and Mail*, May 24, 2012. https://www.theglobeandmail.com/news/national/education/how-to-build-a-healthier-smarter-student/article4209903/.

Barber, Celeste (@celestebarber). "Celeste Barber (@celestebarber)." Instagram. Accessed July 20, 2021. https://www.instagram.com/celestebarber/.

Barnard, David. "Physician as Priest, Revisited." *Journal of Religion and Health* 24, no. 4 (December 1, 1985): 272–86. https://doi.org/10.1007/BF01533009.

Baudrillard, Jean. *Simulacra and Simulation*. Ann Arbor: University of Michigan Press, 1994.

Bayes, Charlotte. "IV Drips Are the Latest Overpriced Bullshit Wellness Fad." *Vice*, August 8, 2019. https://www.vice.com/en/article/zmpjbe/hydration-drip-iv-review -work.

Beck, Julie. "'Americanitis': The Disease of Living Too Fast." *The Atlantic*, March 11, 2016. https://www.theatlantic.com/health/archive/2016/03/the-history-of -neurasthenia-or-americanitis-health-happiness-and-culture/473253/.

Beck, Leslie. "Video: How to Pick a Healthy Snack." *Globe and Mail*. Accessed May 14, 2012. https://www.theglobeandmail.com/life/life-video/how-to-pick-a-healthy-snack /article13101538/.

Belasco, Warren James. *Appetite for Change: How the Counterculture Took on the Food Industry*. New York: Pantheon Books, 1989.

Belling, Catherine. *A Condition of Doubt: The Meanings of Hypochondria*. New York: Oxford University Press, 2012.

Berlant, Lauren. *Cruel Optimism*. Durham, NC: Duke University Press, 2011.

———. "Risky Bigness." In Metzl and Kirkland, *Against Health*, 26–39.

Biss, Eula. "The Illusion of 'Natural.'" *The Atlantic*, September 30, 2014. https://www .theatlantic.com/health/archive/2014/09/the-illusion-of-natural/380836/.

———. *On Immunity: An Inoculation*. Minneapolis: Graywolf, 2014.

Blackwell, Tom. "Firms Back Campaign against Health Bill; Observers Doubt Effort to Stall C-51 Is Grassroots." *National Post* (Toronto), June 16, 2008, A1.

Blaschke, Steffen. "It's All in the Network: A Luhmannian Perspective on Agency." *Management Communication Quarterly* 29, no. 3 (August 2015): 463–68. https://doi .org/10.1177/0893318915584824.

Bloodworth, James. *Hired: Six Months Undercover in Low-Wage Britain*. London: Atlantic Books, 2019.

Bloomfield, Emma Frances. "The Rhetoric of Energy Darwinism: Neoliberal Piety and Market Autonomy in Economic Discourse." *Rhetoric Society Quarterly* 49, no. 4 (August 8, 2019): 320–41. https://doi.org/10.1080/02773945.2019.1634831.

British Columbia Ministry of Health. *BC Health Guide: Helping You and Your Family Stay Healthy*. Edited by Donald W. Kemper, Carrie A. Wiss, and Steven L. Schneider. Boise, ID: Healthwise, 2000.

Brown, Gavin. "Theorizing Ritual as Performance: Explorations of Ritual Indeterminacy." *Journal of Ritual Studies* 17, no. 1 (2003): 3–18. https://www.jstor.org/stable /44368641.

Brown, M. M. "Don't Be the 'Fifth Guy': Risk, Responsibility, and the Rhetoric of Handwashing Campaigns." *Journal of Medical Humanities* 40, no. 2 (June 2019): 211–24. https://doi.org/10.1007/s10912-017-9470-4.

Brownlee, Shannon. *Overtreated: Why Too Much Medicine Is Making Us Sicker and Poorer*. New York: Bloomsbury USA, 2008.

Bunton, Robin, and Alan Petersen, eds. *Foucault, Health and Medicine*. London: Routledge, 2002.

Burke, Amanda. "ACT NOW! The Erosion of Democracy Is Destroying Our Right to Natural Health." Facebook, January 19, 2012. https://www.facebook.com/group.php ?gid=14988003341&v=info.

Burke, Kenneth. *Attitudes toward History*. 3rd ed. With a New Afterword. Berkeley and Los Angeles: University of California Press, 1984.

———. *Language as Symbolic Action*. Berkeley and Los Angeles: University of California Press, 1966.

———. *Permanence and Change: An Anatomy of Purpose*. 2nd rev. ed. Los Altos: University of California Press, 1954.

———. *The Philosophy of Literary Form*. Berkeley and Los Angeles: University of California Press, 1974.

Cairns, Kate, Josée Johnston, and Norah MacKendrick. "Feeding the 'Organic Child': Mothering through Ethical Consumption." *Journal of Consumer Culture* 13, no. 2 (July 1, 2013): 97–118. https://doi.org/10.1177/1469540513480162.

Campbell, Brian, dir. *The Dr. Oz Show*. Episode 80, "Toxic Home: Oz Reveals Most Common Unknown Toxins in Your Home." Starring Mehmet Oz. Aired on CBS, January 19, 2010.

Canadian Association of Naturopathic Doctors. "Common Questions: Naturopathic Visits." Accessed June 5, 2020. https://www.cand.ca/common-questions-naturopathic -visits/.

———. "What Exactly Is Alternative Medicine? How Does Naturopathy Fit In?" Accessed June 5, 2020. https://www.cand.ca/what-exactly-is-alternative-medicine-how-does -naturopathy-fit-in/.

Caulfield, Timothy A. *The Cure for Everything: Untangling Twisted Messages about Health, Fitness, and Happiness*. Boston: Beacon, 2012.

———. *Is Gwyneth Paltrow Wrong about Everything? How the Famous Sell Us Elixirs of Health, Beauty & Happiness*. Boston: Beacon, 2015.

CBC. "Licence to Deceive." *Marketplace*, March 13, 2015. https://www.cbc.ca/player/play /2658659258.

Cederström, Carl, and André Spicer. *The Wellness Syndrome*. Cambridge: Polity, 2015.

Chan, Andrew. "'La Grande Bouffe': Cooking Shows as Pornography." *Gastronomica* 3, no. 4 (2003): 46–53. https://doi.org/10.1525/gfc.2003.3.4.46.

Charland, Maurice. "Constitutive Rhetoric: The Case of the Peuple Québécois." *Quarterly Journal of Speech* 73, no. 2 (May 1, 1987): 133–50. https://doi.org/10.1080 /00335638709383799.

Chase, Kenneth R. "Constructing Ethics through Rhetoric: Isocrates and Piety." *Quarterly Journal of Speech* 95, no. 3 (2009): 239–62. https://doi.org/10.1080 /00335630903140622.

Cheek, Julianne, and Sam Porter. "Reviewing Foucault: Possibilities and Problems for Nursing and Health Care." *Nursing Inquiry* 4, no. 2 (1997): 108–19. https://doi .org/10.1111/j.1440-1800.1997.tb00084.x.

Clare, Eli. *Brilliant Imperfection: Grappling with Cure*. Durham, NC: Duke University Press, 2017.

Clarke, Adele E., Janet K. Shim, Laura Mamo, Jennifer Ruth Fosket, and Jennifer R. Fishman. "Biomedicalization: Technoscientific Transformations of Health, Illness, and U.S. Biomedicine." *American Sociological Review* 68, no. 2 (2003): 161–94. https://doi.org/10.2307/1519765.

Cleveland Clinic. Health Essentials. "What Is Ashwagandha?" May 5, 2021. https:// health.clevelandclinic.org/what-is-ashwagandha/.

Cliffe, Nicole (@Nicole_Cliffe). "The person who came up with 'wellness' as a product adjective is probably living in a castle carved out of gold right now." Twitter, March 26, 2015. https://twitter.com/Nicole_Cliffe/status/58120 6965885399040 (site discontinued; available at http://www.colleenderkatch.com/2018/04/20/archivecliffetweet).

Composed Nutrition. "Composed Nutrition." Accessed June 9, 2020. https://www .composednutrition.com.

———. "Disclaimer." Accessed June 9, 2020. https://www.composednutrition.com /disclaimer.

———. "FAQ." Accessed July 17, 2021. https://www.composednutrition.com/frequently -asked-questions.

Conrad, Peter. *The Medicalization of Society: On the Transformation of Human Conditions into Treatable Disorders.* Baltimore: Johns Hopkins University Press, 2007.

———. "Wellness as Virtue: Morality and the Pursuit of Health." *Culture, Medicine and Psychiatry* 18, no. 3 (September 1, 1994): 385–401. https://doi.org/10.1007/BF01379232.

Cooper, Lane. *The Rhetoric of Aristotle.* 1st ed. Englewood Cliffs, NJ: Pearson, 1960.

Crary, Jonathan. *24/7: Late Capitalism and the Ends of Sleep.* New York: Verso Books, 2013.

Crawford, Robert. "Healthism and the Medicalization of Everyday Life." *International Journal of Health Services* 10, no. 3 (1980): 365–88. https://doi.org/10.2190/3H2H -3XJN-3KAY-G9NY.

Crook, William G. *The Yeast Connection and the Woman.* Jackson, TN: Professional Books/Future Health, 1995.

Crowe, Julie Homchick. "Toxically Clean: Homophonic Expertise, Goop, and the Ideology of Choice." *Rhetoric of Health & Medicine* 4, no. 2 (n.d.): 187–217. https://doi .org/10.5744/rhm.2021.2004.

Davis, Georgiann, and Erin L. Murphy. "Intersex Bodies as States of Exception: An Empirical Explanation for Unnecessary Surgical Modification." *Feminist Formations* 25, no. 2 (2013): 129–52. https://doi.org/10.1353/ff.2013.0022.

Davis, Lennard J. *Enforcing Normalcy: Disability, Deafness, and the Body.* New York: Verso Books, 1995.

Delaney, Brigid. *Wellmania: Extreme Misadventures in the Search for Wellness.* Berkeley: Greystone Books, 2018.

DeRango-Adem, Adebe. "Self-Care Is a Radical Act, But Not in the Way We're Practising It Right Now." *Flare,* November 30, 2017. https://www.flare.com/living/self-care -is-a-radical-act/.

Derkatch, Colleen. *Bounding Biomedicine: Evidence and Rhetoric in the New Science of Alternative Medicine.* Chicago: University of Chicago Press, 2016.

———. "'Wellness' as Incipient Illness: Dietary Supplements in a Biomedical Culture." *Present Tense* 2, no. 2 (2012). https://www.presenttensejournal.org/volume-2 /wellness-as-incipient-illness-dietary-supplements-in-a-biomedical-culture/.

Derkatch, Colleen, and Philippa Spoel. "Public Health Promotion of 'Local Food': Constituting the Self-Governing Citizen-Consumer." *Health* 21, no. 2 (March 1, 2017): 154–70. https://doi.org/10.1177/1363459315590247.

Dickinson, Annette, and Douglas MacKay. "Health Habits and Other Characteristics of Dietary Supplement Users: A Review." *Nutrition Journal* 13, no. 1 (February 6, 2014). https://doi.org/10.1186/1475-2891-13–14.

Dietary Supplement Health and Education Act of 1994. Public Law No. 103-417.

Dumit, Joseph. *Drugs for Life: How Pharmaceutical Companies Define Our Health.* Durham, NC: Duke University Press, 2012.

———. *Picturing Personhood.* Princeton, NJ: Princeton University Press, 2004.

Edbauer, Jenny. "Unframing Models of Public Distribution: From Rhetorical Situation to Rhetorical Ecologies." *Rhetoric Society Quarterly* 35, no. 4 (September 1, 2005): 5–24. https://doi.org/10.1080/02773940509391320.

Ehrenfeld, Dan. "Ecological Investments and the Circulation of Rhetoric: Studying the 'Saving Knowledge' of Dr. Emma Walker's Social Hygiene Lectures." In *Methodologies for the Rhetoric of Health & Medicine,* edited by Lisa Meloncon and J. Blake Scott, 41–60. New York: Routledge, 2017.

Ehrenreich, Barbara. *Natural Causes: An Epidemic of Wellness, the Certainty of Dying, and Killing Ourselves to Live Longer.* New York: Twelve, 2018.

Elliott, Carl. *Better than Well: American Medicine Meets the American Dream.* New York: Norton, 2003.

———. *White Coat, Black Hat: Adventures on the Dark Side of Medicine.* Boston: Beacon, 2010.

Elwyn, Glyn, and Adrian Edwards. "Evidence-Based Patient Choice?" In *Evidence-Based Patient Choice: Inevitable or Impossible?,* edited by Adrian Edwards and Glyn Elwyn, 3–18. New York: Oxford University Press, 2001.

EZ Lifestyle. "About Us." Accessed February 1, 2020. https://ez-lifestyle.com/about-us.

———. "Dream EZ Sleeping Pills & Natural Sleep Aids in Canada." Accessed January 26, 2020. https://ez-lifestyle.com/en-ca/products/dream-ez.

———. "Fuel EZ Natural Energy Supplements & Boosters in Canada." Accessed January 26, 2020. https://ez-lifestyle.com/en-ca/products/fuel-ez.

———. "Over EZ Hangover Cure & Prevention Pills in Canada." Accessed January 26, 2020. https://ez-lifestyle.com/en-ca/products/over-ez.

Foucault, Michel. *The History of Sexuality: An Introduction.* New York: Vintage, 1990.

"From Body Mechanics to Mindfulness, Amazon Launches Employee-Designed Health and Safety Program Called WorkingWell Across U.S. Operations." *Business Wire.* May 17, 2021. https://www.businesswire.com/news/home/20210517005300/en/From-Body-Mechanics-to-Mindfulness-Amazon-Launches-Employee-Designed-Health-and-Safety-Program-called-WorkingWell-Across-U.S.-Operations.

Frost, Samantha. *Biocultural Creatures: Toward a New Theory of the Human.* Durham, NC: Duke University Press, 2016.

Gardner, John. "Let's Send That to the Lab: Technology and Diagnosis." In *Social Issues in Diagnosis: An Introduction for Students and Clinicians,* edited by Annemarie Goldstein Jutel and Kevin Dew, 151–64. Baltimore: Johns Hopkins University Press, 2014.

Gault, Matthew. "Amazon Introduces Tiny 'ZenBooths' for Stressed-Out Warehouse Workers." *Vice,* May 27, 2021. https://www.vice.com/en/article/wx5nmw/amazon-introduces-tiny-zenbooths-for-stressed-out-warehouse-workers.

George, Ann. *Kenneth Burke's "Permanence and Change": A Critical Companion.* Columbia: University of South Carolina Press, 2018.

Gibney, Alex, dir. *Billions.* Episode 15, "Optimal Play." Written by Brian Koppelman, David Levien, and Andrew Ross Sorkin. Featuring Paul Giamatti, Damien Lewis, and Maggie Siff. Aired March 5, 2017, on Showtime.

Glasbergen, Randy. "Due to unusually high call volume, this conversation will be really loud." Glasbergen Cartoon Service. Accessed July 10, 2021. https://glasbergen.b-cdn .net/wp-content/gallery/service/toon-1870.gif.

Globe and Mail. "Video: BBQ Basics: 4 Tips to Get Your BBQ Ready for Grilling Season." Accessed June 28, 2021. https://www.theglobeandmail.com/life/life-video/video-4-tips -to-get-your-bbq-ready-for-grilling-season/article11278538/.

Goop. "Goop Beauty GOOPGENES Marine Collagen Superpowder—5-Stick Pack." Accessed June 4, 2021. https://goop.com/ca-en/goop-beauty-goopgenes-marine -collagen-superpowder-5-stick-pack/p/.

Goop (@goop). "GOOPGENES: What's inside? A combination of wild marine collagen, ceramides, astaxanthin, and aloe. We focused on getting the very best. . . ." Instagram photo. Accessed June 4, 2021. https://www.instagram.com/p/Bo7sZPeApoG/?hl=en.

"The Great Debate: Should You Replace Your Hormones?" *The Oprah Winfrey Show.* Aired January 15, 2009.

Gunter, Jennifer. "Jennifer Gunter (@DrJenGunter) / Twitter." Twitter. Accessed February 5, 2020. https://twitter.com/drjengunter.

Guo, Xiaoyan, Noreen Willows, Stefan Kuhle, Gian Jhangri, and Paul J. Veugelers. "Use of Vitamin and Mineral Supplements among Canadian Adults." *Canadian Journal of Public Health* 100, no. 5 (September 1, 2009): 357–60. https://doi.org/10.1007 /BF03405270.

Guthman, Julie. *Weighing In: Obesity, Food Justice, and the Limits of Capitalism.* California Studies in Food and Culture 32. Berkeley: University of California Press, 2011.

Hacking, Ian. *Mad Travelers: Reflections on the Reality of Transient Mental Illnesses.* Cambridge, MA: Harvard University Press, 1998.

Hadler, Norton M. *Worried Sick: A Prescription for Health in an Overtreated America.* Chapel Hill: University of North Carolina Press, 2012.

Hanson, Alan. "Goop and the Anxiety of Wellness—Digg." *Digg,* June 16, 2017. https:// digg.com/2017/goop-summit.

Haraway, Donna. *Staying with the Trouble: Making Kin in the Chthulucene.* Durham, NC: Duke University Press, 2016.

Hargreaves Heap, Shaun, Martin Hollis, Bruce Lyons, Robert Sugden, and Albert Weale. *The Theory of Choice: A Critical Guide.* Oxford: Blackwell, 1992.

Health Canada. "About Natural Health Products." Organizational descriptions, November 26, 2010. https://www.canada.ca/en/health-canada/services/drugs-health -products/natural-non-prescription/regulation/about-products.html.

———. "2.6 Efficacy Evidence Recommendations | Pathway for Licensing Natural Health Products Used as Traditional Medicines." May 18, 2012. https://www.canada.ca/en /health-canada/services/drugs-health-products/natural-non-prescription/legislation -guidelines/guidance-documents/pathway-licensing-traditional-medicines.html.

———. "2.7 Safety Evidence for Traditional Medicines | Pathway for Licensing Natural Health Products Used as Traditional Medicines." May 18, 2012. https://www.canada .ca/en/health-canada/services/drugs-health-products/natural-non-prescription /legislation-guidelines/guidance-documents/pathway-licensing-traditional -medicines.html.

Healthline. "12 Proven Health Benefits of Ashwagandha." November 3, 2019. https:// www.healthline.com/nutrition/12-proven-ashwagandha-benefits.

Herek, Stephen, dir. *Bill & Ted's Excellent Adventure*. Los Angeles: Orion Pictures International, 1989.

Hodge, Brent, dir. *A User's Guide to Cheating Death*. Los Gatos, CA: Netflix, 2017.

———. *A User's Guide to Cheating Death*. Los Gatos, CA: Netflix, 2018.

———. *A User's Guide to Cheating Death*. Los Gatos, CA: Netflix, 2019.

Hurley, Dan. *Natural Causes: Death, Lies, and Politics in America's Vitamin and Herbal Supplement Industry*. New York: Broadway Books, 2006.

Hyde, Abbey, Jean Nee, Etaoine Howlett, Jonathan Drennan, and Michelle Butler. "Menopause Narratives: The Interplay of Women's Embodied Experiences with Biomedical Discourses." *Qualitative Health Research* 20, no. 6 (June 2010): 805–15. https://doi.org/10.1177/1049732310363126.

Hyde, Michael J. *Perfection: Coming to Terms with Being Human*. Waco, TX: Baylor University Press, 2010.

INBLOOM Nutrition (@tobeinbloom). "Elevate the every day with whole-food ingredients and full-spectrum herbal blends. Our formulas are inspired by the powerful properties of. . . ." Instagram photo, May 11, 2021. https://www.instagram.com/p/COaczISJP_Z/.

———. "INBLOOM Nutrition." Instagram. Accessed July 20, 2021. https://www.instagram.com/tobeinbloom/.

———. "It really is this easy [smiley face emoji with tongue out] / SHAKE, SHAKE, SHAKE / Because INBLOOM powders are made from whole foods, plants, and herbs, they perform. . . ." Instagram photo. Accessed May 12, 2021. https://www.instagram.com/p/COxuZ1mpZ-W/.

———. "Our products are an example of what you can make when you work with nature, the right way. Take essential elements for example. . . ." Instagram photo, May 11, 2021. https://www.instagram.com/p/COwHP5xJMlb/.

———. "We're all on our own wellness journeys but together, we're a community being INBLOOM." Instagram photo, April 8, 2021. https://www.instagram.com/p/CNaAee3JwWY/.

Irving, Greg, Ana Luisa Neves, Hajira Dambha-Miller, Ai Oishi, Hiroko Tagashira, Anistasiya Verho, and John Holden. "International Variations in Primary Care Physician Consultation Time: A Systematic Review of 67 Countries." *BMJ Open* 7, no. 10 (October 1, 2017): e017902. https://doi.org/10.1136/bmjopen-2017-017902.

Jack, Jordynn. "'The Piety of Degradation': Kenneth Burke, the Bureau of Social Hygiene, and Permanence and Change." *Quarterly Journal of Speech* 90, no. 4 (2004): 446–68. https://doi.org/10.1080/0033563042000302180.

Jensen, Robin E. "An Ecological Turn in Rhetoric of Health Scholarship: Attending to the Historical Flow and Percolation of Ideas, Assumptions, and Arguments." *Communication Quarterly* 63, no. 5 (October 20, 2015): 522–26. https://doi.org/10.1080/01463373.2015.1103600.

———. "Theorizing Chemical Rhetoric: Toward an Articulation of Chemistry as a Public Vocabulary." *Journal of Communication* 71, no. 3 (June 1, 2021): 431–53. https://doi.org/10.1093/joc/jqab011.

Jutel, Annemarie Goldstein. *Diagnosis: Truths and Tales*. Toronto: University of Toronto Press, 2019.

———. *Putting a Name to It: Diagnosis in Contemporary Society*. Baltimore: Johns Hopkins University Press, 2011.

Kannan, Viji Diane, Laura M. Gaydos, Adam J. Atherly, and Benjamin G. Druss. "Medical Utilization among Wellness Consumers." *Medical Care Research and Review* 67, no. 6 (December 1, 2010): 722–36. https://doi.org/10.1177/1077558710370706.

Kaori Gurley, Lauren. "Amazon Denies Workers Pee in Bottles. Here Are the Pee Bottles." *Vice*, March 25, 2021. https://www.vice.com/en/article/k7amyn/amazon -denies-workers-pee-in-bottles-here-are-the-pee-bottles.

Kardashian, Kim (@kimkardashian). "Loving the New @sugarbearhair Vegan Women's Multi gummies for total body wellness! They pair great with their hair vitamins and taste. . . ." Instagram photo, December 13, 2018. https://www .instagram.com/p/BrV1lkEnMOd/.

Kelly, Jack. "Social Media Savaged Amazon's New 'Dystopian' and 'Black Mirror' Wellness Zen Meditation Booths for Warehouse Workers." *Forbes*. Accessed July 29, 2021. https://www.forbes.com/sites/jackkelly/2021/05/29/social-media-savaged -amazons-new-dystopianand-black-mirror---zen-booths/.

Kelly, Kevin. "What Is the Quantified Self?" Quantified Self. 2007. https://web.archive.org /web/20111101100244/http://quantifiedself.com/2007/10/what-is-the-quantifiable-self/.

Keränen, Lisa. "Addressing the Epidemic of Epidemics: Germs, Security, and a Call for Biocriticism." *Quarterly Journal of Speech* 97, no. 2 (April 29, 2011): 224–44. https://doi.org/10.1080/00335630.2011.565785.

———. "How Does a Pathogen Become a Terrorist? The Collective Transformation of Risk into Bio(in)Security." In Leach and Dysart-Gale, *Rhetorical Questions of Health and Medicine*, 77–96.

Kimmerer, Robin Wall. *Braiding Sweetgrass: Indigenous Wisdom, Scientific Knowledge, and the Teachings of Plants*. Minneapolis: Milkweed Editions, 2013.

Kirkey, Sharon. "The Delusion of Detoxing: There's No Evidence to Support Holiday Cleanses, Experts Say." *National Post*, December 27, 2018. https://nationalpost.com /health/the-delusion-of-detoxing-theres-no-evidence-to-support-holiday-cleanses -experts-say.

Kirmayer, Laurence J. "Mind and Body as Metaphors: Hidden Values in Biomedicine." In *Biomedicine Examined*, edited by Margaret Lock and Deborah Gordon, 57–93. Culture, Illness and Healing. Dordrecht: Springer Netherlands, 1988. https://doi.org /10.1007/978-94-009-2725-4_4.

Klein, Richard. "What Is Health and How Do You Get It?" In Metzl and Kirkland, *Against Health*, 15–25.

Klingbeil, Kurt. "Stop Bill C-51: Petition." Care2, September 10, 2008. https://www .thepetitionsite.com/en-ca/.

Klippenstein, Ken. "Documents Show Amazon Is Aware Drivers Pee in Bottles and Even Defecate En Route, Despite Company Denial." *The Intercept*, March 25, 2021. https://theintercept.com/2021/03/25/amazon-drivers-pee-bottles-union/.

Kolata, Gina. "Hormone Studies: What Went Wrong?" *New York Times*, April 22, 2003. https://www.nytimes.com/2003/04/22/science/hormone-studies-what-went-wrong .html.

Kosova, Weston, and Pat Wingert. "Live Your Best Life Ever! Wish Away Cancer! Get A Lunchtime Face-Lift! Eradicate Autism! Turn Back The Clock! Thin Your Thighs! Cure Menopause! Harness Positive Energy! Erase Wrinkles! Banish Obesity! Live Your Best Life Ever!" *Newsweek* 153, no. 23 (2009).

Kraft, Frederic B., and Phillips W. Goodell. "Identifying the Health Conscious Consumer." *Journal of Health Care Marketing* 13, no. 3 (Fall 1993): 18–25.

Larocca, Amy. "How 'Wellness' Became an Epidemic." *The Cut*, June 27, 2017. https://www.thecut.com/2017/06/how-wellness-became-an-epidemic.html.

Latimer, Heather. "Bio-Reproductive Futurism: Bare Life and the Pregnant Refugee in Alfonso Cuarón's *Children of Men*." *Social Text* 29, no. 3 (108) (2011): 51–72. https://doi.org/10.1215/01642472-1299965.

Leach, Joan, and Deborah Dysart-Gale, eds. *Rhetorical Questions of Health and Medicine*. Lanham, MD: Lexington Books, 2011.

Leah Michele (@leamichele). "WELLNESS." Instagram. Accessed July 19, 2021. https://www.instagram.com/stories/highlights/17898973402152054/.

Leung, Wency. "Stiff Joints, Grey Hair: Pandemic-Induced Isolation, Grief and Anxiety Aged You—but It's Not Too Late to Reverse the Effects." *Globe and Mail*, July 26, 2021. https://www.theglobeandmail.com/canada/article-the-pandemic-aged -you-but-you-can-still-reverse-the-effects/.

Levenstein, Harvey. *Fear of Food: A History of Why We Worry about What We Eat*. Chicago: University of Chicago Press, 2012.

Levinovitz, Alan. *Natural: How Faith in Nature's Goodness Leads to Harmful Fads, Unjust Laws, and Flawed Science*. Boston: Beacon, 2020.

Lexchin, Joel. *Doctors in Denial: Why Big Pharma and the Canadian Medical Profession Are Too Close for Comfort*. Toronto: James Lorimer, 2017.

Lindsay O'Reilly Nutrition. Accessed June 9, 2020. https://www.lindsayoreillyrd.com.

Lock, Margaret. "Anomalous Ageing: Managing the Postmenopausal Body." *Body & Society* 4, no. 1 (March 1, 1998): 35–61. https://doi.org/10.1177/1357034X98004 001003.

Logan, Dana W. "The Lean Closet: Asceticism in Postindustrial Consumer Culture." *Journal of the American Academy of Religion* 85, no. 3 (September 1, 2017): 600–628. https://doi.org/10.1093/jaarel/lfw091.

Long, Katherine Anne. "Amazon, Contractors Settle Wage-Theft Lawsuit by Seattle-Area Drivers for $8.2 Million." *Seattle Times*, March 19, 2021. https://www .seattletimes.com/business/amazon/amazon-contractors-settle-wage-theft-lawsuit -by-seattle-area-drivers-for-8-2-million/.

Longhetti, Chloe-Lee. "That's Some Pocket Money! Roxy Jacenko's Six-Year-Old Daughter Pixie Curtis Earns $600 for a Single Sponsored Instagram Post." *Daily Mail*, September 27, 2017. http://www.dailymail.co.uk/~/article-4923898/index .html.

Lourie, Bruce, and Rick Smith. *Toxin Toxout: Getting Harmful Chemicals Out of Our Bodies and Our World*. Toronto: Vintage Canada, 2013.

Love, Shayla. "The Dark Truths behind Our Obsession with Self-Care." *Vice*, December 11, 2018. https://www.vice.com/en_us/article/zmdwm4/the-young-and-the-uncared-for -v25n4.

Lowenberg, June S., and Fred Davis. "Beyond Medicalisation-Demedicalisation: The Case of Holistic Health." *Sociology of Health & Illness* 16, no. 5 (1994): 579–99. https://doi.org/10.1111/1467-9566.ep11348024.

Luhmann, Niklas. "The Autopoiesis of Social Systems." *Sociocybernetic Paradoxes* 6, no. 2 (1986): 172–92.

———. "The Concept of Society." *Thesis Eleven* 31, no. 1 (February 1, 1992): 67–80. https://doi.org/10.1177/072551369203100106.

Lupton, Deborah. "M-Health and Health Promotion: The Digital Cyborg and Surveillance Society." *Social Theory & Health* 10, no. 3 (August 1, 2012): 229–44. https://doi.org/10.1057/sth.2012.6.

———. *The Quantified Self.* Oxford: Polity Press, 2016.

Lynch, John. "'Prepare to Believe': The Creation Museum as Embodied Conversion Narrative." *Rhetoric and Public Affairs* 16, no. 1 (2013): 1–28. https://doi.org/10.14321/rhetpublaffa.16.1.0001.

MacKendrick, Norah. *Better Safe than Sorry: How Consumers Navigate Exposure to Everyday Toxics.* Berkeley: University of California Press, 2018.

Majdik, Zoltan P. "A Computational Approach to Assessing Rhetorical Effectiveness: Agentic Framing of Climate Change in the Congressional Record, 1994–2016." *Technical Communication Quarterly* 28, no. 3 (July 3, 2019): 207–22. https://doi.org/10.1080/10572252.2019.1601774.

Martin, Emily. "The End of the Body?" *American Ethnologist* 19, no. 1 (1992): 121–40. https://doi.org/10.1525/ae.1992.19.1.02a00070.

Mayo Clinic. "Bioidentical Hormones: Are They Safer?" Accessed June 28, 2021. https://www.mayoclinic.org/diseases-conditions/menopause/expert-answers/bioidentical-hormones/faq-20058460.

McGreavy, Bridie. "Resilience as Discourse." *Environmental Communication* 10, no. 1 (2016): 104–21. https://doi.org/10.1080/17524032.2015.1014390.

Melman, Jeff, dir. *Grey's Anatomy.* Episode 15, "Into You Like a Train." Written by Shonda Rhimes and Krista Vernoff, featuring Ellen Pompeo, Sandra Oh, and Katherine Heigl. Aired on ABC, August 31, 2006.

Meme Generator. "Conspiracy Keanu—What If an Unusually High Call Volume Is Really the Usual Call Volume?" Accessed July 10, 2021. https://memegenerator.net/instance/64856186/conspiracy-keanu-what-if-an-unusually-high-call-volume-is-really-the-usual-call-volume.

Metabolic Renewal. " Overview." Accessed June 2, 2020. https://metabolicrenewal.com/overview.html.

Metzl, Jonathan M., and Anna Kirkland, eds. *Against Health: How Health Became the New Morality.* New York: New York University Press, 2010.

Molina, Brett. "Does Your Kid Have a 'finsta' Account? Why It's a Big Deal." *USA Today.* Accessed July 17, 2021. https://www.usatoday.com/story/tech/talkingtech/2017/10/20/does-your-kid-have-finsta-account-why-its-big-deal/783424001/.

Motta, Matthew, Timothy Callaghan, and Steven Sylvester. "Knowing Less but Presuming More: Dunning-Kruger Effects and the Endorsement of Anti-Vaccine Policy Attitudes." *Social Science & Medicine* 211 (August 2018): 274–81. https://doi.org/10.1016/j.socscimed.2018.06.032.

Moynihan, Ray, and Alan Cassels. *Selling Sickness: How the World's Biggest Pharmaceutical Companies Are Turning Us All into Patients.* New York: Nation Books, 2005.

Mull, Amanda. "Americans Have Baked All the Flour Away: The Pandemic Is Reintroducing the Nation to Its Kitchens." *The Atlantic,* May 12, 2020. https://www.theatlantic.com/health/archive/2020/05/why-theres-no-flour-during-coronavirus/611527/.

My VIOME Results. Accessed July 17, 2021. https://www.youtube.com/watch?v
=ESUDgXMwkzM.

Naftulin, Julia. "Oprah's Best and Worst Health Advice: Vaccines, Meditation, Diet—
Insider." February 20, 2020. https://www.insider.com/oprah-winfrey-best-worst-health
-advice-2020-2#suzanne-somers-told-oprah-viewers-she-injected-herself-with-human
-growth-hormones-to-look-more-youthful-doctors-say-the-practice-can-be-dangerous-8.

The Nap Ministry. "About." January 5, 2018. https://thenapministry.wordpress.com/about/.

The Nap Ministry (@TheNapMinistry). "It is our right to rest. #thenapministry." Twitter,
August 19, 2019. https://twitter.com/TheNapMinistry/status/1163511408815820800.

The Nap Ministry (@thenapministry). "Public Service Announcement for the
weekend. . . ." Instagram photo, January 30, 2021. https://www.instagram.com/p
/CKrHhO5l6Zr.

Natrol. "Melatonin For Sleep." Accessed January 26, 2020. https://www.natrol.com
/benefits/benefitssleep/.

———. *What Is Healthy Sleep?* YouTube video, 2017. https://www.youtube.com/watch?v
=Rkvp7O5CeFI&feature=emb_logo.

Newmaster, Steven G., Meghan Grguric, Dhivya Shanmughanandhan, Sathishkumar
Ramalingam, and Subramanyam Ragupathy. "DNA Barcoding Detects Contamination and Substitution in North American Herbal Products." *BMC Medicine* 11,
no. 222 (October 11, 2013): 1–13. https://doi.org/10.1186/1741-7015-11-222.

Nichter, Mark, and Jennifer Jo Thompson. "For My Wellness, Not Just My Illness:
North Americans' Use of Dietary Supplements." *Culture, Medicine and Psychiatry*
30, no. 2 (June 1, 2006): 175–222. https://doi.org/10.1007/s11013-006-9016-0.

Nicotra, Jodie. "Assemblage Rhetorics: Creating New Frameworks for Rhetorical
Action." In *Rhetoric, Through Everyday Things*, edited by Scot Barnett and Casey
Boyle, 185–96. Tuscaloosa: University of Alabama Press, 2016.

Nisly, Nicole L., Brian M. Gryzlak, M. Bridget Zimmerman, and Robert B. Wallace.
"Dietary Supplement Polypharmacy: An Unrecognized Public Health Problem?"
Evidence-Based Complementary and Alternative Medicine 7, no. 1 (2010): 107–13.
https://doi.org/10.1093/ecam/nem150.

Northrup, Christiane. *The Wisdom of Menopause: Creating Physical and Emotional
Health and Healing during the Change.* 4th ed. New York: Bantam, 2021.

Oreskes, Naomi, and Erik M. Conway. *Merchants of Doubt: How a Handful of Scientists
Obscured the Truth on Issues from Tobacco Smoke to Global Warming.* New York:
Bloomsbury USA, 2010.

Paltrow, Gwyneth (@gwynethpaltrow). "I think pretty much everything in my medicine
cabinet is non-toxic and clean by our standards at @goop. We work hard to make
and curate. . . ." Instagram photo, August 26, 2020. https://www.instagram.com/p
/CEWs3r2D_4V/?hl=en.

Parker, Stephen. *Bertolt Brecht: A Literary Life.* New York: Bloomsbury USA, 2014.

Parsons, Talcott. *The Social System.* Glencoe, IL: Free Press, 1951.

Perceptive Health. "Hidden Food Sensitivities." August 1, 2019. https://www
.perceptivehealth.ca/news/2018/3/8/hidden-food-sensitivities.

Perelman, Chaïm. *The Realm of Rhetoric.* Notre Dame, IN: University of Notre Dame
Press, 1982.

Perelman, Chaïm, and Lucie Olbrechts-Tyteca. *The New Rhetoric: A Treatise on Argumentation*. Notre Dame, IN: University of Notre Dame Press, 1969.

Petersen, Alan, Mark Davis, Suzanne Fraser, and Jo Lindsay. "Healthy Living and Citizenship: An Overview." *Critical Public Health* 20, no. 4 (December 1, 2010): 391–400. https://doi.org/10.1080/09581596.2010.518379.

Pezzullo, Phaedra C. *Toxic Tourism: Rhetorics of Pollution, Travel, and Environmental Justice*. Rhetoric, Culture, and Social Critique. Tuscaloosa: University of Alabama Press, 2007.

Picard, André. "Legislation Worthy of Our Support." *Globe and Mail*, April 17, 2008. https://www.theglobeandmail.com/life/health-and-fitness/legislation-worthy-of-our -support/article719193/.

Porter, Roy. *Quacks: Fakers & Charlatans in Medicine*. Charleston, SC: Tempus, 2003.

Precision Analytical. "DUTCH: Dried Urine Test for Comprehensive Hormones." Accessed March 3, 2022. https://dutchtest.com/wp-content/uploads/2021/06 /DUTCH-Complete-Female-Sample-Report-Ref062521.pdf.

Quantified Self. "Homepage." Accessed July 18, 2021. https://quantifiedself.com/.

Rappaport, Roy Abraham. *Ritual and Religion in the Making of Humanity*. New York: Cambridge University Press, 1999.

Reagle, Joseph M., Jr. *Hacking Life: Systematized Living and Its Discontents*. Cambridge, MA: MIT Press, 2019.

Reeve, Donna. "Biopolitics and Bare Life: Does the Impaired Body Provide Contemporary Examples of Homo Sacer?" In *Arguing about Disability: Philosophical Perspectives*, edited by Kristjana Kristiansen, Simo Vehmas, and Tom Shakespeare, 203–17. London: Routledge, 2008.

Reich, Jennifer A. *Calling the Shots: Why Parents Reject Vaccines*. New York: New York University Press, 2016.

Renew Life Canada. "Renew Life® CleanseSMART®, Full Body Cleanse, 30 Day Program." Accessed February 5, 2020. https://www.renewlife.ca/product/cleanse smart-full-body-cleanse-30-day-kit/.

———. "Renew Life® First Cleanse, 15 Day Program." Accessed February 7, 2020. https://www.renewlife.ca/product/first-cleanse-15-day-kit/.

———. "Renew Life® Rapid Cleanse, 7 Day Kit." Accessed February 5, 2020. https://www.renewlife.ca/product/rapid-cleanse-7-day-kit/.

Rescue Remedy. "RESCUE® On the Go." Accessed February 1, 2020. https://www .rescueremedy.com/en-ie/brand/rescue-on-the-go.

———. "Discover The RESCUE® Range." Accessed March 3, 2022. https://www .rescueremedy.com/en-au/range/.

———. "Rescue Remedy." Youtube video. Accessed February 1, 2020. https://www .youtube.com/channel/UCUoGoK1wv9ZOGCO2pdJpdOA/featured.

———. "RESCUE Remedy® Dropper." Accessed January 26, 2020. https://www .rescueremedy.com/en-au/rescue-range/rescue-remedy/rescue-remedy-dropper.

———. "RESCUE Remedy®—Our Every Day Essentials." Accessed May 10, 2020. https://www.rescueremedy.com/en-au/rescue-range/rescue-remedy.

———. *Rescue Remedy Mother and Exam*. YouTube video, 2015. https://www.youtube.com /watch?v=78ogyLq5Ero.

———. *Rescue Remedy Mother and Interview*. YouTube video, 2015. https://www.youtube .com/watch?v=3FKhg4uUHKI.

————. *Rescue Remedy TVC Mother, Bride and Exam.* YouTube video, 2015. https://www
.youtube.com/watch?v=piGobeI_9mE.

————. *Rescue Remedy TVC Mother, Bride and Interviewee.* YouTube video, 2015.
https://www.youtube.com/watch?v=_5pnxZLrY2U.

REVIV. Accessed December 22, 2021. https://web.archive.org/web/20190211035207
/http://revivme.com/.

REVIV. "Become the Best Version of You." Accessed February 1, 2020. https://revivme.com/.

————. "IV Therapies." Accessed January 26, 2020. https://revivme.com/iv-therapies/.

————. "Royal Flush Deluxe IV." Accessed February 1, 2020. https://revivme.com
/therapies/royal-flush/.

————. "Ultraviv Recovery IV Therapy." Accessed January 26, 2020. https://revivme.com
/therapies/ultraviv/.

Rickert, Thomas. *Ambient Rhetoric: The Attunements of Rhetorical Being.* Pittsburgh:
University of Pittsburgh Press, 2013.

Riedl, Sue. "Video: Chef Basics: How to Make the Perfect Pancake." *Globe and Mail.*
Accessed June 28, 2021. https://www.theglobeandmail.com/life/life-video/video
-chef-basics-how-to-make-the-perfect-pancake/article11527835/.

Rocky Mountain Analytical. "RMA FST™-IgG Food Sensitivity Test." Accessed July 29,
2021. https://rmalab.com/test/rma-fst-igg-food-sensitivity-test/.

Rose, Nikolas. *The Politics of Life Itself: Biomedicine, Power, and Subjectivity in the
Twenty-First Century.* Princeton, NJ: Princeton University Press, 2007.

Rosteck, Thomas, and Michael Leff. "Piety, Propriety, and Perspective: An Interpretation and Application of Key Terms in Kenneth Burke's Permanence and Change."
Western Journal of Speech Communication: WJSC 53, no. 4 (Fall 1989): 327–41.
https://doi.org/10.1080/10570318909374312.

Rozga, Mary R., Judith S. Stern, Kimber Stanhope, Peter J. Havel, and Alexandra G.
Kazaks. "Dietary Supplement Users Vary in Attitudes and Sources of Dietary
Supplement Information in East and West Geographic Regions: A Cross-Sectional
Study." *BMC Complementary and Alternative Medicine* 13, no. 1 (July 30, 2013): 200.
https://doi.org/10.1186/1472-6882-13-200.

Ruth, Cory. "Welcome!" The Women's Dietitian. Accessed July 16, 2021. https://www
.thewomensdietitian.com.

Toronto Metropolitan University (formerly Ryerson University). "Ryerson Recharge:
Prioritizing Work to Support Your Wellbeing." Accessed July 11, 2021. https://www
.ryerson.ca/covid-19/updates/2020/08/ryerson-recharge-prioritizing-work-to
-support-your-wellbeing/.

Schechner, Richard. *Performance Studies: An Introduction.* 4th ed. London: Routledge,
2020.

Schuster, Tonya L., Marnie Dobson, Maritza Jauregui, and Robert H. I. Blanks.
"Wellness Lifestyles I: A Theoretical Framework Linking Wellness, Health Lifestyles, and Complementary and Alternative Medicine." *Journal of Alternative and
Complementary Medicine* 10, no. 2 (April 1, 2004): 349–56. https://doi.org/10.1089
/10755530432306247.

Scott, J. Blake. "Kairos as Indeterminate Risk Management: The Pharmaceutical
Industry's Response to Bioterrorism." *Quarterly Journal of Speech* 92, no. 2 (May 1,
2006): 115–43. https://doi.org/10.1080/00335630600816938.

———. *Risky Rhetoric: AIDS and the Cultural Practices of HIV Testing.* Carbondale: Southern Illinois University Press, 2003.

"Secrets to Healthier Aging." *Dr. Oz: The Good Life: Feel Younger,* January 2020.

Segal, Judy Z. *Health and the Rhetoric of Medicine.* Carbondale: Southern Illinois University Press, 2005.

———. "Rhetoric of Health and Medicine." In *The Sage Handbook of Rhetorical Studies,* edited by Kirt H. Wilson and Rosa A. Eberly, 227–46. Thousand Oaks, CA: Sage, 2008.

———. "What, in Addition to Drugs, Do Pharmaceutical Ads Sell? The Rhetoric of Pleasure in Direct-to-Consumer Advertising for Prescription Pharmaceuticals." In Leach and Dysart-Gale, *Rhetorical Questions of Health and Medicine,* 9–32.

Seigel, Marika. *The Rhetoric of Pregnancy.* Chicago: University of Chicago Press, 2014.

@shegotawildhair. "[Gray-hair emojis] It's about WAY more than the growth of your hair. It's the growth of WHO YOU ARE. The internal transformation that happens over. . . ." Instagram photo. Accessed May 26, 2021. https://www.instagram.com/p/CObqfZHsok9/.

Shotwell, Alexis. *Against Purity: Living Ethically in Compromised Times.* Minneapolis: University of Minnesota Press, 2016.

Smith, Rick, and Bruce Lourie. *Slow Death by Rubber Duck: How the Toxic Chemistry of Everyday Life Affects Our Health.* Toronto: Knopf Canada, 2009.

Smith, Walter George. *The Wellness Prescription.* Belleville, ON: Epic Press, an imprint of Essence Publishing, 1999.

Somers, Suzanne. *Ageless: The Naked Truth about Bioidentical Hormones.* New York: Three Rivers, 2006.

———. *I'm Too Young for This! The Natural Hormone Solution to Enjoy Perimenopause.* New York: Harmony Books, 2013.

———. "Newsweek Attack—Huh? The Truth About Bioidentical Hormones vs. Synthetic." *Suzanne's Blog.* Accessed October 7, 2017. www.suzannesomers.com/Blog/post/Newsweek-Attack-Huh.aspx.

———. *The Sexy Years: Discover the Hormone Connection; The Secret to Fabulous Sex, Great Health, and Vitality, for Women and Men.* Foreword by Robert A. Greene, MD. New York: Harmony, 2005.

———. *Suzanne Somers' Fast and Easy: Lose Weight the Somersize Way with Quick, Delicious Meals for the Entire Family!* New York: Three Rivers, 2004.

Sontag, Susan. *Illness as Metaphor.* New York: Vintage, 1979.

Spoel, Philippa, and Colleen Derkatch. "Constituting Community through Food Charters: A Rhetorical-Genre Analysis." *Canadian Food Studies / La Revue Canadienne Des Études Sur l'alimentation* 3, no. 1 (April 4, 2016): 46–70. https://doi.org/10.15353/cfs-rcea.v3i1.144.

———. "Resilience and Self-Reliance in Canadian Food Charter Discourse." *Poroi* 15, no. 1 (January 7, 2020): 1–28. https://doi.org/10.13008/2151-2957.1298.

Spoel, Philippa, Roma Harris, and Flis Henwood. "The Moralization of Healthy Living: Burke's Rhetoric of Rebirth and Older Adults' Accounts of Healthy Eating." *Health: An Interdisciplinary Journal for the Social Study of Health, Illness and Medicine* 16, no. 6 (November 2012): 619–35. https://doi.org/10.1177/1363459312441009.

———. "Rhetorics of Health Citizenship: Exploring Vernacular Critiques of Government's Role in Supporting Healthy Living." *Journal of Medical Humanities* 35, no. 2 (June 1, 2014): 131–47. https://doi.org/10.1007/s10912-014-9276-6.

Stambler, Danielle Mollie. "Eating Data: The Rhetorics of Food, Medicine, and Technology in Employee Wellness Programs." *Rhetoric of Health & Medicine* 4, no. 2 (2021): 158–86. https://doi.org/10.5744/rhm.2021.2003

Statistics Canada. "Health Fact Sheets: Use of Nutritional Supplements." June 20, 2015. http://www.statcan.gc.ca/pub/82-625-x/2017001/article/14831-eng.htm.

Stephenson, Barry. *Ritual: A Very Short Introduction.* New York: Oxford University Press, 2015.

Stokols, D. "Establishing and Maintaining Healthy Environments: Toward a Social Ecology of Health Promotion." *American Psychologist* 47, no. 1 (1992): 6–22. https://doi.org/10.1037//0003-066x.47.1.6.

"Stop C-51 Forever." The Official Stop C-51 Website. March 1, 2015. https://web.archive.org/web/20150301223618/http://www.stopc51.com/.

Stormer, Nathan, and Bridie McGreavy. "Thinking Ecologically about Rhetoric's Ontology: Capacity, Vulnerability, and Resilience." *Philosophy & Rhetoric* 50, no. 1 (2017): 1–25. https://doi.org/10.5325/philrhet.50.1.0001.

Thaler, Kylie, Angela Kaminski, Andrea Chapman, Tessa Langley, and Gerald Gartlehner. "Bach Flower Remedies for Psychological Problems and Pain: A Systematic Review." *BMC Complementary and Alternative Medicine* 9 (May 26, 2009): 16. https://doi.org/10.1186/1472-6882-9-16.

Tiedemann, Marlisa. "Bill C-51: An Act to amend the Food and Drugs Act and to make consequential amendments to Other Acts." 39th Parliament, 2nd session, 2008. Legislative summary 39-2-LS-602-E. Parliament of Canada. Research publications. April 21, 2008. Rev. July 24, 2008. https://lop.parl.ca/sites/PublicWebsite/default/en_CA/ResearchPublications/LegislativeSummaries/392LS602E.

Tsing, Anna Lowenhaupt. "Blasted Landscapes (and the Gentle Arts of Mushroom Picking)." In *The Multispecies Salon*, edited by Eben Kirksey, 87–110. Durham, NC: Duke University Press, 2014.

———. *The Mushroom at the End of the World: On the Possibility of Life in Capitalist Ruins.* Princeton, NJ: Princeton University Press, 2015.

Turner, Victor. *From Ritual to Theatre: The Human Seriousness of Play.* New York: Performing Arts Journal Publications, 1982.

23andMe. "Health + Ancestry Service." Accessed June 8, 2020. https://www.23andme.com/en-ca/dna-health-ancestry.

US Food and Drug Administration. "Questions and Answers on Dietary Supplements." Accessed June 30, 2020. https://www.fda.gov/food/information-consumers-using-dietary-supplements/questions-and-answers-dietary-supplements.

Van De Wall, Virginia. "We Tried Those Kardashian-Approved SugarBearHair Vitamins and Here's What Happened." *Life & Style*, March 17, 2017. https://www.lifeandstylemag.com/posts/sugarbearhair-vitamins-reviews-kardashians-127265/.

VanDerWerff, Emily. "How to Bake Bread: On the Existential Comforts of Coaxing Yeast out of Air, Kneading, Proofing, Baking, and Sharing." *Vox*, May 19, 2020. https://www.vox.com/the-highlight/2020/5/19/21221008/how-to-bake-bread-pandemic-yeast-flour-baking-ken-forkish-claire-saffitz.

VEGAMOUR. "The Science of VEGAMOUR." Accessed May 27, 2021. https://vegamour.com/pages/science.

VEGAMOUR (@vegamour). "VEGAMOUR." Instagram. Accessed May 27, 2021. https://www.instagram.com/vegamour/.

———. "Your hair thanks you." Instagram story. Accessed July 20, 2021. https://www.instagram.com/vegamour/.

Viome. "Customized, Precision Supplements with Health Intelligence." Accessed June 28, 2021. https://beta.viome.com/products/hi-supplements.

———. "Gut Intelligence Test™." Accessed June 11, 2020. https://beta.viome.com/products/gut-intelligence.

———. "Gut Microbiome Testing, Health Supplements & Probiotics." Accessed June 28, 2021. https://beta.viome.com/.

———. "Terms & Conditions." Accessed June 29, 2021. https://beta.viome.com/terms.

———. "Viome's Health Intelligence™ Service." Accessed June 11, 2020. https://beta.viome.com/products/health-intelligence.

Viome App Tour Video. Accessed June 11, 2021. https://www.youtube.com/watch?v=AmNX_qymP_k.

Walker, Kenneth, and Lauren E. Cagle, eds. "Resilience Rhetorics in Science, Technology, and Medicine." Special issue, *Poroi* 15, no. 1 (2020).

Watt, D., S. Verma, and L. Flynn. "Wellness Programs: A Review of the Evidence." *CMAJ: Canadian Medical Association Journal* 158, no. 2 (January 27, 1998): 224–30.

Welch, H. Gilbert, Lisa Schwartz, and Steve Woloshin. *Overdiagnosed: Making People Sick in the Pursuit of Health.* Boston: Beacon, 2011.

Wellman, Mariah L. "What It Means to Be a Bodybuilder: Social Media Influencer Labor and the Construction of Identity in the Bodybuilding Subculture." *Communication Review* 23, no. 4 (October 1, 2020): 273–89. https://doi.org/10.1080/10714421.2020.1829303.

Wells, Katherine, and James Hamblin. "Listen: You Are Worthy of Sleep." *The Atlantic.* Accessed July 11, 2021. https://www.theatlantic.com/health/archive/2020/04/you-are-worthy-of-sleep/610996/.

Whorton, James. "Civilisation and the Colon: Constipation as the 'Disease of Diseases.'" *BMJ: British Medical Journal* 321, no. 7276 (December 23, 2000): 1586–89. http://dx.doi.org/10.1136/bmj.321.7276.1586.

———. *Inner Hygiene: Constipation and the Pursuit of Health in Modern Society.* Oxford: Oxford University Press, 2000.

Wolf, Gary. "Know Thyself: Tracking Every Facet of Life, from Sleep to Mood to Pain, 24/7/365." *Wired,* June 22, 2009. https://www.wired.com/2009/06/lbnp-knowthyself/.

Wolf, Joan B. "Against Breastfeeding (Sometimes)." In Metzl and Kirkland, *Against Health,* 83–90.

World Health Organization. "Burn-out an 'Occupational Phenomenon': International Classification of Diseases." Accessed January 15, 2020. https://www.who.int/news/item/28-05-2019-burn-out-an-occupational-phenomenon-international-classification-of-diseases.

———. "ICD-11—Mortality and Morbidity Statistics." Accessed January 15, 2020. https://icd.who.int/browse11/l-m/en#/http%3a%2f%2fid.who.int%2ficd%2fentity%2f129180281.

Zimmer, Ben. "Wellness." *New York Times Magazine,* April 16, 2010. https://www.nytimes.com/2010/04/18/magazine/18FOB-onlanguage-t.html.

www.ingramcontent.com/pod-product-compliance
Ingram Content Group UK Ltd.
Pitfield, Milton Keynes, MK11 3LW, UK
UKHW041439130525
458414UK00002B/16